PROTHROMBIN AND RELATED COAGULATION FACTORS

# BOERHAAVE SERIES
# FOR POSTGRADUATE
# MEDICAL EDUCATION
# Nr. 10

PROCEEDINGS OF BOERHAAVE COURSES
ORGANIZED BY
THE FACULTY OF MEDICINE, UNIVERSITY OF LEIDEN
THE NETHERLANDS

# PROTHROMBIN AND RELATED COAGULATION FACTORS

EDITED BY

H. C. HEMKER M.D., PH. D. AND J. J. VELTKAMP M.D.

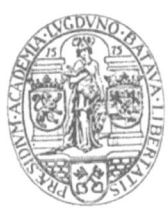

1975

LEIDEN UNIVERSITY PRESS

ISBN-13: 978-94-010-1929-3     e-ISBN-13:978-94-010-1927-9
DOI:10.1007/978-94-010-1927-9

Jacket design: E. Wijnans

# FOREWORD

One of the most fascinating tools at the disposal of the molecular biologist is the medical clinic. The responsibilities of those who provide health care do not stop when they give optimal care to the individual patient and train their successors adequately. They also are under the obligation to obtain maximal information from every case they treat in order to reach a better understanding of the underlying illness in order to improve therapeutic results in the next patient. Fundamental research in pathological material is therefore a medical must as well as an opportunity for scientific work.

The scientist working in this field can profit from nature's unasked for experiments, which are encountered by his medical colleagues in their clinical material. There are many examples of subjects of study – for instance hemoglobins and immunoglobulins – which started in a medical context and gradually developed into a field of prime interest for the molecular biologist.

The study of blood coagulation is one of the younger areas of this kind. When we started our investigations in this field twelve years ago, a serious biochemist who did not look upon blood coagulation with horror, would have been hard to find. Today, scores of workers are making it one of the most fascinating subjects in molecular biology. Not only because scientific results have a good chance of being converted into medical profit, but also because blood coagulation is a system that can serve as a model for biological amplification, lipid protein interactions, regulation in proenzyme-enzyme conversion, and still yields other items of basic interest.

The discovery of the proteins induced by vitamin K absence (PIVKAs) in 1963 evolved from a very practical medical problem indeed, viz. the control of anticoagulant treatment. When first reported at the Gleneagles Conference of the International Committee for the Nomenclature of Blood Clotting Factors, it was looked upon as one of those things that made oral anticoagulation so difficult, but we ourselves were among the only to hope that it might shed light on the mode of action of vitamin K.

At present, due to the work of numerous colleagues, many of whom have contributed to this book, and many of whom have become friends, it is universally recognized that the PIVKAs are of fundamental interest for the molecular biology of vitamin K action.

Research on the vitamin K-dependent coagulation factors is now developing rapidly. This book is not meant to be more than a snapshot of the state of the art at this particular moment. As such, we hope it will prove useful to everyone interested in the field.

Why a snapshot taken just now should be of value, was not immediately apparent ahead of times. As it happened, however, some major advances were reported at this conference, such as the nature of the change brought about in the prothrombin precursor by the vitamin K-dependent system and the primary structure of prothrombin.

Department of Biochemistry
Biomedical Centre
Medical Faculty, Maastricht

H. C. Hemker

Department of Haematology,
University Hospital, Leiden

J. J. Veltkamp

# CONTENTS

PART FOUR

PIVKA VII, IX AND X

# CONTRIBUTORS

B. M. Bas, Central Clinical-Chemical Laboratory, Hospital 'De Goddelijke Voorzienigheid', Sittard, The Netherlands.

E. A. Beck, Central Hematology Laboratory, Inselspital and University of Berne, School of Medicine, Berne, Switzerland.

R. Benarous, Hôpital Universitaire Necker-Enfants Malades, Département d'Hémato, logie, Paris, France.

C. Boyer, Service Central d'Immunologie et Hématologie, Hôpital Beaujon, Clichy, France.

M. Brozovic, Coagulation Laboratory, Epidemiology and Medical Care Unit and Haematology Department, Northwick Park Hospital, Harrow.

H. Claeys, Department of Molecular Biology, University of Aarhus, Århus, Denmark.

N. Cesbron, Service Central d'Immunologie et Hématologie, Hôpital Beaujon, Clichy, France.

D. Collen, Laboratory of Blood Coagulation, Medical Research Department, University of Leuven, Belgium.

P. P. Devilee, Department of Biochemistry, Medical Faculty Maastricht, Maastricht The Netherlands.

C. T. Esmon, Department of Biochemistry, College of Agricultural and Life Sciences, University of Wisconsin, Madison, Wisconsin, U.S.A.

E. Fressinaud, Institut de Pathologie Cellulaire, Hôpital de Bicêtre, Le Kremlin-Bicêtre France.

A. Girolami, University of Padua Medical School, Institute of 'Semeiotica Medica'-Padua, Italy.

S. N. Gitel, Department of Internal Medicine, The Jewish Hospital of St. Louis, St. Louis, Missouri.

J. S. de Graaf, Laboratory of Cardiovascular and Blood Coagulation Biochemistry, Department of Internal Medicine, University Hospital, Leiden, The Netherlands.

M.-C. Guillin, Service Central d'Immunologie et Hématologie, Hôpital Beaujon, Clichy, France.

H. C. Hemker, Department of Biochemistry, Medical Faculty Maastricht, Maastricht, The Netherlands.

R. A. Henriksen, Department of Biological Chemistry, Division of Biology and Biomedical Sciences, Washington University, St. Louis, Missouri, U.S.A.

D. J. Howarth, Coagulation Laboratory, Epidemiology and Medical Care Unit and Haematology Department, Northwick Park Hospital, Harrow.

C. M. Jackson, Department of Biological Chemistry, Division of Biology and Biomedical Sciences, Washington University, St. Louis, Missouri, U.S.A.

F. Josso, Hôpital Universitaire Necker-Enfants Malades, Département d'Hématologie, Paris, France.

M. J. P. Kahn, Service d'Immunologie et de Transfusion Sanguine, Laboratoire de Physiologie Générale, Hôpital Universitaire Saint-Pierre, Université Libre de Bruxelles, Belgique.

B. H. M. Kop-Klaassen, Department of Biochemistry, Medical Faculty Maastricht, Maastricht, The Netherlands.

M. J. Larrieu, Institut de Pathologie Cellulaire, Hôpital de Bicêtre, Le Kremlin-Bicêtre, France.

J. M. Lavergne, Hôpital Universitaire Necker-Enfants Malades, Département d'Hématologie, Paris, France.

M. J. Lindhout, Department of Biochemistry, Medical Faculty Maastricht, Maastricht, The Netherlands.

S. Magnusson, Department of Molecular Biology, University of Aarhus, Århus, Denmark.

K. G. Mann, Hematology Research, Mayo Clinics, Rochester, Minnesota, U.S.A.

F. Markwardt, Institute of Pharmacology and Toxicology, Medical Academy Erfurt, Erfurt, DDR.

D. Menache, Service Central d'Immunologie et Hématologie, Hôpital Beaujon, Centre Hospitalo Universitaire Xavier Bichat, Clichy, France.

D. Meyer, Institut de Pathologie Cellulaire, Hôpital de Bicêtre, Le Kremlin-Bicêtre, France.

J. Monasterio de Sanchez, Medical Faculty of Barcelona, Barcelona, Spain.

A. D. Muller, Department of Biochemistry, Medical Faculty Maastricht, Maastricht, The Netherlands.

A. T. van Oosterom, Haemostasis and Thrombosis Research Unit, Division of Haematology, Department of Internal Medicine, University Hospital, Leiden, The Netherlands.

W. G. Owen, Department of Pathology, College of Medicine, University of Iowa, Iowa City, Iowa, U.S.A.

T. E. Petersen, Department of Molecular Biology, University of Aarhus, Århus, Denmark.

H. Prydz, Institute of Medical Biology, University of Tromsø, Tromsø, Norway.

J. Rouvier, Laboratory of Blood Coagulation, Medical Research Department, University of Leuven, Belgium.

S. S. Shapiro, The Cardeza Foundation, Jefferson Medical College, Philadelphia, Pennsylvania, U.S.A.

L. SOTTRUP-JENSEN, Department of Molecular Biology, University of Aarhus, Århus, Denmark.

J. STENFLO, Department of Clinical Chemistry, University of Lund, Malmö General Hospital, Malmö, Sweden.

J. W. SUTTIE, Department of Biochemistry, College of Agricultural and Life Sciences, University of Wisconsin-Madison, Madison, Wisconsin, U.S.A.

A. C. W. SWART, Laboratory of Cardiobiochemistry, Department of Medicine, University of Leiden, The Netherlands.

J. TRIGINER, Hôpital Universitaire Necker-Enfants Malades, Département d'Hématologie, Paris, France.

M. VERSTRAETE, Laboratory of Blood Coagulation, Medical Research Department, University of Leuven, Belgium.

J. M. VAN DER VOORT-BEELEN, Department of Biochemistry, Medical Faculty Maastricht, Maastricht, The Netherlands.

This symposion was organized in cooperation with the "Inter Limburgs Post Universitair Centrum" (Maastricht, the Netherlands). Financial support was obtained from Janssen Pharmaceutica (Beerse, Belgium) and Merck, Sharp & Dohme B.V. (Haarlem, the Netherlands).

PART ONE

# PROTHROMBIN

# HISTORICAL DEVELOPMENT OF THE PROTHROMBIN CONCEPT

E. A. BECK

## INTRODUCTION: WHAT CAN WE LEARN FROM HISTORY OF MEDICINE?

This lecture about historical aspects of blood coagulation as part of a postgraduate course for practising physicians needs some special introductory comments. First, I am myself a practising hematologist with some experimental interests and a rather scanty background in history of medicine. Although I wrote my M.D. thesis in 1965 about the history of the socalled classical coagulation theory I did never find the time to read all the important original reports which constitute the framework of our present-day knowledge. Therefore, I must ask from you not to expect an exhaustive documentation of famous or neglected work on prothrombin, whatever its past or present merit may be.

One main aspect has puzzled me in preparing this talk, i.e. the problem of *impact of discovery*. While we are sitting here to learn about recent developments of research on hemostasis and thrombosis and how to transmit our newly acquired knowledge to the benefit of our patients we tend to look at today's accumulating information as the result of a rational and continuous development. I intend to use this historic review about certain developments in coagulation research, especially the development of a prothrombin (precursor) concept, as a means to demonstrate our own uncertain position within the *dimension of time*. This time dimension is clearly not identical for all of us: some are struggling in research laboratories to unmask more and more of Nature's secrets, others check results of basic research by the epidemiological approach on laboratory animals or patients, while the third and largest part of our profession has to decide in a rather arbitrary fashion which of the available '*knowledge*' should be considered as part of our diagnostic and therapeutic considerations. We should, however, learn from historical reading that what seems rational at a given time appears as partial truth or pure nonsense somewhat later. On the other hand, 'truth' may be bypassed many times and the whole process of human discovery is excessively wasteful. I have therefore chosen a few stations of discovery from the general area of early studies of blood coagulation to corroborate my previous, rather harsh statements. Background reading on the history of research in the area of blood coagulation, hemostasis and thrombosis is accessible in many excellent and more complete reviews (e.g. Morawitz 1905, Biggs and Macfarlane 1962, Owen et al. 1968, Schröer 1974).

## SEARCH FOR CAUSES OF BLOOD COAGULATION

### Physical causes of blood coagulation

The difference between liquid and coagulated blood is readily apparent and has therefore been a topic of scientific speculation for a very long time. Without any knowledge about the intricate systems which control biochemical activation of enzyme-substrate systems it was sensible to study or simply reason on the following formula:

$$\text{Liquid Blood} + X \text{ (or } - X?) = \text{Clotted Blood}$$

Some effects which were supplemented for X either experimentally or by logic deduction are shown in table 1. These theories are based on the com-

Table 1. Physical causes of blood coagulation

---

*Cold environment:* Aristoteles and many others

*Stasis and separation of blood elements:*
  Malpighi (1686)
  A. von Haller (1757)
  Schröder van der Kolk (1820)
  and many others

*Contact with air:*
  Hewson (1772)
  Virchow (1845)
  and many others

*Disintegration of blood cells with release of 'fibrin':*
  – fibrin nucleus of red cells: E. Home (1817), G. Hayem (1889)
  – fibrin from platelets: K. Bürker (1904)

*Release of gas from blood:*
  – ammonia: Richardson (1858)
  – $CO_2$: Thackrah (1819), A. Schmidt (1861)

---

mon assumption that fibrin, a fibrous substance responsible for gelation of blood, preexists in blood. 'X' simply represents a change from the natural environment of circulating blood. Thus, the effect of cooling was, as an example of deductive thinking, simply compared with freezing of water.

## EVOLUTION OF THE 'PRECURSOR' CONCEPT

A radical step forward was achieved by speculating somewhat differently: A change in environment (X) does not affect fibrin directly but a 'profibrin' or 'fibrinogen'. Malpighi (1686) did not yet reach this conclusion when he showed that cooling of blood delayed rather than accelerated blood coagulation. He was much more interested in the observation of the socalled 'inflammatory crust' which formed on top of certain clotted blood samples obtained from patients with fever or other 'inflammatory' disorders. (The 'inflammatory crust' actually corresponds to an accelerated sedimentation rate of red cells associated with reactive hyperfibrinogenemia, i.e. the blood separates into a solid cell-containing clot, whereas some plasma clots on top of the cells.)

An entirely novel approach of the problem was chosen in 1836 by Buchanan. He used socalled 'fibriniferous' liquids, i.e. exudates from hydroceles and other sources, which would not coagulate spontaneously, even upon prolonged standing. Coagulation was, however, rapidly induced when serum from fresh blood clots was added to the exudate. Buchanan concluded that disrupted white cells released a coagulating substance (1836), but he also mentioned the possibility of enzyme action as part of the process (1845). His ideas still did not conceive a transition of precursors and might be summarized as follows:

Fibrin (liquid) $+$ X (cellular breakdown? enzyme?) $\rightarrow$ Fibrin clot

The concept of 'fibrinogen' is often attributed to Virchow (e.g. Schröer 1974). Virchow also used exudates where he believed to observe the transition of soluble fibrin into a homogeneous gel, probably through the action of oxygen.

When putrefaction of exudates started upon prolonged preservation, clottability was reduced or completely lost. Virchow clearly described this change as follows: 'There is no reason to call this (decaying) substance fibrin (Faserstoff); indeed, should one look for a name, then it might be at most suitable to call it fibrinogen' (1847, translated from German). Virchow, therefore, had not discovered the precursor of fibrin but rather proteolytic degradation of fibrinogen. Denis (1859), however, tried to isolate 'fibrin' from blood plasma and came to the following conclusion: 'I believe that I should repeat once more that I do not mean to define a liquid fibrin, plasma fibrin, but rather a substance which is not at all fibrous and which is the origin of fibrin, i.e. clottable lymph, a substance which I would like to call 'sérofibrine', and which one might also designate 'fibrinogène', if such a word would be admissible' (translated from French).


### DEVELOPMENT OF METHODS TO STUDY BLOOD IN ITS LIQUID STATE

Buchanan was successful in demonstrating clot-promoting activity in serum by use of a stable, liquid 'substrate' which, as we know today, contained fibrinogen. However, it was far more difficult to study the coagulation system directly on blood or blood components since fresh blood would invariably clot more or less rapidly when taken out of its natural environment. Malpighi (1686) had shown that *cooling* did delay the process, but studies of blood coagulation at low temperature do not reflect physiological conditions. One change of environment responsible for acceleration of clotting was 'surface contact'. Thus, Hewson (1772), Brücke (1857) and many others showed that blood would remain liquid for prolonged periods when ligated vascular segments were studied. While these experiments showed a lack of clot-promoting 'surface contact' by an intact vessel wall they failed to explain the sequence of events as soon as blood was removed from the vessel segments.

Hewson was especially interested in the role of oxygen. He observed the bright red color of oxygenated blood and tried to reproduce the color change by adding various salts, including nitrates. To his astonishment, concentrated salt solutions, irrespective of their oxidising properties, *inhibited* clotting. Many authors used *neutral salts*, especially magnesium sulphate, throughout the 19th century to separate incoagulable plasma from blood cells. This procedure allowed the separation of certain plasma constituents, but blood coagulation was initiated only after *dilution* of 'salt plasma'. Furthermore, it was not shown at which level clotting was prevented.

The main difference between exudates and whole blood was thought to be the amount of cellular materials (cf. table 1). Indeed, if cells were removed from blood, e.g. by sedimentation in the cold, the supernatant plasma would clot at a much slower rate than whole blood. However, *cell-free plasma*, in contrast to exudates, would always spontaneously clot. Cell separation was, therefore, not a satisfactory method to obtain stable plasma samples. (The clot-promoting properties of substances derived from disintegrated cells will be discussed later.)

The specific action of *calcium ions* was discovered independently by Arthur and Pagès (1890) and Pekelharing (1891). Arthur and Pagès used oxalate to bind calcium and compared blood coagulation with formation of cheese: 'Cheese formation is therefore a general phenomenon which, based on chemical transformation of an albuminoid substance through the influence of an enzyme, leads to the formation of an insoluble, calcium-containing component, caséum' (translated from French). The term 'hémato-caséum' was proposed for fibrin. Although Pekelharing introduced *citrate* as a calcium-binding anticoagulant the implication of this discovery for blood transfusion was not immediately recognised.

## ALEXANDER SCHMIDT

The scene of blood coagulation research was entered in the second half of the 19th century by a powerful and contradictory figure, the first scientist to devote his entire lifetime to coagulation research: Alexander Schmidt. In 1861 he isolated from serum a socalled 'fibrinoplastic' substance which, as he then claimed, was not an enzyme and formed, together with fibrinogen, the fibrin clot. Ten years later, he and his students started the characterisation of the 'Fibrinferment' which was thought to interact with fibrinogen and 'Paraglobulin' (a substance released from white cells) to form fibrin (Schmidt 1872 and 1876). The 'Fibrinferment' was later called 'thrombin' by Schmidt (1892) because its injection into experimental animals caused lethal thrombosis (Köhler 1877). Hammarsten (1877) supported the view that the 'Fibrinferment' was an enzyme but could not confirm the necessity of a third element in its interaction with purified fibrinogen.

Schmidt had clearly recognised the biologically dangerous properties of active thrombin and therefore postulated the existence of an inactive precursor, *prothrombin* (1892, p. 202). Table 2 summarizes the main concepts of his rather complicated and fluctuating coagulation schemes. It is noteworthy that Schmidt also recognised the necessity of inhibitors ('cytoglobulins') limiting the spreading of the coagulation process in vivo.

*Table* 2. Chemistry of coagulation: concepts of Alexander Schmidt

---

a. Fibrinogen + Fibrinoplastic substance (from serum, no enzyme) ⟶ Fibrin (1861)

b. Fibrinogen + Paraglobulin (from white cells) + Fibrinferment ⟶ Fibrin (1872, 1876)

c. Summary (1892, 1895):

Fibrinferment = *Thrombin* (causing lethal thrombosis in experimental animals)

Precursor = *Prothrombin* (released from various organs and white cells)

1. Plasma disrupts blood cells, release of 'zymoplastic substances'

2. Zymoplastic substances + prothrombin→ thrombin

3. thrombin + fibrinogen + neutral salts→ fibrin

4. process controlled in vivo by 'cytoglobulins' (inhibitors)

---

By describing the outline of Schmidt's work one would assume that his scientific impact must have been enormous. This was clearly not the case. Schmidt was a man of many ideas, a stimulating teacher and certainly open to criticism (Wöhlisch 1954). However, his last work (Schmidt 1895) which appeared one year after his death is written in a rather defensive style. Perhaps, too many of his results had to be revoked. His nomenclature was complicated and clumsy, with the exception of the two still accepted terms 'thrombin' and 'prothrombin'. Morawitz (1905) finally gave full credit to the work and personality of Schmidt. I am very unhappy about the thought that scientists with a personality similar to that of Alexander Schmidt may live, work and be neglected in a similar way right now.


ACTIVATION OF PROTHROMBIN: THE CLASSICAL COAGULATION THEORY


The accelerating effects of extracts from blood cells or tissues on the whole process of blood coagulation was previously mentioned. However, it was not clear in what way such extracts acted and whether they were an essential constituent of the system. The reader of reports on studies of such substances which later became known as 'thrombokinase' (thromboplastin) will be confused by a host of synonyms such as 'cell globulin, cellular or tissue fibrinogen, nucleohistone, nucleoalbumin, zymogen, tissue nucleoproteid, coagulin, paraglobulin, fibrinoplastic or zymoplastic substances etc.'

(Morawitz 1905). To shorten a very long story: Fuld (1902) suggested that muscle extracts were responsible for accelerated clotting of goose plasma (which otherwise clots very slowly), independent of thrombin action. Fuld and Spiro (1904) confirmed this idea by demonstrating that the simultaneous addition of liver extract and calcium to purified fibrinogen did not produce clotting, whereas clotting of plasma was markedly accelerated. Their conclusion was *summarised* by Morawitz (1905, p. 370, fig. 1), a scheme which is virtually never reproduced in modern reviews.

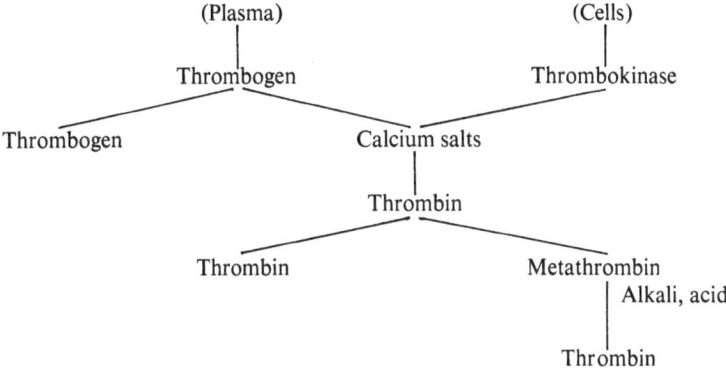

*Fig. 1.* Chemistry of blood coagulation: Concept of Fuld (1902, 1903), Fuld and Spiro (1904).
Cellular saline extracts accelerate conversion of thrombogen (prothrombin). Thrombin is rapidly inactivated in serum (metathrombin).

Morawitz, who is uniformly quoted as the founder of the 'classical coagulation theory', has been very modest and unequivocal about his own contributions: he showed, among other important studies on blood coagulation, that saline extraction would yield 'thrombokinase' from almost any tissue (Morawitz 1903). Thrombokinase appeared to combine with prothrombin (or thrombogen). In his review, Morawitz (1905) summarized the ideas of Fuld and Spiro (1904) and his own as follows: 'Plasma of circulating blood contains fibrinogen, calcium salts and probably also thrombogen. The formed elements, especially the blood platelets, when irritated by foreign contact, release on the outside of blood vessels thrombokinase into the plasma. Thrombokinase now forms, together with thrombogen and calcium salts, thrombin'. (Im Plasma des zirkulierenden Blutes finden sich Fibrinogen, Kalksalze und wahrscheinlich auch Thrombogen. Ausserhalb der Gefässe geben die geformten Elemente, besonders die Blutplättchen, durch die Berührung mit Fremdkörpern gereizt, Thrombokinase in das Plasma ab. Die Thrombokinase bildet nun mit dem Thrombogen und den Kalksalzen zusammen Thrombin.)

## WHAT HAPPENED THEREAFTER?

With our present-day concept of blood coagulation we are most willing to accept the classical coagulation scheme as a sound conquest of arduous research. Not so coagulation scientists after 1905, including Morawitz (1925). It is far beyond the goal of this presentation to retrace even the most important later studies on the prothrombin concept. Table 3 summari-

*Table* 3.  Summary of some additional concepts after 1905

a. Thrombozyme + Thrombogen + Fibrinogen = Fibrin (Nolf 1908)
                      Contact, Calcium

b. Proserozyme ──────────────→ Serozyme
   Serozyme + Cytozyme ──────────→ Thrombin
   Thrombin + Fibrinogen ─────────→ Fibrin (Bordet 1920)

c. Enzyme nature of thrombin doubted (Morawitz 1925)

d. Prothrombin + Calcium = Thrombin, reaction prevented by heparin.
   Thromboplastin neutralizes heparin and, therefore, formation of thrombin is possible (Howell 1935)

zes a few of the subsequently developed concepts. In conclusion, as Morawitz (1925) and many other critical scientists state in their later publications, the elucidation of the conversion of prothrombin to thrombin and of earlier and later phases of blood coagulation entirely depended on the development of adequate methods. One decisive step was the preparation of stable 'thromboplastin' by Quick (1935, 1936) which made the accurate measurement of prothrombin activation possible. The development of techniques for purification and structure analysis of prothrombin is described elsewhere in this volume. The 'prothrombin story' can only teach us again what Isaac Newton stated in 1672: 'For the best and safest method of philosophizing seems to be, first to inquire diligently into the properties of things, and of establishing those properties by experiments, and then to proceed more slowly to hypotheses for the explanation of them. For hypotheses should be subservient only in explaining the properties of things, but not assumed in determining them unless so far as they may furnish experiments.'

REFERENCES

1. *Aristoteles: Meteorologica*. With an English Translation by H. D. P. Lee. Loeb's Classical Library, Harvard Press, Boston, Vol. 4, chap. 7, p. 335 and chap. 10, p. 365 (1952).
2. Arthus, M. and C. Pagès, Nouvelle théorie chimique de la coagulation du sang. *Arch. Physiol. norm. path.* 22:739 (1890).
3. Beck, E. A., *Die klassische Blutgerinnungstheorie*. Thesis (M.D.), Zurich 1965.
4. Biggs, R. and R. G. Macfarlane, *Human blood coagulation* and its disorders. Third edition. Blackwell, Oxford (1962).
5. Bordet, J., Considérations sur les théories de la coagulation du sang. *Ann. Inst. Pasteur* 34: 561 (1920).
6. Brücke, E., Ueber die Ursache der Gerinnung des Blutes. *Arch. Path. Anat.* 12: 81 and 172 (1857).
7. Bürker, K., Blutplättchen und Blutgerinnung. *Pflügers Arch. ges. Physiol.* 102: 36 (1904).
8. Buchanan, A., Contributions to the physiology and pathology of the animal fluids. *Lond. Med. Gaz.* 18: 51 (1836).
9. Buchanan, A., On the coagulation of the blood and other fibriniferous liquids. *Lond Med. Gaz.* (N.S.) p. 617 (1845).
10. Denis, P. S., *Mémoire sur le sang*. J. Baillière, Paris (1859).
11. Fuld, E., Ueber das Zeitgesetz des Fibrinferments. *Beitr. chem. Physiol. Path.* (Hofmeister's) 2: 514 (1902).
12. Fuld, E., Ueber die Vorbedingungen der Blutgerinnung sowie über die Gerinnbarkeit des Fluorplasmas. *Zbl. Physiol.* 17: 529 (1903).
13. Fuld, E. and K. Spiro, Der Einfluss einiger gerinnungshemmender Agentien auf das Vogelplasma. *Beitr. chem. Physiol. Path.* (Hofmeister's) 5: 171 (1904).
14. von Haller, A., Elementa physiologiae corporis humani, vol. 2, p. 284. *Lausanne*, (1757-1763).
15. Hammarsten, O., Zur Lehre von der Faserstoffgerinnung. *Pflügers Arch. ges. Physiol.* 14: 211 (1877).
16. Hayem, G., *Du sang et de ses altérations anatomiques*. G. Masson, Paris (1889).
17. Hewson, W., *An experimental inquiry into the properties of blood*. Cadell, London, 2nd ed. (1772).
18. Home, E., On the changes the blood undergoes in the act of coagulation. *Philosoph. Trans. Roy. Soc.* (London) 108: 172 (1818).
19. Howell, W. H., Theories of blood coagulation. *Physiol. Rev.* 15: 435 (1935).
20. Köhler, A., *Ueber Thrombose und Transfusion, Eiter und septische Infection und deren Beziehung zum Fibrinferment*. Thesis (M.D.), Dorpat (1877), quoted from Schmidt (1892).
21. Malpighi, M., *De polypo cordis dissertatio*. In: *Opera omnia*, London (1686). Quoted from a reprint published by Almqvist and Wiksells, Stockholm, p. 123 (1956).
22. Morawitz, P., Beiträge zur Kenntnis der Blutgerinnung. *Dtsch. Arch. klin. Med.* 79: 1 (1903).
23. Morawitz, P., Die Chemie der Blutgerinnung. *Ergebn. Physiol.* 4: 307 (1905); English Translation: *The chemistry of blood coagulation*. R. Hartmann and P. F. Guenther. C. C. Thomas, Springfield, Ill., (1958).
24. Morawitz, P., Blutgerinnung. In: *Handbuch der Biochemie des Menschen und der Tiere*. C. Oppenheimer, Ed., vol. 4, p. 44 (1925).
25. Newton, I., Reply to a letter from P. Pardie. *Phil. Trans-Roy. Soc.* 85: 4014 (1672).
26. Nolf, P., Contribution à l'étude de la coagulation du sang. Les facteurs primordiaux, leur origine. *Arch. int. Physiol.* 6: 1 (1908).

27. Owen, C. A., E. J. W. Bowie, P. Didisheim, and J. H. Thompson, *The diagnosis of bleeding disorders*. Churchill, London (1969). The first chapter 'Introduction and Historical Perspective' contains biographic notes and some photographs of several authors quoted in the present review.
28. Pekelharing, G. A., Ueber die Bedeutung der Kalksalze für die Gerinnung des Blutes. *Internat. Beitr. wiss. Med.* (Festschrift R. Virchow) 1: 433 (1891).
29. Quick, A. J., The prothrombin in hemophilia and in obstructive jaundice (abstract) *J. biol. Chem.* 73: 109 (1935).
30. Quick, A. J., On various properties of thromboplastin (aqueous tissue extracts). *Amer. J. Physiol.* 114: 282 (1936).
31. Richardson, B., *The cause of the coagulation of blood*. Churchill, London (1858).
32. Schmidt, A., Ueber den Faserstoff und die Ursache seiner Gerinnung. *Arch. Anat. Physiol.* (Reichert-DuBois-Reymonds), p. 545 and 675 (1861).
33. Schmidt, A., Neue Untersuchungen über die Faserstoffgerinnung. *Pflügers Arch. ges. Physiol.* 6: 413 (1872).
34. Schmidt, A., *Die Lehre von den fermentativen Gerinnungserscheinungen*. Matthiessen, Dorpat (1876).
35. Schmidt, A., *Zur Blutlehre*. Vogel, Leipzig (1892).
36. Schmidt, A., *Weitere Beiträge zur Blutlehre*. Bergmann, Wiesbaden (1895).
37. Schroeder van der Kolk, J. L., *Sistens sanguinis coagulantis historiam, cum experimentis ad eam illustrandam institutis*. Groningen (1820).
38. Schröer, H., *Die Entwicklung der Hämostaseologie*. In: *Einführung in die Geschichte der Hämatologie*. Thieme, Stuttgart, p. 80 (1974).
39. Thackrah, C. T., *An inquiry into the nature and properties of the blood, as existent in health and diseases*. Cox, London (1819).
40. Virchow, R., Zur pathologischen Physiologie des Blutes. *Arch. path. Anat. Physiol.* 1: 547 (1847).
41. Virchow, R., *Ueber den Faserstoff* (1845/46). In: *Gesammelte Abhandlungen zur wissenschaftlichen Medizin*. Frankfurt a.M. (1856).
42. Wöhlisch, E., Die Blutgerinnung: Forschung und Faktoren. *Schweiz. med. Wschr.* 29: 774 (1954).

# THE PRIMARY STRUCTURE OF PROTHROMBIN, THE ROLE OF VITAMIN K IN BLOOD COAGULATION AND A THROMBIN CATALYZED 'NEGATIVE FEED-BACK' CONTROL MECHANISM FOR LIMITIMG THE ACTIVATION OF PROTHROMBIN

STAFFAN MAGNUSSON, LARS SOTTRUP-JENSEN, TORBEN ELLEBAEK PETERSEN AND HENDRIK CLAEYS

There are several reasons for wanting to know the structure of prothrombin. One is that thrombin is a proteolytic enzyme with highly restricted specificity towards fibrinogen and a few other physiological substrates such as plasma transglutaminase (Factor XIII), Factor V, Factor VIII and prothrombin. We need to know the structure of thrombin in order to understand its selective specificity towards these substrates and also to understand its interactions with the inhibitors antithrombin-III, heparin and hirudin, none of which seems to inhibit the pancreatic serine proteinases which are close evolutionary congeners of thrombin.

A second reason for wanting to know the structure of prothrombin is that unlike the pancreatic serine proteinase zymogens, which are only slightly larger than their corresponding active enzymes, prothrombin is nearly twice as big as its active enzyme thrombin. This fundamental difference between prothrombin on the one hand and trypsinogen, the chymotrypsinogens A and B, and proelastase on the other hand raises several questions about the activation mechanism, the evolutionary relationship, and the function of the rather large protein that constitutes the 'Pro'-piece of prothrombin. Again we cannot hope to give rational answers to any of these questions without knowing the structure of prothrombin and being able to design experiments based on this knowledge.

A third reason for determining the structure of prothrombin is the fact that prothrombin is the most easily available of those proteins which are known to require vitamin K for their biosynthesis, and one would expect to find out, during the course of a structural investigation of prothrombin, what sort of unusual structure is present in prothrombin as a result of vitamin K action. We wish to report here the complete primary structure of thrombin, of neoprothrombin-S, neoprothrombin-T, as well as of the A-fragment and the S-fragment from the 'Pro' piece of prothrombin.


MATERIALS AND METHODS


*Bovine thrombin* was purified to homogeneity in starch gel electrophoresis and had a specific activity of 2100 NIH-U/mg dry weight (Magnusson, 1965 and 1970).

*Bovine prothrombin* was isolated as described earlier (Magnusson, 1965a and 1970) and has a specific activity of 1400-1450 NIH-U/mg when tested in a two-stage system using highly purified and stable fibrinogen (fraction I-4 of Blombäck and Blombäck, 1956) as substrate, and excluding acacia gum, and using standard NIH-thrombin for calibration of the standard curve. This specific activity in our hands corresponds to 2350-2450 U/mg using the 15 second unit standard and acacia gum (Ware and Seegers, 1949).

*Activation of prothrombin*

When 2.6-2.9 g of the prothrombin preparations used was dissolved at a high concentration of 70-200 mg/ml in a buffer of pH 7.5 which was 40-100 m$M$ in tris-chloride buffer and 20-50 m$M$ in EDTA, the prothrombin was almost quantitatively converted in 20-30 minutes at room temperature to a mixture of A-fragment (A for N-terminal alanine), S-fragment (S for N-terminal serine), thrombin, neoprothrombin-S and a small amount of neoprothrombin-T (T for N-terminal threonine). See figure 1. These fragments were separated on a 5 × 65 cm column of DEAE-Sephadex A-50 equilibrated with the above mentioned buffer but 0.08 $M$ in chloride concentration and eluting with a linear ionic strength gradient obtained by adding sodium chloride to raise the chloride concentration to 0.48 $M$ (Saundry, R. H., Magnusson, S. and Hartley, B. S., unpublished results, 1969). The results are shown in figure 2. Fractions 220-340 contain a mixture of neoprothrombin-T and active thrombin. The term neoprothrombin is used to indicate that this protein contains the thrombin structure and that is is derived from prothrombin by a limited proteolysis which does *not* lead to activation but to a modified zymogen in analogy with the chymotryp-sinogen-neochymotrypsinogen-chymotrypsin system (Magnusson and Murano, 1974). The isolation from prothrombin preparations of a protein having the same starch gel electrophoretic mobility as thrombin, but lacking

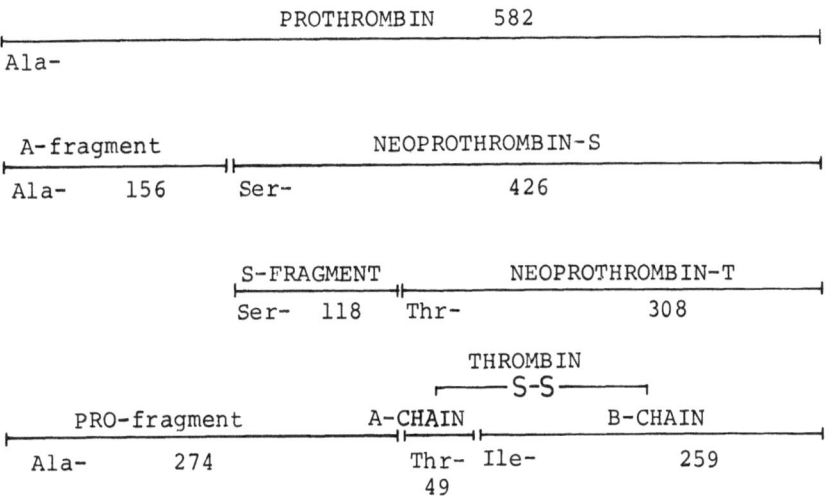

Fig. 1. Suggested nomenclature for prothrombin and its activation products. Numbers indicate the total number of amino acid residues in the fragments. Ala-, Ser-, Thr-, Ile- indicate the N-terminal amino acid residues.

thrombin activity was first reported in 1961 (Magnusson, 1962) and independently by Asada et al. (1961). Fractions 540-600 contain the N-terminal activation fragment, called the A-fragment. Fractions 610-685 contain three variants of the S-fragment.

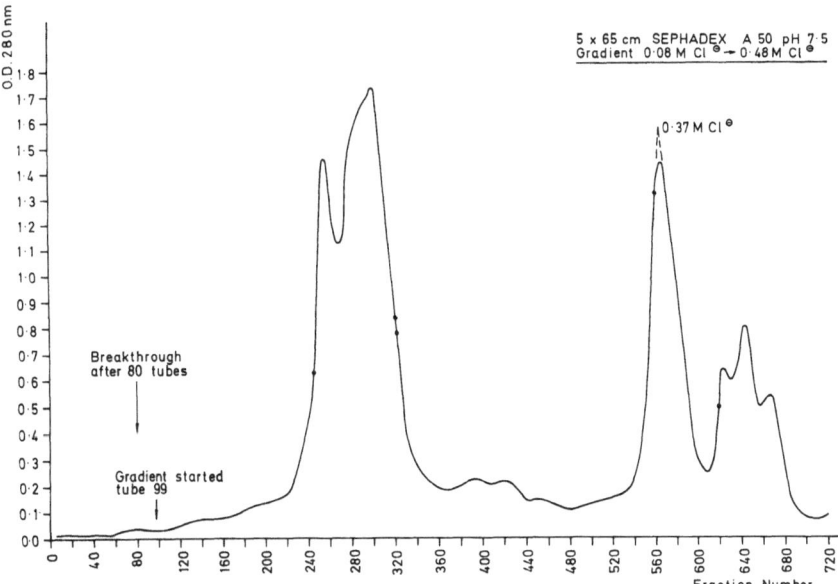

Fig. 2. Separation of prothrombin activation mixture.

*Sequence methods*

The amino acid composition of peptide hydrolysates was analyzed by a semiquantitative screening method using highvoltage electrophoresis on paper at pH 2.1. Pure samples were analyzed quantitatively according to Spackman, Moore and Stein, using Locarte amino acid analyzers.

Amino acid sequences were determined by sequential degradation with phenyl*iso*thiocyanate according to Edman and the N-terminal amino acid at each step was identified by chromatography of its DNS-derivative on poly-amide layers.

In some cases the amino acid sequence was also determined by mass spectrometry of acetylated and permethylated derivatives in collaboration with Howard Morris and Anne Dell at the University Chemical Laboratory, Cambridge, England.

*Detection of glycopeptides*

Throughout this work carbohydrate peptides have been detected because they contained glucosamine, which is seen in the amino acid analysis and because they give a brown or black colour on acid hydrolysis because of 'humin' formation. No hexosamines other than glucosamine have been seen. This is in agreement with our earlier data for the carbohydrate composition of prothrombin (Magnusson, 1965a).

RESULTS

The amino acid sequence determination of the two chains of thrombin was started in collaboration with B. S. Hartley in 1967 at the Laboratory of Molecular Biology, Cambridge, England.

*The A-chain of thrombin*

The sequence of the A-chain of 49 residues was reported, except for some of the amides, in 1968 (Magnusson, 1968).

*The B-chain of thrombin*

Preliminary results of the sequence determination of the B-chain have been reported previously (Magnusson, 1971). This work has now been completed by investigating a plasmic digest of native thrombin, a peptic digest of neoprothrombin-T, and a cyanogen bromide degradation of neoprothrombin-S.

*1. The plasmic digest* of native thrombin provided no new important information for the sequence work, but showed that fragments corresponding in size to the so-called β- and γ-thrombins described by Lundblad (1971), Lanchantin et al. (1965) and Mann et al. (1973) could be obtained from our thrombin preparations by a very short incubation with a small amount of plasmin.

```
1                                                    10
Thr-Ser-Glu-Asp-His-Phe-Gln-Pro-Phe-Phe-

-Asn-Glu-Lys-Thr-Phe-Gly-Ala-Gly-Glu-Ala-

-Asp-Cys-Gly-Leu-Arg-Pro-Leu-Phe-Glu-Lys-

-Lys-Gln-Val-Gln-Asp-Glu-Thr-Gln-Lys-Glu-

-Leu-Phe-Glu-Ser-Tyr-Ile-Glu-Gly-Arg
```

*Fig.* 3. Amino acid sequence of the A-chain of thrombin. 49 residues. M.w. = 5721.

*2. The peptic digest of neoprothrombin-T.* Several peptic peptides were isolated and sequenced, which proved that in neoprothrombin-T the potential A- and B-chains of thrombin are directly connected in sequence such that the C-terminal Arg-49 of the A-chain is bound to the N-terminal Ile-16 of the B-chain. These peptic peptides were as follows:

```
A-46 A-47 A-48 A-49 B-16 B-17 B-18  B-19  B-20  B-21  B-22  B-23
Ile - Glu - Gly - Arg - Ile - Val - Glu - Gly - Gln - Asp - Ala - Glu
Ile - Glu - Gly - Arg - Ile - Val - Glu - Gly - Gln - Asp
Ile - Glu - Gly
                      Arg - Ile - Val - Glu - Gly - Gln - Asp - Ala - Glu
                      Arg - Ile - Val - Glu - Gly - Gln - Asp
```

From this peptic digest information was also obtained which identifies the three intra-chain disulphide bridges of the B-chain as well as the single inter-chain disulphide bridge that connects the A-chain and B-chain. It also confirmed the overlap Lys-126 to Gln-127. The peptic digest also provided sequence and overlap evidence for residues 65I to 68 in the carbohydrate binding region.

*3. Cyanogen bromide degradation of neoprothrombin-S* was followed by reduction with dithiothreitol, alkylation with ¹⁴C-iodo-acetate and blocking

of free amino groups by citraconic anhydride. The resulting peptides were
separated on a column of Sephadex G-75 in 0.15 $M$ NH$_4$HCO$_3$ at pH 8.3.
Pool II, containing the B-chain CNBr-fragment Leu-85 to Met-180 was

```
 16   17   18   19   20   21   22   23   24   25   26   27   28   29   30   31
Ile-Val-Glu-Gly-Gln-Asp-Ala-Glu-Val-Gly-Leu-Ser-Pro-Trp-Gln-Val-

 32   33   34   35   36  36A   37   38   39   40   41   42   43   44   45   46
-Met-Leu-Phe-Arg-Lys-Ser-Pro-Gln-Glu-Leu-Leu-Cys-Gly-Ala-Ser-Leu-

 47   48   49   50   51   52   53   54   55   56   57   58   59   60   61   62
-Ile-Ser-Asp-Arg-Trp-Val-Leu-Thr-Ala-Ala-His-Cys-Leu-Leu-Tyr-Pro-

 63   64   65  65A  65B  65C  65D  65E  65F  65G  65H  65I   66   67   68   69
-Pro-Trp-Asx-Lys-Asn-Phe-Thr-Val-Asp-Asp-Leu-Leu-Val-Arg-Ile-Gly-

 70   71   72   73   74   75   76   77   78   79   80   81   82   83   84  84A
-Lys-His-Ser-Arg-Thr-Arg-Tyr-Glu-Arg-Lys-Val-Glu-Lys-Ile-Ser-Met-

 85   86   87   88   89   90   91   92   93   94   95   96   97   98   99  99A
-Leu-Asp-Lys-Ile-Tyr-Ile-His-Pro-Arg-Tyr-Asn-Trp-Lys-Glu-Asn-Leu-

100  101  102  103  104  105  106  107  108  109  110  111  112  113  114  115
-Asp-Arg-Asp-Ile-Ala-Leu-Leu-Lys-Leu-Lys-Arg-Pro-Ile-Glu-Leu-Ser-

116  117  118  119  120  121  122  123  124  125  126  127  128 128A128B128C
-Asp-Tyr-Ile-His-Pro-Val-Cys-Leu-Pro-Asp-Lys-Gln-Thr-Ala-Ala-Lys-

129  130  131  132  133  134  135  136  137  138  139  140  141  142  143  144
-Leu-Leu-His-Ala-Gly-Phe-Lys-Gly-Arg-Val-Thr-Gly-Trp-Gly-Asn-Arg-

145  146  147 147A147B147C147D147E 148  149  150  151  152  153  154  155
-Arg-Glu-Thr-Trp-Thr-Thr-Ser-Val-Ala-Glu-Val-Gln-Pro-Ser-Val-Leu-

156  157  158  159  160  161  162  163  164  165  166  167  168  169  170  171
-Gln-Val-Val-Asn-Leu-Pro-Leu-Val-Glu-Arg-Pro-Val-Cys-Lys-Ala-Ser-

172  173  174  175  176  177  178  179  180  181  182  183  184 184A185  186
-Thr-Arg-Ile-Arg-Ile-Thr-Asn-Asp-Met-Phe-Cys-Ala-Gly-Tyr-Lys-Pro-

187  188 188A188B188C188D189  190  191  192  193  194  195  196  197  198
-Gly-Glu-Gly-Lys-Arg-Gly-Asp-Ala-Cys-Glu-Gly-Asp-Ser-Gly-Gly-Pro-

199  200  201  202  203 203A203B204  205  206  207  208  209  210  211  212
-Phe-Val-Met-Lys-Ser-Pro-Tyr-Asn-Asn-Arg-Trp-Tyr-Gln-Met-Gly-Ile-

213  214  215  216  217  219  220  221 221A222  223  224  225  226  227  228
-Val-Ser-Trp-Gly-Glu-Gly-Cys-Asp-Arg-Asn-Gly-Lys-Tyr-Gly-Phe-Tyr-

229  230  231  232  233  234  235  236  237  238  239  240  241  242  243  244
-Thr-His-Val-Phe-Arg-Leu-Lys-Lys-Trp-Ile-Gln-Lys-Val-Ile-Asp-Arg-

245 245A245B
-Leu-Gly-Ser
```

*Fig.* 4. Amino acid sequence of the B-chain of thrombin. 259 residues. M.w. 29683 +
carbohydrate. The chymotrypsin numbering system is used to facilitate homology comparison.

digested with trypsin. The peptide Glu-146 to Arg-173 was then subdigested with elastase to resolve the sequence of this region. Pool I, containing the entire S-fragment, the entire A-chain of thrombin and residues Ile-16 to Met-32 in the B-chain of thrombin was subdigested with chymotrypsin. The information obtained helped establish the sequence of neoprothrombin-S. The complete amino acid sequence of the B-chain of thrombin is shown in figure 4. The numbering system for chymotrypsin is used. The carbohydrate of thrombin is bound to Asn-65B as shown in figure 5. The positions of the four disulphide bridges of thrombin are given in figure 6.

```
A-fragment 74-82
                      CHO ·· ·
                     /
     -Tyr-Arg-Gly-ASN-Val-SER-Val-Thr-Arg-


A-fragment 98-106
                      CHO - ·
                     /
     -Pro-Glu-Ile-ASN-Ser-THR-Thr-His-Pro-


Thrombin B-chain
                      CHO -· ·
                     /
     -Trp-Asx-Lys-ASN-Phe-THR-Val-Asp-Asp-
      64   65  65A 65B 65C 65D 65E 65F 65G
```

*Fig. 5.* Carbohydrate attachment sites in prothrombin: Asn-77 and Asn-101 in the A-fragment (numbers as in fig. 8) and Asn-65B in the B-chain of thrombin (numbers as in fig. 4).

| A-fragment | | S-fragment | | Thrombin | |
|---|---|---|---|---|---|
| Cys-18 | to Cys-23 | Cys-15 | to Cys-93 | Cys-A22 | to Cys-122 |
| Cys-48 | to Cys-61 | Cys-36 | to Cys-76 | Cys-42 | to Cys-58 |
| Cys-66 | to Cys-144 | Cys-64 | to Cys-88 | Cys-168 | to Cys-182 |
| Cys-87 | to Cys-127 | | | Cys-191 | to Cys-220 |
| Cys-115 | to Cys-139 | | | | |

*Fig. 6.* Disulphide bridges in prothrombin. (Numbers for A-fragment as fig. 8, S-fragment as fig. 7, A-chain as fig. 3, and B-chain as fig. 4).

There is a total of 12 disulphide bridges, 5 in the A-fragment, 3 in the S-fragment, and 4 in thrombin. Three of the four bridges in thrombin are internal in the B-chain and the fourth connects the A-chain to the B-chain.

*The S-fragment from the 'Pro'-piece*

From the S-fragment the following digests were investigated:

1. Reduced, carboxymethylated S-fragment was digested with trypsin. The resulting peptides were separated on a column of DEAE-cellulose using a linear ionic strength gradient of 0.02 to 0.5 $M$ NH$_4$HCO$_3$ pH 8.3, and further purified on paper. Some peptides were subdigested with thermolysin, chymotrypsin or pepsin.
2. Native S-fragment was digested with thermolysin at pH 6.5. The resulting peptides were separated on paper. The three disulphide bridges were isolated from this digest and identified by diagonal electrophoresis using either performic acid to oxidize cystines to cysteic acids, or reduction and carboxymethylation.
3. Reduced, carboxymethylated S-fragment was digested with elastase, and the peptides were separated on paper. Some information regarding the S-fragment sequence was also obtained from chymotryptic and tryptic digests of neoprothrombin-S, that had been reduced, citraconylated and carboxymethylated.
5. For the sequence 107-113 partial acid hydrolysis was employed under conditions (1 m$M$ HCl, 110°C, 24 h) that specifically released aspartic acid.

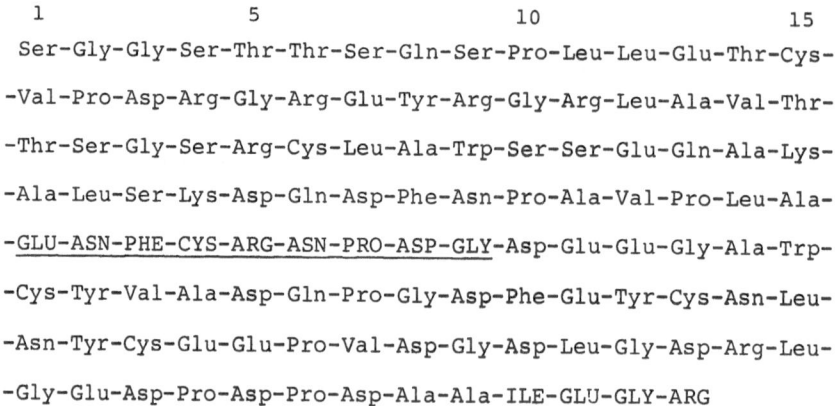

```
  1                 5                    10                       15
Ser-Gly-Gly-Ser-Thr-Thr-Ser-Gln-Ser-Pro-Leu-Leu-Glu-Thr-Cys-
-Val-Pro-Asp-Arg-Gly-Arg-Glu-Tyr-Arg-Gly-Arg-Leu-Ala-Val-Thr-
-Thr-Ser-Gly-Ser-Arg-Cys-Leu-Ala-Trp-Ser-Ser-Glu-Gln-Ala-Lys-
-Ala-Leu-Ser-Lys-Asp-Gln-Asp-Phe-Asn-Pro-Ala-Val-Pro-Leu-Ala-
-GLU-ASN-PHE-CYS-ARG-ASN-PRO-ASP-GLY-Asp-Glu-Glu-Gly-Ala-Trp-
-Cys-Tyr-Val-Ala-Asp-Gln-Pro-Gly-Asp-Phe-Glu-Tyr-Cys-Asn-Leu-
-Asn-Tyr-Cys-Glu-Glu-Pro-Val-Asp-Gly-Asp-Leu-Gly-Asp-Arg-Leu-
-Gly-Glu-Asp-Pro-Asp-Pro-Asp-Ala-Ala-ILE-GLU-GLY-ARG
```

*Fig.* 7. Amino acid sequence of the S-fragment from the 'Pro' part of prothrombin. Residues numbered 1-118. M.w. = 12775. The underlined sequence is the nonapeptide duplicated in the A-fragment (see fig. 8).

From these data the complete amino acid sequence of the S-fragment was deduced and is shown in figure 7. The three internal disulphide bridges of the S-fragment are listed in figure 6. We have found no carbohydrate in the S-fragment.

*The A-fragment from the 'Pro'-piece*

The following digests of the A-fragment were investigated:

1. A-fragment reduced with dithiothreitol and carboxymethylated with $^{14}$C-iodoacetate was digested with trypsin. Peptides were separated on a column of Sephadex G-25 in 50 mM NH$_3$ and further purified on paper by electrophoresis and chromatography, except for fractions containing larger peptides which were first purified on a column of DEAE-cellulose in buffers giving a gradient from pH 9.0 to 4.0.

2. Native A-fragment was digested with thermolysin at pH 6.5. Peptides were separated on a column of Sephadex G-25 in pyridinium acetate at pH 5.95 (125 mM in pyridine) and further purified on paper. The five disulphide bridges were isolated from this digest using diagonal electrophoresis.

3. A-fragment was degraded with cyanogen bromide and then reduced and carboxymethylated. The two main fragments were separated on a column of Sephadex G-75 in 50 mM NH$_3$. The fractions obtained were subdigested with chymotrypsin and the resulting peptides purified on paper.

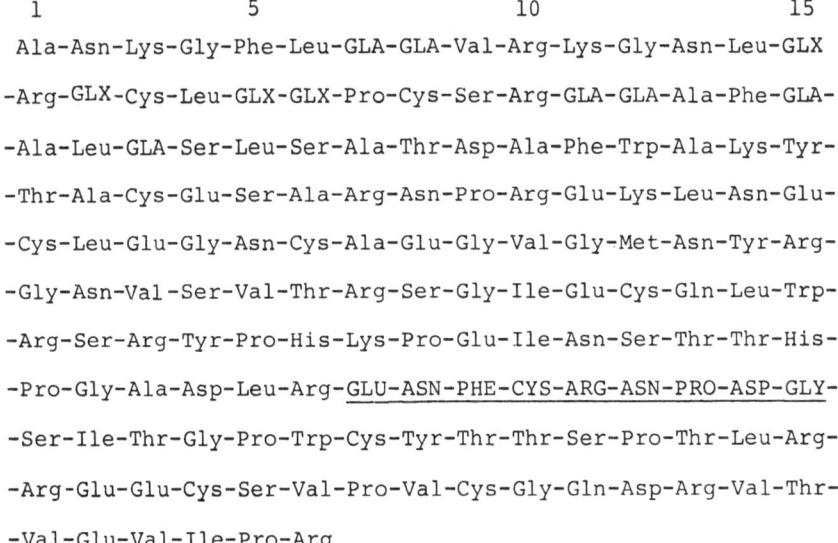

| 1 | 5 | 10 | 15 |
|---|---|----|----|

Ala-Asn-Lys-Gly-Phe-Leu-GLA-GLA-Val-Arg-Lys-Gly-Asn-Leu-GLX

-Arg-GLX-Cys-Leu-GLX-GLX-Pro-Cys-Ser-Arg-GLA-GLA-Ala-Phe-GLA-

-Ala-Leu-GLA-Ser-Leu-Ser-Ala-Thr-Asp-Ala-Phe-Trp-Ala-Lys-Tyr-

-Thr-Ala-Cys-Glu-Ser-Ala-Arg-Asn-Pro-Arg-Glu-Lys-Leu-Asn-Glu-

-Cys-Leu-Glu-Gly-Asn-Cys-Ala-Glu-Gly-Val-Gly-Met-Asn-Tyr-Arg-

-Gly-Asn-Val-Ser-Val-Thr-Arg-Ser-Gly-Ile-Glu-Cys-Gln-Leu-Trp-

-Arg-Ser-Arg-Tyr-Pro-His-Lys-Pro-Glu-Ile-Asn-Ser-Thr-Thr-His-

-Pro-Gly-Ala-Asp-Leu-Arg-GLU-ASN-PHE-CYS-ARG-ASN-PRO-ASP-GLY-

-Ser-Ile-Thr-Gly-Pro-Trp-Cys-Tyr-Thr-Thr-Ser-Pro-Thr-Leu-Arg-

-Arg-Glu-Glu-Cys-Ser-Val-Pro-Val-Cys-Gly-Gln-Asp-Arg-Val-Thr-

-Val-Glu-Val-Ile-Pro-Arg

*Fig.* 8. Amino acid sequence of the A-fragment from the 'Pro' part of prothrombin. Residues numbered 1-156. M.w. = 17533 + carbohydrate + GLA-substituents. GLA-residues 7, 8, 26, 27, 30 and 33 are substituted Glu-residues carrying extra negative charges and therefore indicated GLA in the Fig. (compare the nomenclature Cys, Cya for cysteine and cysteic acid). At least two of the GLX-residues 15, 17, 20 and 21 also carry one more negative charge than can be accounted for by all four GLX-residues being GLU.

4. Reduced and carboxymethylated A-fragment was purified on a column of Sephadex G-50 in 0.3 $M$ NH$_4$HCO$_3$ at pH 8.5. The major part of the material was digested with elastase and the resulting peptides separated on a column of DEAE-cellulose at pH 8.3 using a gradient of NH$_4$-HCO$_3$ from 20 m$M$ to 1.0 $M$, and further purified on paper.

In all four digests some larger peptides have been subdigested with other enzymes.

The complete amino acid sequence of the A-fragment is shown in figure 8. The five internal disulphide bridges are listed in figure 6.

The A-fragment contains two carbohydrate attachment sites at Asn-77 and Asn-101 as shown in figure 5.

We found in 1972 (Magnusson, 1972) that the tryptic peptides 4-10 (-Gly-Phe-Leu-Glu-Glu-Val-Arg-) and 4-11 (-Gly-Phe-Leu-Glu-Glu-Val-Arg-Lys-) had electrophoretic mobilities at pH 6.5, which could only be accounted for by one or two extra acidic groups. These peptides did not contain carbohydrate and prothrombin does not contain co-valently bound phosphorus. Since the electrophoretic mobilities of these peptides indicated that the substituent extra acidic groups were almost completely neutralized at pH 2.1 we concluded that they were probably carboxyl groups. Amino acid analysis charts of hydrolysates from these peptides were also found to contain two unknown peaks close to the positions of carboxymethylcysteine and aspartic acid respectively (Magnusson et al., 1974).

Electrophoretic mobility data indicated that glutamic acid residues 7, 8, 26, 27, 30 and 33 carried extra negative charges. Mass spectrometry of acetylated and permethylated derivatives of peptide 14-31 showed the presence of one extra methyl group on each of Glx-residues 26, 27 and 30, as well as patterns indicating that the methylated Glu had been formed by decarboxylation. Labelling experiments with CD$_3$I in the permethylation step showed that only two of the three to four methyl groups introduced by the derivatization procedure came from the methyl iodide. The assignment of the exact structure of this glutamic acid derivative cannot be made with certainty until the mechanism of derivative formation has been studied in further detail.* On hydrolysis in 6 $M$ HCl at 110°C for 20 hours the glutamic acid derivative in the native peptide is more or less completely degraded to glutamic acid.

---

* Note added in proof: Later experiments proved that all ten Glx-residues in positions 7, 8, 15, 17, 20, 21, 26, 27, 30 and 33 were γ-carboxy-glutamic acid residues (Magnusson, S., Sottrup-Jensen, L., Petersen, T. E., Morris, H. R. & Dell, A. (1974) *FEBS Letters 44*, 189-193).

| | Thrombin (275-323 + 324-582) | | | Neoprothrombin-S (157-582) |
| | A-chain (275-323) | B-chain (324-582) | Total* (275-582) | |
|---|---|---|---|---|
| Asp | 3 | 14 | 17 | 30 |
| Asn | 1 | 9 | 10 | 15 |
| Asx | – | 1 | 1 | 1 |
| Thr | 3 | 11 | 14 | 19 |
| Ser | 2 | 14 | 16 | 25 |
| Glu | 8 | 13 | 21 | 32 |
| Gln | 4 | 8 | 12 | 16 |
| Pro | 2 | 14 | 16 | 25 |
| Gly | 4 | 21 | 25 | 37 |
| Ala | 2 | 12 | 14 | 24 |
| ½Cys | 1 | 7 | 8 | 14 |
| Val | 1 | 20 | 21 | 26 |
| Met | – | 5 | 5 | 5 |
| Ile | 1 | 14 | 15 | 16 |
| Leu | 3 | 24 | 27 | 36 |
| Tyr | 1 | 10 | 11 | 15 |
| Phe | 6 | 7 | 13 | 16 |
| Trp | – | 9 | 9 | 11 |
| Lys | 4 | 20 | 24 | 26 |
| His | 1 | 6 | 7 | 7 |
| Arg | 2 | 20 | 22 | 30 |
| Total | 49 | 259 | 308 | 426 |
| M.w. | 5721 | 29683 + CHO | 35404 + CHO | 48143 + CHO |

* same as neoprothrombin-T, which has Mol.wt. 35386 + CHO.

*Fig.* 9. Amino acid compositions calculated from the amino acid sequences. Molecular weights calculated from the amino acid sequences; do not include the carbohydrate and GLA-substituents. Numbers in brackets indicate positions of the respective fragments in total prothrombin sequence.

The amino acid compositions of the two thrombin chains, thrombin, neoprothrombin-T and neoprothrombin-S are given in figure 9A; those of the A-fragment, the S-fragment, the total Pro and prothrombin in figure 9B.

DISCUSSION

*Homology of B-chain with the pancreatic serine proteinases*
The fact that the B-chain of thrombin contains all the necessary structural

|  | Prothrombin (1-582) | Total Pro-fragment (1-274) | A-fragment (1-156) | S-fragment (157-274) |
|---|---|---|---|---|
| Asp | 34 | 17 | 4 | 13 |
| Asn | 25 | 15 | 10 | 5 |
| Asx | 1 | – | – | – |
| Thr | 29 | 15 | 10 | 5 |
| Ser | 36 | 20 | 11 | 9 |
| Glu | 43–45 | 22–24 | 11–13 | 11 |
| Gln | 18 | 6 | 2 | 4 |
| Gla | 8–10 | 8–10 | 8–10 | – |
| Pro | 35 | 19 | 10 | 9 |
| Gly | 48 | 23 | 11 | 12 |
| Ala | 34 | 20 | 10 | 10 |
| ½Cys | 24 | 16 | 10 | 6 |
| Val | 35 | 14 | 9 | 5 |
| Met | 6 | 1 | 1 | – |
| Ile | 20 | 5 | 4 | 1 |
| Leu | 46 | 19 | 10 | 9 |
| Tyr | 19 | 8 | 4 | 4 |
| Phe | 20 | 7 | 4 | 3 |
| Trp | 14 | 5 | 3 | 2 |
| Lys | 31 | 7 | 5 | 2 |
| His | 9 | 2 | 2 | – |
| Arg | 45 | 23 | 15 | 8 |
| Total | 582 | 274 | 156 | 118 |
| M.w. | 65658 + 3 CHO + GLA- subst. | 29290 + 2 CHO + GLA- subst. | 17533 + 2 CHO + GLA- subst. | 12775 |

requirements for a serine proteinase has been apparent for some time (Magnusson, 1971; Hartley, 1970). This fact has only been stressed further by the completion of the sequence determination of thrombin. The three internal disulphide bridges in the B-chain occur in both chymotrypsins A and B, trypsin and elastase.

The internal disulphide bridge that connects the A- and B-chains of thrombin is homologous with the interchain bridge in chymotrypsin at least as far as the half-cystine sequence in the B-chains of these two proteins are concerned.

### Homology of thrombin with haptoglobin

It has been recognized almost since the start of the primary structure work on the β-chain of haptoglobin (Barnett et al., 1970 and 1972) that the se-

quence of this chain is homologous with those of the pancreatic serine proteinases and of the thrombin B-chain to such an extent that haptoglobin and
the serine proteinases must be considered to have evolved from a common
ancestor despite the fact that haptoglobin is not itself a proteolytic enzyme.
Since no sequence homology was observed between the α-chain of haptoglobin (Black and Dixon, 1970) and the A-chain of chymotrypsin, workers
in the haptoglobin field have not excluded the possibility that the two chains
of haptoglobin might be synthesized separately and then joined by the inter-
chain disulphide bridge in a secondary step. However, a comparison of the
interchain disulphide bridge sequences in thrombin and haptoglobin (fig. 10)
shows homology not only between the B- and β-chains in this region, but
also between the A- and α-chains. Since thrombin is derived by limited proteolysis from a single-chain zymogen it appears likely that the two-chain

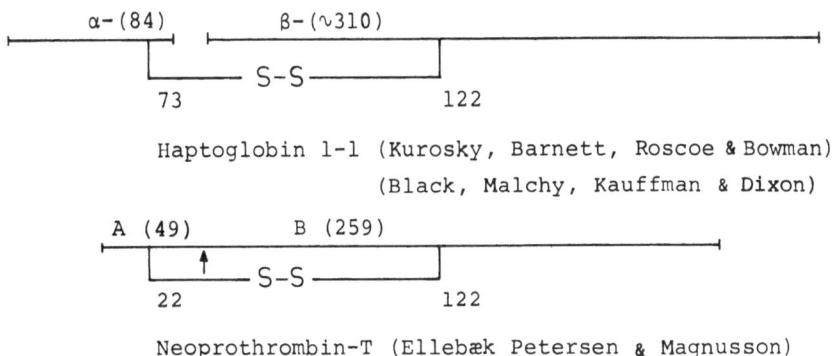

Fig. 10. Homologies in haptoglobin (α and β-chains) and neoprothrombin-T. Numbers in
brackets indicate the total number of amino acid residues in the respective chains. In
haptoglobin 1-1 the inter-chain disulphide bridge connects Cys-73 in the α-chain with Cys-
122 in the β-chain; in thrombin Cys-22 in the A-chain with Cys-122 in the B-chain. For the
β-chain of haptoglobin and the B-chain of thrombin the chymotrypsin numbering system
is used. HP = haptoglobin; NPTT = neoprothrombin-T.

structure of haptoglobin may well be derived in a similar fashion from a single-chain precursor protein. The limited proteolytic process might involve a loss of about 16 amino acid residues from the area between the potential chains of haptoglobin.

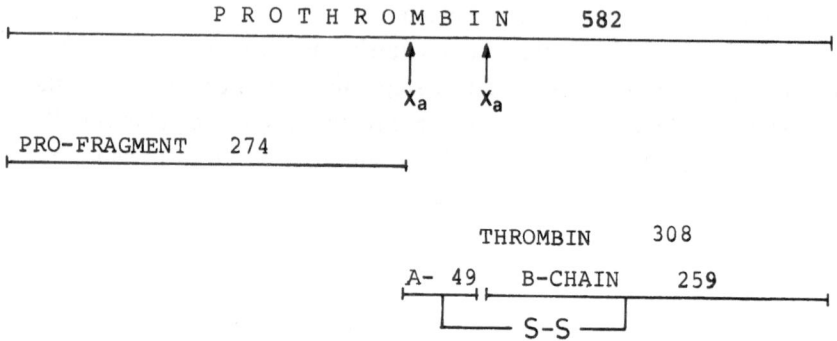

*Fig.* 11. Factor $X_a$ digestion of prothrombin (formation of active thrombin). In the Factor $X_a$-catalyzed $Ca^{2+}$-phospholipid, Factor V-dependent activation of prothrombin two peptide bonds are split producing the 'Pro'-fragment (1-274) and the two-chain thrombin (275-323 + 324-582).

*Activation of prothrombin by Factor $X_a$. Substrate specificity of Factor $X_a$*
When prothrombin is activated to thrombin at least the two peptide bonds indicated in figure 11 are split to produce active thrombin. Recent evidence (Owen et al., 1974; Kisiel and Hanahan, 1974) indicates that these two peptide bonds are the only two that are cleaved by Factor $X_a$. It turns out that the amino acid sequences of these two regions in prothrombin (fig. 12) are very similar and contain identical residues in positions P1, P2, P3, P4 and P'3. It appears reasonable to assume that this sequence has been conserved because it satisfies the substrate specificity requirements for Factor $X_a$. We are now trying to develop specific substrates and inhibitors for Factor $X_a$ based on this sequence.*

---

* Note added in proof: The substrate Tos-L-Ile-L-Glu-Gly-L-Arg-pNA (Novo, Copenhagen, Denmark) has been synthesized. It was cleaved by highly purified bovine Factor $X_a$ (gift from Dr. P. Esnouf, Oxford, England). This substrate was also cleaved rapidly by trypsin. The rate of splitting by thrombin was about 2-5% of that by Factor $X_a$ (T. E. Petersen, L. Sottrup-Jensen and S. Magnusson, in prep.). Russell's viper venom, urokinase, and streptokinase-plasminogen complex did not split the substrate. Abbreviations: Tos, *p*-toluene-sulphonyl; pNA, *p*-nitroanilide.

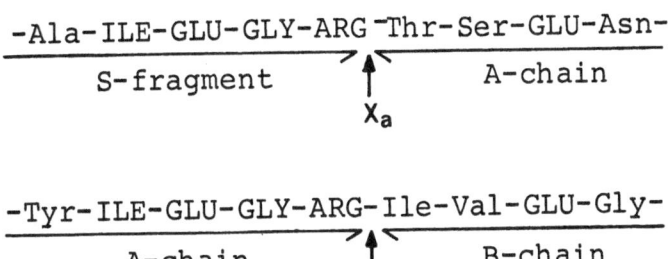

Fig. 12. Amino acid sequences of the two Factor $X_a$-cleavage sites in prothrombin.

*Thrombin-catalyzed conversion of prothrombin to neoprothrombin-S. A mechanism for 'inactivation' of prothrombin by thrombin*

A 'modified' prothrombin in the sense that the material had very different activation properties from prothrombin was first isolated and characterized in 1961 with regard to gel electrophoretic mobility, amino acid composition and sialic acid content (Magnusson, 1962; Magnusson, 1965b). This material (TEAE-peak I material) was found to be essentially inactive in the two-stage test system for prothrombin activity but could be very slowly activated by supplying the test system with serum. Other groups have made similar observations (Asada et al., 1961; Shulman and Hearon, 1963; Papahadjopoulos et al., 1964; Lechner and Deutsch, 1965; Aronson and Ménaché, 1966). Seegers et al. (1967) found that a similar product could be obtained by thrombin-catalyzed cleavage of prothrombin. This has recently been confirmed by Esmon et al. (1974).

A comparison of the published amino acid composition of the TEAE-peak I material from 1961 with that of neoprothrombin-S as calculated from our present sequence data shows only minor differences (1-4%) except in the case of a few amino acid residues where e.g. loss on hydrolysis, incomplete hydrolysis or loss on reaction of lysine with hexose could account for the differences. Thus, it is clear that the TEAE-peak I material is identical to neoprothrombin-S.

In view of the highly restricted specificity of thrombin toward protein substrates generally the presence of a thrombin-sensitive substrate region in the prothrombin structure is not likely to be unimportant physiologically. Therefore we want to propose the following general model for the activation of prothrombin. In the *first reaction*, which is catalyzed by Factor $X_a$ (fig. 11) a small percentage of the prothrombin molecules are *activated* by conversion to thrombin. When the resulting thrombin activity is sufficiently high the *second reaction* takes over. In this second reaction which is catalyzed

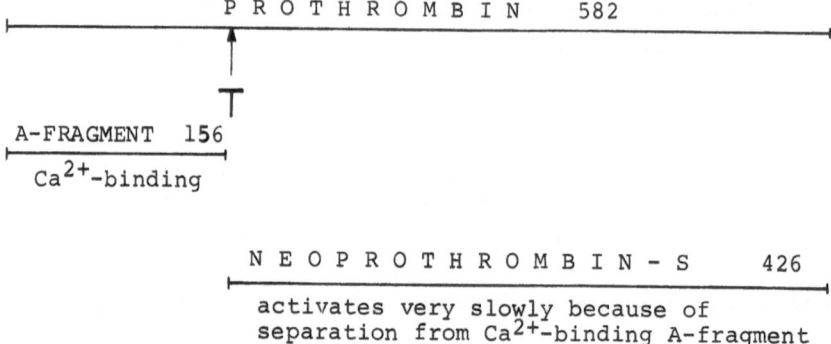

Fig. 13. Thrombin digestion of prothrombin (prevention of fast activation of remaining prothrombin). In the thrombin-catalyzed 'inactivation' of prothrombin one peptide bond is split producing the A-fragment (1-156) and neoprothrombin-S (157-582).

by thrombin (fig. 13) the remaining prothrombin molecules are *'inactivated'* by conversion to neoprothrombin-S. This proposed control mechanism would help explain the long-known fact that under 'physiological' conditions of coagulation, although the system is essentially depleted of prothrombin activity, only a small percentage of the total potential can be demonstrated as active thrombin. Thus, one important function of the large 'Pro' part of prothrombin is probably to provide the necessary structural basis for this built-in control mechanism for modulation of the degree of activation.

*Internal homologies in the A- and S-fragments*

The two 'Pro'-fragments A and S have a nonapeptide amino acid sequence in common, namely the sequence: -Glu-Asn-Phe-Cys-Arg-Asn-Pro-Asp-Gly-, which occurs in position 112-120 in the A-fragment and position 61-69 in the S-fragment (fig. 7, 8, 14 and 15). When the two fragments were aligned with regard to this sequence it turned out that each fragment contains one homologous region of 83 residues where 31 amino acid residues are identical in the two fragments. The identity includes all six half-cystines (fig. 14). The disulphide bridges in this region are also identically placed (fig. 6 and 15), forming a 'kringle'[1]-like pattern. It is interesting to note that although the two carbohydrate attachment sites in the A-fragment are placed in this very homologous region, the corresponding parts of the S-fragment have sequences (-Arg-Leu-Ala- instead of -Asn-Val-Ser-, and -Asp-Gln-Asp- instead of -Asn-Ser-Thr-) which do not fit the two common sequences

1. a classical shape of Scandinavian cakes.

```
A:   Ala-Asn-Lys-Gly-Phe-Leu-Gla-Gla-Val-Arg-Lys-Gly-Asn-Leu-Glx-Arg-Glx-Cys-Leu-Glx-
S:

A:   -Glx-Pro-Cys-Ser-Arg-Gla-Gla-Ala-Phe-Gla-Ala-Leu-Gla-Ser-Leu-Ser-Ala-Thr-Asp-Ala-
S:

A:   -Phe-Trp-Ala-Lys-Tyr-Thr-Ala-Cys-Glu-Ser-Ala-Arg-Asn-Pro-Arg-Glu-Lys-Leu-Asn-Glu-
S:                                             Ser-Gly-Gly-Ser-Thr-Thr-Ser-GlN-Ser-
                                                                        CHO
           62
A:   -Cys-Leu-Glu-Gly-Asn-Cys-Ala-Glu-Gly-Val-Gly-Met-Asn-Tyr-Arg-Gly-ASN-Val-Ser-Val-
S:   -Pro-Leu-Leu-Glu-Thr-Cys-Val-Pro-Asp-Arg-Gly-Arg-Glu-Tyr-Arg-Gly-Arg-Leu-Ala-Val-
           11

A:   -Thr-Arg-Ser-Gly-Ile-Glu-Cys-GlN-Leu-Trp-Arg-Ser-Arg-Tyr-Pro-His-Lys-Pro-Glu-Ile-
S:   -Thr-Thr-Ser-Gly-Ser-Arg-Cys-Leu-Ala-Trp-Ser-Ser-Glu-GlN-Ala-Lys-Ala-Leu-Ser-Lys-
        CHO
A:   -ASN-Ser-Thr-Thr-His-Pro-Gly-Ala-Asp-Leu-Arg-Glu-Asn-Phe-Cys-Arg-Asn-Pro-Asp-Gly-
S:   -Asp-GlN-Asp-Phe-Asn-Pro-Ala-Val-Pro-Leu-Ala-Glu-Asn-Phe-Cys-Arg-Asn-Pro-Asp-Gly

A:   -Ser-Ile-Thr-Gly-Pro-Trp-Cys-Tyr-Thr-Thr-Ser-Pro-Thr-Leu-Arg-Arg-Glu-Glu-Cys-Ser-
S:   -Asp-Glu-Glu-Gly-Ala-Trp-Cys-Tyr-Val-Ala-Asp-GlN-Pro-Gly-Asp-Phe-Glu-Tyr-Cys-Asn-

A:   -Val-Pro-Val-Cys-Gly-GlN-Asp-Arg-Val-Thr-Val-Glu-Val-Ile-Pro-Arg
S:   -Leu-Asn-Tyr-Cys-Glu-Glu-Pro-Val-Asp-Gly-Asp-Leu-Gly-Asp-Arg-Leu-Gly-Glu-Asp-Pro-

A:
S:   Asp-Pro-Asp-Ala-Ala-Ile-Glu-Gly-Arg
```

*Fig.* 14. Alignment of the amino acid sequences of the A-fragment (156 residues, numbers 1-156 in prothrombin) and the S-fragment (118 residues, numbers 157-274 in prothrombin). The alignment is based on the two nonapeptide sequences that are identical in the two fragments (see fig. 7 and 8). All positions where the two fragments have identical residues have been underlined. Residues numbered 62 and 11 indicate the beginning of the two 'kringle' regions.

-Asn-X-Ser- and -Asn-X-Thr- that normally code for the attachment of glucosamine-containing carbohydrate units in glycoproteins (Marshall, 1972). The 'kringle' region in the A-fragment contains two histidine residues (His-96 and His-105), whereas the S-fragment contains no histidine residues. The high degree of internal homology indicates that a partial gene duplication has taken place in this region during the evolution of prothrombin. The C-terminal end of the S-fragment which contains one of the two Factor $X_a$-specific sites (fig. 12) in prothrombin is not part of the 'kringle'-loop region, and is not duplicated in the A-fragment (fig. 14 and 15). This agrees with the fact that the peptide bond 156-157 that connects the A-fragment to the S-fragment is not susceptible to cleavage by Factor $X_a$.

The N-terminal region of the A-fragment (residues 1-51) is unique to the A-fragment and is not duplicated in the S-fragment (fig. 14 and 15). This is the only region where we have observed modified glutamic acid residues

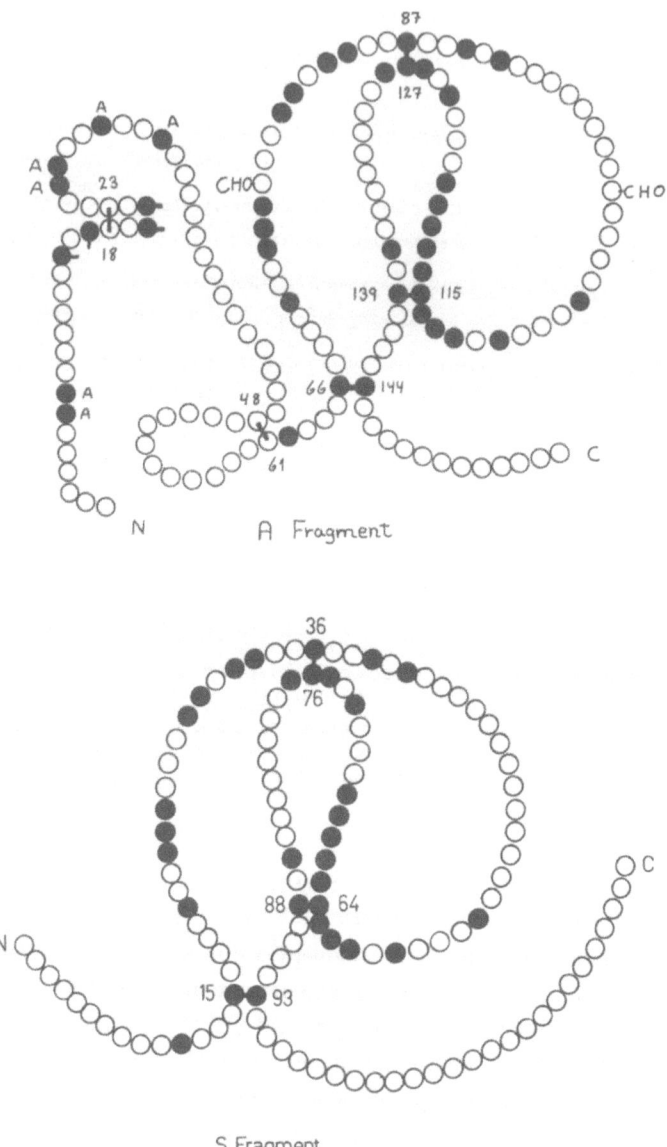

Fig. 15. Each ring represents one amino acid residue. Filled rings represent identical residues in the two 'kringle' loop regions (residues 62-144 in the A-fragment and 11-93 in the S-fragment). Connected rings represent disulphide bridges. Numbers indicate positions of Cys-residues. Filled rings marked 'A' indicate Gla-residues. Filled rings with a bar ( ● ) indicate Glu- or Gla-residues. N and C indicate N- and C-terminal amino acid residues. CHO indicates attachment sites (Asn-77 and Asn-101) for carbohydrate in the A-fragment.

and it appears that this region contains all of the vitamin K-dependent structure of prothrombin. The sequence of this region accounts for our peptide Gly-Phe-Leu-Glx-Glx-Val-Arg-Lys (residues 4-11) (Magnusson, 1972) as well as for Nelsestuen and Suttie's barium citrate adsorbable peptide, the amino acid composition of which fits approximately with residues 12-42 in our structure. Nelsestuen and Suttie (1973) found no barium citrate adsorbable peptide in digests of dicoumarol prothrombin. Stenflo (1974) found that dicoumarol prothrombin has no extra charges on residues 4-11. These findings together with our own data indicate that the function of vitamin K in prothrombin biosynthesis is to cause a postsynthetic modification of at least six, possibly all ten, glutamic acid residues in the region 1-35 to make them more acidic, thus accounting for the fact that normal prothrombin is a strongly calcium-binding protein (Ganrot and Niléhn, 1968). There is at present no convincing evidence to indicate that any other region of prothrombin is modified by vitamin K. Consequently, it also seems likely that this is the only region which strongly binds calcium ions and presumably therefore also phospholipid (Gitel et al, 1973).

*Homology between prothrombin and Factors X and IX. Role of vitamin K in blood coagulation*

Prothrombin consists of a single polypeptide chain of 582 amino acid residues. Evidence for the N-terminal 13-14 amino acid residues as well as for some other parts of the Factor X and Factor IX structures has recently been presented by Fujikawa et al. (1972, 1974). Their evidence shows that Factor X consists of two chains; the N-terminal end of the light chain is homologous with the vitamin K-dependent calcium-binding region of the A-fragment in prothrombin. The heavy chain corresponds in homology and function as a serine proteinase to the thrombin part of the prothrombin structure. The two chains of Factor X are held together by a disulphide bridge. Even after activation of Factor X to Factor $X_a$ this disulphide bridge connects the active serine proteinase chain with the light chain. The latter apparently contains the vitamin K-dependent calcium-binding region. Factor IX consists of a single polypeptide chain. Its N-terminal end is also homologous with the vitamin K-dependent calcium-binding region of prothrombin. The activated Factor $IX_a$ consists of two chains. The light chain, apparently carrying the vitamin K-dependent calcium-binding region, is attached by a disulphide bridge to the heavy chain serine proteinase part just as in Factor $X_a$. It is logical to conclude from this information that the role of vitamin K in blood coagulation is to provide the enzymes Factor $X_a$ and Factor $IX_a$ as well as their respective substrates prothrombin and Factor X with a strongly calcium-binding structure such that these otherwise quite hydrophilic proteins can be 'anchored' to the surface of phospholipid micelles. This leads to a high local concentration of *both enzyme and substrate* in the two activation reactions which are known to be phospholipid dependent, namely the activation of Factor X and the activation of prothrombin. Therefore the consequence of the vitamin K-dependent structural modification of these factors is that the rate of thrombin formation becomes much more rapid than if it were to occur in plasma where the concentrations of Factors IX, X and prothrombin are too low to give rapid activation (cf. e.g. Barton and Hanahan, 1969).

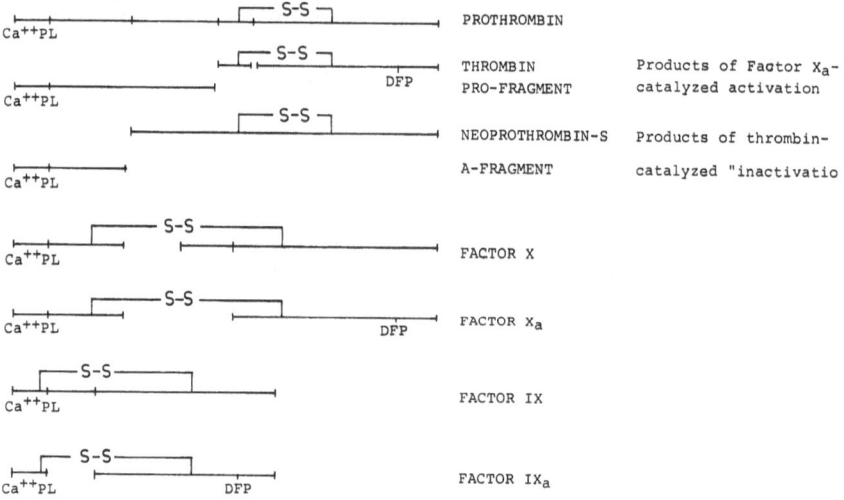

*Fig.* 16. General structures of Factors IX, $IX_a$, X, $X_a$, prothrombin and thrombin. Vitamin K-dependent calcium-($Ca^{++}$) and phospholipid-(PL) binding region is part of the structures of prothrombin (but *not* of thrombin), Factors IX, $IX_a$, X and $X_a$.

DFP indicates position of active site serine residues in the B-chain of thrombin and the heavy chains of Factors $X_a$ and $IX_a$. These chains are homologous.

The light chains of Factors $X_a$ and $IX_a$ are homologous in their N-terminal part with the N-terminal of the A-fragment from the 'Pro'-part of prothrombin.

Chain lengths are proportional to the number of amino acid residues. (Factor IX and X data from Fujikawa et al. 1972 and 1974).

A major structural difference between Factors $IX_a$, $X_a$ and thrombin, which are all three serine proteinases ('sophisticated trypsins'), is that thrombin lacks the disulphide bridge that connects the enzyme region (A-chain + B-chain) with the calcium-phospholipid-binding region (A-fragment) (see fig. 16). Therefore thrombin is detached from the phospholipid micelles and acts as a plasma enzyme, while Factors $X_a$ and $IX_a$ remain phospholipid-bound. In that sense they can be regarded as membrane-bound enzymes. Considering the rate of thrombin formation which is thus achieved it is not surprising that it has been of evolutionary advantage to 'build in' an extra piece of structure in prothrombin (the S-fragment) which has no counter-parts in the structures of Factors X and IX. The presence of this extra structure makes it possible to split off the calcium-phospholipid-binding region (the A-fragment) without obtaining active thrombin. Because the resulting neoprothrombin-S has lost the calcium-phosphate-binding region, it (fig. 13) becomes unavailable to Factor $X_a$ and is not further converted to thrombin (Magnusson, 1962 and 1965b). In this manner the formation of too much of the final product (thrombin) has been safeguarded against, without impairing the speed of initial thrombin generation. It might be argued against this theory of the thrombin-dependent negative feed-back control of prothrombin activation that since neoprothrombin-S still con-tains both of the two Factor $X_a$-susceptible regions from the original pro-thrombin molecule it would be as good a substrate as prothrombin itself for Factor $X_a$. However, the fact that the calcium-phospholipid-binding region has been lost with the A-fragment, means that a physical separation of neoprothrombin-S (in plasma) and Factor $X_a$ (on the phospholipid) is achieved. Therefore neoprothrombin-S is not an intermediate in the activa-tion of prothrombin but only a product of the thrombin-catalyzed 'shut-off' reaction. This 'negative feed-back' control mechanism probably also serves the purpose of preventing general dissemination of clotting throughout the vascular system by limiting the activation of prothrombin in space so that it occurs only on phospholipid micelles made available as the result of tissue damage or other abnormal processes. A second corollary of the negative feed-back control is that proteolytic enzyme inhibitors which act only on thrombin would only cause the system to produce more thrombin until the inhibitor is overcome and a level of active (noninhibited) thrombin has been reached, which is sufficient to start the shutting-off reaction and convert the remaining prothrombin to neoprothrombin-S, thus 'inactivating' it.

*Acknowledgements*
We wish to thank Laila Brøns, Lene Kristensen, Lone Christensen, and Margit Skriver for technical assistance, and the Danish Science Research Council and the U.S. National Heart And Lung Institute (grant number 1 RO 1 HL 16238-01 HEM) for financial support. L.S. wishes to thank the Svend Coles Frederiksen Foundation; H.C. wishes to thank the Nationaal Fonds voor Wetenschappelijk Onderzoek for a fellowship.

## REFERENCES

1. Aronson, D. L. and D. Ménaché, *Biochem.* 5, 2635 (1966).
2. Asada, T., Y. Masaki, K. Kitahara, R. Nagayama, T. Hatashita and I. Yanagisawa, *J. biochem.* 49, 721 (1961).
3. Barnett, D. R., T.-H. Lee and B. H. Bowman, *Nature* 225, 938 (1970).
4. Barnett, D. R., T.-H. Lee and B. H. Bowman, *Biochem.* 11, 1189 (1972).
5. Barton, P. G. and D. J. Hanahan, *Biochim. biophys. Acta* 187, 319 (1969).
6. Black, J. A. and G. H. Dixon, *Canad. J. Biochem.* 48, 133 (1970).
7. Blombäck, B. and M. Blombäck, *Arkiv Kemi* 10, 415 (1956).
8. Esmon, C. T., W. G. Owen and C. M. Jackson, *J. biol. Chem.* 249, 606 (1974).
9. Fujikawa, K., M. H. Coan, D. L. Enfield, K. Titani, L. H. Ericsson and E. W. Davie, *Proc. nat. Acad. Sci.* 71, 427 (1974).
10. Fujikawa, K., M. E. Legaz and E. W. Davie, *Biochem.* 11, 4892 (1972).
11. Ganrot, P. O. and J. E. Niléhn, *Scand. J. clin. Lab. Invest.* 21, 238 (1968).
12. Gitel, S. N., W. G. Owen, C. T. Esmon and C. M. Jackson, *Proc. nat. Acad. Sci.* 70, 1344 (1973).
13. Hartley, B. S., *Phil. Trans.* B. 257, 77 (1970).
14. Kisiel, W. and D. J. Hanahan, *Biochem. biophys. Res. Commun.* 59, 570 (1974).
15. Lanchantin, G. F., J. A. Friedmann and D. W. Hart, *J. biol. Chem.* 240, 3276 (1965).
16. Lechner, K. and E. Deutsch, *Thrombos. Diathes. haemorrh.* 13, 314 (1965).
17. Lundblad, R. L., *Biochem.* 10, 2501 (1971).
18. Magnusson, S., *Thrombos. Diath. haemorrh.* 7, Suppl. 1, 229 (1962).
19. Magnusson, S., *Arkiv Kemi* 24, 349 (1965).
20. Magnusson, S., *Arkiv Kemi* 23, 285 (1965a).
21. Magnusson, S., *Arkiv Kemi* 24, 217 (1965b).
22. Magnusson, S., *Biochem. J.* 110, 25p (1968).
23. Magnusson, S., In *Methods in enzymology* 19, 157. Academic Press, New York. Eds.: G. E. Perlmann and L. Lorand (1970).
24. Magnusson, S., In *The enzymes* (Ed.: P. Boyer), Vol. III, 227. Academic Press, New York (1971).
25. Magnusson, S., *Folia Haemat. (Lpz.)* 98, 385 (1972).
26. Magnusson, S., *Thrombos. Diathes. haemorrh.* Suppl. 54, 31 (1973).
27. Magnusson, S. and G. Murano, Report of the Task Force on Nomenclature of Thrombin and Thrombin-Like Enzymes, Their Peptide Chains and Zymogens Thereof, page 279-81 in *Thrombosis:* Pathogenesis and Clinical Trials. Editors: E. Deutsch, K. Lechner, K. M. Brinkhous, S. Hinnom. Schattauer Verlag, Stuttgart (1974).
28. Magnusson, S., L. Sottrup-Jensen, T. E. Petersen, P. Klemmensen and Kouba, E. Wayne State University Blood Symposium (Jan. 1973). *Thrombos. Diathes. haemorrh.* Suppl. 57, 153 (1974).
29. Mann, K. G., R. Yip, C. M. Heldebrant and D. N. Fass, *J. biol. Chem.* 248, 1868 (1973).
30. Marshall, R. D., *Ann. Rev. Biochem.* 41, 673 (1972).
31. Nelsestuen, G. L. and J. W. Suttie, *Proc. nat. Acad. Sci.* 70; 3366 (1973).
32. Owen, W. G., C. T. Esmon and C. M. Jackson, *J. biol. Chem.* 249, 594 (1974).
33. Papahadjopoulos, D., C. Hougie and D. J. Hanahan, *Biochem.* 3, 264 (1964).
34. Seegers, W. H., E. Marciniak, R. K. Kipfer and K. Yasunaga, *Arch. Biochem.* 121, 372 (1967).
35. Shulman, N. R. and J. Z. Hearon, *J. biol. Chem.* 238, 155 (1963).
36. Stenflo, J., *J. biol. Chem.* 249, 5527 (1974).
37. Ware, A. G. and W. H. Seegers, *Amer. J. clin. Path.* 19, 471 (1949).

# THE CONVERSION OF PROTHROMBIN INTO THROMBIN[1]

KENNETH G. MANN[2]

The approach our laboratory has taken in order to assess the events which occur during the process of prothrombin activation represent a rather classical physical-organic approach to the description of reactionmechanism. This approach can be summarized in four primary steps: 1) The identification of products and reactants; 2) kinetics of activation; 3) isolation and characterization of intermediates; 4) studies of the partial reaction of isolated individual intermediates. Further, since our ultimate aim is to establish a biochemical mechanism which is representative of the process which occurs when the zymogen prothrombin is activated in blood, an additional restriction is placed on our interpretation; we must have a means of establishing that the processes observed in isolated purified systems are representative of the events which occur in a complete system. For this reason, in addition to studies in purified systems, we have attempted to follow the process of prothrombin activation in activation systems which more closely approximate whole blood.

## THE REACTANT AND PRODUCT

Prothrombin has been isolated from many mammalian sources, and studied by numerous laboratories. With the exception of the recently characterized rat proenzyme, which has a molecular weight of about 90,000 (1), most mammalian prothrombins studied have a molecular weight of the order of

1. This research was supported by Grants HL 15381 and HL 16150 from the National Heart Lung Institute, and by the Mayo Foundation.
2. Recipient of a Camille and Henry Dreyfus Foundation Teacher/Scholar Grant; Established Investigator, American Heart Association.
3. Abbreviations used: DodSO$_4$, sodium dodecyl sulfate; DFP, diisopropylfluorophosphate; TAME, tosyl-L-arginine methylester.

47

70,000. On the other hand, the product of the activation process, α-thrombin (2) as it has been isolated from human, equine, canine porcine and bovine sources, has a molecular weight of about 40,000, and is composed of two chains: one of molecular weight 6,000 (the A-chain); the other of molecular weight 33,000 (the B-chain). Largely through the efforts of Staffan Magnusson (3, 4), sequence data obtained on bovine thrombin indicates that it is homologous to the other proteases of the serine protease family. In addition to α-thrombin, at least two principal degradation products exist, β and γ-thrombin. These degradation products, while present in most commercial thrombins, are not produced during the rapid activation of prothrombin, and I shall not discuss this further in the context of this talk. Henceforth, when I refer to thrombin in this discussion, I refer to α-thrombin, which is the 40,000 molecular weight molecule.


## THE INTERMEDIATES OF PROTHROMBIN ACTIVATION

The molecular weight difference between prothrombin and thrombin (approximately 30,000) indicates that the activation process occurrs with the deletion of about 42% of the molecule as 'pro' fragments. In our initial studies of prothrombin activation (5, 6, 7), we made use of the molecular weight change which we knew to exist between the product and the reactant in assessing changes. In short, in our earliest crude experiments which made use of dilute defibrinated plasma and 25% sodium citrate as activators of prothrombin, we observed, by means of kinetic studies of product formation using sodium dodecyl sulfate electrophoresis (DodSO$_4$) (8) that a variety of single chain intermediates were produced prior to the formation of thrombin activity. In our initial work, we observed three intermediates that occurred prior to the formation of thrombin activity, and later studies (9, 10, 11) led to the identification of the fourth component. Since these components were identified in terms of their apparent molecular weights relative to prothrombin in DodSO$_4$ gels, this technique has provided the primary means of identification of the intermediates, and also has provided the nomenclature system we use for the intermediates of activation. They are numbered from 1 through 4 in terms of their decreasing molecular weights relative to prothrombin. Following our initial studies, which made use of a relatively crude activation system, similar studies were performed using isolated factor X which had been activated to factor Xa by a variety of means, including Russell's viper venom, insolubilized trypsin (12), and purified tissue-factor-

factor VII[4]. In these studies of prothrombin activation, as well as those performed with the snake venom factor Xa analogues, tiger snake venom and Taipan venom (13) identical activation intermediates were produced from prothrombin when the system was evaluated by the $DodSO_4$ electrophoretic technique. Intermediates of prothrombin activation were subsequently isolated by conventional chromatographic techniques, and characterized in terms of their molecular weight, using both sedimentation equilibrium and gel filtration in 6 M guanidinium chloride (9, 10, 11).

*Table* 1.

| Component | Molecular Weight[a] | NH$_2$ Terminal[b] |
| --- | --- | --- |
| Prothrombin | 70,000 | Ala |
| Intermediate 1 | 51,000 | Ser |
| Intermediate 2 | 41,000 | Thr |
| Intermediate 3 | 23,000 | Ala |
| Intermediate 4 | 13,000 | Ser |
| α-thrombin | 39,000 | Thr, Ile |

a. Value determined by exact technique
b. Determined using the quantitative procedure of Stark and Smyth (28).

Table 1 presents the molecular weight data obtained for prothrombin, prothrombin activation intermediates, and thrombin, as well as their amino terminal amino acids. During the course of these initial studies, it was observed that while all the intermediates depicted in table 1 were observed on factor Xa activation of prothrombin, in addition, intermediate 1 and intermediate 3 were produced as the sole products of thrombin treatment of prothrombin. This observation has been extremely useful in the identification of the product-precursor relationships of each component in the activation system.

Activation studies have also been conducted with human, canine, equine, and porcine prothrombin. Examination of intermediate and product formation for these prothrombins reveals the presence of the same components produced on activation of bovine prothrombin[5].

4. Obtained from and through the courtesy of Dr. Yale Nemerson.
5. In the case of canine prothrombin, two species of proenzyme are isolated, which differ slightly in molecular size. The smaller dog prothrombin has a molecular weight of about 68,000, and differs by virtue of a deletion at the carboxyl terminal.

BIOLOGICAL RELEVANCE OF THE INTERMEDIATES

The fact that the same prothrombin activation intermediates have been identified in DodSO$_4$ electrophoretic systems, regardless of the source of prothrombin or the source of activator, indicates that there are relatively few degrees of freedom in terms of the cleavages which occur during the activation of prothrombin in purified systems. However, it is reasonable to ask whether or not the same intermediates are produced under the conditions in which prothrombin is normally activated in the biological system, that is, whole blood.

It is worth stating here that there is obviously no completely satisfactory system one can construct in order to assess the biological relevance of the intermediates. However, one can approach the question by attempting to reconstitute activation systems which approximate the complexity of the real one. We have prepared two derivatives of prothrombin which are fully active, and which generate the same products as unmodified prothrombin upon activation in purified systems. These two labeled prothrombins, fluorescein-prothrombin (14) and [$^3$H]-sialyl prothrombin (15, 16) have been evaluated in terms of their activation in whole plasma using both thromboplastin-calcium and cephalin-calcium as activators. The activation studies conducted with these two labeled prothrombins indicate that all the intermediates which are identified in table 1 from purified-system studies are produced when prothrombin is activated in whole plasma. Thus, the components listed in table 1 are probably representative of the products of the activation process in vivo.

PARTIAL REACTIONS OF THE PROTHROMBIN ACTIVATION PROCESS

The ordering of product precursor relationships during prothrombin activation has been investigated in my laboratory by making use of both factor Xa and thrombin as activators for prothrombin, and for each intermediate of prothrombin activation (9, 10, 11). These steps, as evaluated from studies of partial reaction, may be summarized as follows: prothrombin, in the presence of factor Xa or thrombin, gives rise to intermediate 1 and intermediate 3. Intermediate 1 is a precursor of thrombin and subsequently, on activation with factor Xa, gives rise to intermediate 2 and intermediate 4. Intermediate 4 is a secondary 'pro'-fragment, while intermediate 2 is a precursor of thrombin. Activation of intermediate 2 with factor Xa gives rise to the two chain α-thrombin structure.

Physical and chemical studies of prothrombin, the intermediates produced during activation, and thrombin, when combined with the knowledge of the consecutive steps of the reaction process, have allowed us to construct a structural model for prothrombin which places each intermediate within the proenzyme structure. Our model for prothrombin produced in this manner is presented in figure 1. The structural model is consistent with all the partial activation studies, as well as the physical and chemical studies of the pro-thrombin intermediates. We have confirmed placement of each intermediate within the prothrombin molecule depicted in figure 1 by amino acid sequence studies (17) which are continuing in progress and most recently, by immuno-chemical studies using antisera directed against each fragment (18). Carbo-hydrate chain placement has been deduced from quantitative determination of the carbohydrate content within each fragment of prothrombin activation[6] (19).

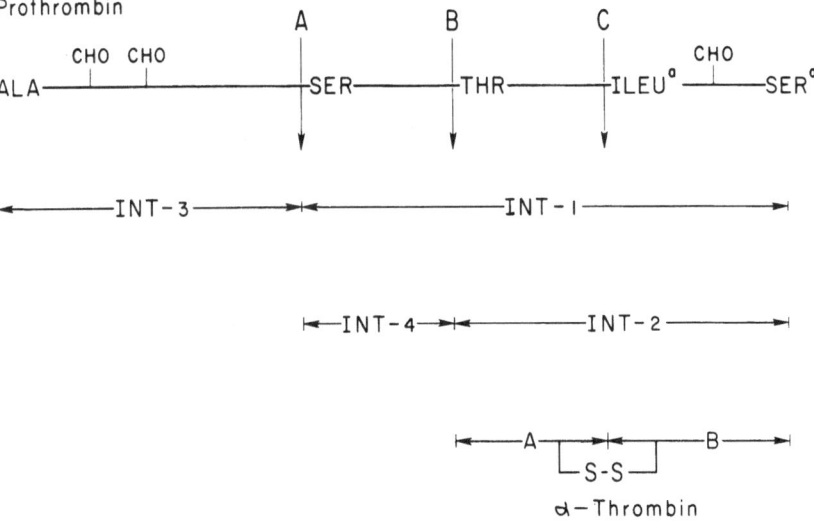

Fig. 1. Schematic structural model for prothrombin. 'CHO' represents a carbohydrate side chain. A, B, C represent cleavages which occur during activation (Modified from Reference 17).

6. Identification and quantitative determinations of all neutral and amino sugars, as well as sialic acid in prothrombin recently completed in our laboratory lead us to conclude that there are three carbohydrate chains in prothrombin, rather than four as proposed by Nelsestuen and Suttie (29).

OTHER INTERMEDIATES

During the course of our work, an intriguing experiment performed by Stenn and Blout (20) indicated that prothrombin, when activated in the presence of thrombin inhibitors, yielded a fragment composed of the entire 'pro' end of the molecule, i.e., intermediate 3 covalently linked to intermediate 4. This intermediate would not be observed if thrombin were present because of the lability of the bond between intermediate 3 and intermediate 4 to thrombin. Their observation was confirmed recently by Esmon, et al (21), and has been in part confirmed in this laboratory. In our studies, the inclusion of Diisopropylfluorophosphate (DFP) in factor Xa, calcium, phospholipid activation systems results in limited consumption of prothrombin. If more complex activation systems are constructed *vis* [³H]-sialyl prothrombin, whole serum, thromboplastin and calcium, we can show production of the intermediate 3-4 fragment. This new 'pro' fragment (intermediate 3-4) is produced in DFP inhibited systems at a rate equivalent to the rate of intermediate 3 production. Following removal of DFP, all the intermediate 3-4 produced is converted to intermediate 3 and intermediate 4 by the addition of thrombin. In contrast, in all activation systems which have been studied in the presence of hirudin as the thrombin inhibitor, the conversion of prothrombin to any product is totally eliminated. While hirudin does not appear to inhibit factor Xa esterolytic activity,[7] we have not been able to secure adequate quantitities of the material to investigate thoroughly its other (possible) interactions with factor Xa or prothrombin.

The present state of the data suggests that cleavage B of figure 1 can be elicited by factor Xa prior to cleavage A. However, even in DFP-inhibited systems, cleavage A is still occurring. From our data obtained with [³H]-sialyl prothrombin, activated in serum-thromboplastin, we would conclude that cleavage A and cleavage B are occurring at equivalent rates in DFP-inhibited systems.

CALCIUM-BINDING BY PROTHROMBIN INTERMEDIATES: POSSIBLE ROLES IN REGULATION OF COAGULATION

The fact that calcium greatly accelerates the rate of prothrombin activation implies that prothrombin binds calcium. The work of Stenflo, et al., (22, 23,

---

7. Even at hirudin concentration as high as 1 mg/ml, factor Xa esterolytic activity for TAME is not inhibited.

24) and Nelsestuen and Suttie (25) have clearly demonstrated that prothrombin binds calcium, and that, interestingly enough, this calcium binding ability appears to be deleted in the abnormal prothrombin which is elaborated in the plasma of dicumarolized animals. Extensive equilibrium dialysis studies conducted in our laboratory (26, 27) indicate that there are between 10 and 11 calcium binding sites in the prothrombin molecule, half of which have a log $K_a$ of 3.7 and half of which have a log $K_a$ of about 2.5. The strong binding sites (log $K_a$ 3.7) are contained within the intermediate 3 segment of the molecule, while the weak calcium binding sites (log $K_a$ 2.5) are contained within the intermediate 4 segment of the molecule. Thus both 'pro' fragments, intermediate 3 and intermediate 4, represent the calcium binding potential of the prothrombin molecule, and further, both of these fragments mediate aspects of the prothrombin activation process. Intermediate 3, the amino-terminal 'pro' fragment, is a potent inhibitor of the prothrombinase complex, and may serve as a feed-back regulator of this step in blood coagulation. The inhibitory effectiveness of intermediate 3 can be demonstrated in purified systems when calcium and factor Xa alone are supplied as the catalyst, and can also be seen in such complex systems as the plasma clot time, the partial thromboplastin time, the prothrombin time, and the two-stage activation of prothrombin.

Three observations suggest that the intermediate 3 segment of the prothrombin molecule is responsible for the binding of the zymogen to the prothrombinase complex; these are as follows: 1) the abnormal prothrombin isolated from the plasma of dicoumarolized animals is indistinguishable from normal prothrombin in all respects save those of calcium binding and activatibility; 2) the strong calcium binding sites for the prothrombin molecule are contained within the intermediate 3 segment of the molecule; and 3) the intermediate 3 segment is a potent inhibitor of the prothrombinase complex. It is likely that vitamin K plays a role in the formation of the calcium binding sites in the intermediate 3 segment of the molecule.

The intermediate 4 segment of the prothrombin molecule, which contains the remaining weak calcium binding sites, appears to have a regulatory influence on thrombin activity, but at the present time, it is not clear what the biological significance of this regulation is. Intermediate 4 binds tightly to thrombin, and has the effect of potentiating thrombin activity towards synthetic esters such as tosyl-L-arginine methylester (TAME) (7, 27). This activating effect is not seen when intermediate 4 is admixed with other serine proteases, including factor Xa. Intermediate 4 has neither an inhibitory nor activating effect on the activity of thrombin on fibrinogen. Intermediate 4 can be displaced from α-thrombin by the addition of intermediate 2, and can also be displaced by other components which bind α-thrombin, such as soybean trypsin inhibitor. At the present time, we assume that the binding of intermediate 4 to thrombin, and the potentiation of thrombin esterase activity by this route is a phenomenon which may be indicative of an altered proteolytic specificity of thrombin, but we do not understand the biological relevance of this altered esterase activity.

*Table* 2. Rate of Thrombin Formation

| Activator | | Relative Rate* (nmole/minute) | |
|---|---|---|---|
| | II | Intermediate 1 | Intermediate 2 |
| Xa | 1.0 | 0.3 | 6.1 |
| Xa, Ca++ | 37.0 | 0.86 | 2.0 |
| Xa, Ca++ Pl | 110.0 | 0.63 | 6.5 |

* Relative to prothrombin with Xa alone as catalyst.

KINETICS OF PROTHROMBIN ACTIVATION

Studies conducted with prothrombin and each of the thrombin precursor intermediates (intermediate 1 and intermediate 2) are presented in table 2. It will be noted here that a dilemma is presented. The enhancement of the rate of prothrombin activation by calcium and calcium-phospholipid is not exemplified by either of the two intermediates which are produced prior to thrombin formation. The rate of activation of neither intermediate 1 nor intermediate 2 to thrombin is amplified by the addition of calcium or calcium and phospholipid to the activation system (27). Both intermediate 1 and intermediate 2 are furthermore poor substrates when compared to prothrombin in conventional two-stage activation. These data present a dilemma in terms of mechanistic interpretation, since two intermediates which give rise to thrombin during prothrombin activation in complete systems, as well as in partial systems, activate at slower rates than their prothrombin precursor. One interpretation of this could be that the conversion of intermediate 1 to intermediate 2 and then to thrombin, and intermediate 2 to thrombin in the normal catalytic process occurs before these intermediates diffuse away from the lipid bound enzyme complex. Neither intermediate 1 nor intermediate 2 apparently have any tight-binding characteristics with respect to the complete prothrombinase complex; that is, once the $NH_2$-

terminal intermediate 3 segment of the molecule has been deleted, the remaining products no longer have any pronounced affinity for the biological activator. Another interpretation is that our picture of the catalytic activator of prothrombin may not be entirely correct.

Studies of prothrombin activation in a variety of laboratories have indicated that the activation process, in terms of thrombin production as a function of time, shows sigmoidal kinetic behavior. We have also observed this sigmoidal behavior in those activation systems which include calcium, phospholipid and factor Xa as the activator, and in those systems using calcium, phospholipid, factor Xa and factor V; in other words, a complete purified prothrombinase complex. In both systems lag phase kinetics are observed; that is, there is a definite lag following the addition of catalyst (factor Xa) prior to the production of active enzyme (thrombin). Our kinetic studies which made use of purified prothrombin and insolubilized trypsin activated factor Xa indicate that the lag phase of the reaction process is entirely dependent upon the factor Xa concentration, and that once the lag phase has been overcome, the rate of prothrombin activation is independent of the concentration of factor Xa. Table 3 provides some representative

*Table* 3. Kinetic Parameters of Prothrombin Activation

| Factor Xa Concentration | Lag time (minutes) | IIa Formation NIH IIa units/ml/minute |
|---|---|---|
| Bachmann Units | | |
| 0.5 | 0.82 | 6.12 |
| 0.05 | 1.21 | 5.58 |
| 0.02 | 1.89 | 5.14 |

kinetic parameters in terms of duration of lag (time prior to thrombin production) and initial rate of thrombin formation (following the lag phase of the reaction). The rate of the activation process appears to show a dependence only on prothrombin concentration. If one defines the lag phase in prothrombin activation kinetics as a pre-steady state event, one might be able to examine activation intermediates produced during this time, which may be different from those intermediates which we have defined earlier in this paper. Sampling of the activation mixture during the lag phase prior to thrombin formation indicates that at typical enzyme substrate ratios (i.e., 1 to 50 on a mole basis), one can observe no change in the gross prothrombin in the system during the lag phase. Our experiments, while preliminary, suggest that during the lag phase of prothrombin activation, an event which has not yet been adequately described is occurring which involves the formation of the complex activator which eventually converts prothrombin to thrombin. The observation that the lag phase of prothrombin activation is totally dependent only upon factor Xa concentration has led us to examine what the effect of intermediate 3 is on the activation rate of prothrombin in factor Xa, calcium, phospholipid and factor Xa, factor V, calcium, phospholipid activation studies. The addition of intermediate 3 to either activation system results in increased lag times, but no significant changes in the post lag phase initial rate of thrombin formation. In other words, data similar to that presented in table 3 for varying the factor Xa concentration is obtained. At increasing concentrations of intermediate 3 added to either catalytic system, one sees a prolongation of lag phase as a function of intermediate 3 concentration, while the initial rate of thrombin generation is nearly unaffected by the presence of intermediate 3. The prothrombin time, the partial thromboplastin time, and the Bachmann factor Xa assay most probably do not reflect the conversion of a significant amount of the prothrombin present to thrombin, but rather the total amount of time required to convert some small fraction of the prothrombin to thrombin. The inhibitory effectiveness of intermediate 3 as represented by such gross analyses as the prothrombin time and the partial thromboplastin time can probably be respresented in terms of a change in the duration of the lag phase of the activation system.

This last segment is included in this discussion primarily as food for thought. The kinetic studies presented are only a beginning, but they do indicate that the complete picture of prothrombin activation is only partially represented by the simple activation systems which we have presented thus far.

## REFERENCES

1. Morrissey, J. J. and R. E. Olsen, Comparative proteolysis of rat and bovine prothrombins. *Fed. Proc.* 32, 317 Abs. (1973).
2. Mann, K. G., R. Yip, C. M. Heldebrant and D. N. Fass, Multiple active forms of thrombin III. Polypeptide chain location of active site serine and carbohydrate. *J. biol. Chem.* 248, 1868-1875 (1973).
3. Magnusson, S., Thrombin and prothrombin. In: *The Enzymes III*, ed. 3 (P. Boyer ed.) Academic Press, New York. 277-321 (1971).
4. Hartley, B. S., Homologies in Serine Proteases. *Phil. Trans. B* 257, 77-89 (1970).
5. Mann, K. G., C. M. Heldebrant, D. N. Fass, Multiple active forms of thrombin 1. Partial resolution, differential activities, and sequential formation. *J. biol. Chem.* 246, 5994-6001 (1971).

6. Mann, K. G., C. M. Heldebrant, D. N. Fass, Multiple active forms of thrombin II. Mechanism of production from prothrombin. *J. biol. Chem.* 246, 6106-6114 (1971).
7. Heldebrant, C. M. and K. G. Mann, The activation of prothrombin I. Isolation and preliminary characterization of intermediates. *J. biol. Chem.* 248, 3642-3652 (1973).
8. Weber, K. and M. Osborn, The reliability of molecular weight determinations by dodecyl sulfate-polyacrylamide gel electrophoresis. *J. biol. Chem.* 244, 4406-4412 (1969).
9. Mann, K. G., C. M. Heldebrant, D. N. Fass, S. P. Bajaj and R. J. Butkowski, The molecular mechanism of prothrombin activation. Abstracts: The twenty-first annual symposium on blood, Wayne State University, Detroit, Michigan, p. 34 (1973) and *Thrombos. Diathes. haemorrh.* In press (1973).
10. Heldebrant, C. M., R. J. Butkowski, S. P. Bajaj and K. G. Mann, Intermediates of Prothrombin Activation-Physical Studies. *Fed. Proc.* 32, 318 Abs. (1973).
11. Heldebrant, C. M., R. J. Butkowski, S. P. Bajaj and K. G. Mann, The activation of prothrombin II. Partial reactions physical and chemical properties of the intermediates. *J. biol. Chem.* 248, 7149-7163 (1973).
12. Bajaj, S. P. and K. G. Mann, Simultaneous purification of bovine prothrombin and factor X. Activation of prothrombin by trypsin-activated factor X. *J. biol. Chem.* 248, 7739-7741 (1973).
13. Mann, K. G., C. M. Heldebrant, D. N. Fass, S. P. Bajaj and R. J. Butkowski, *Mechanism of prothrombin activation.* III Congress, International Society on Thrombosis and Haemostasis, Washington, D. C., 122 (1973).
14. Fass, D. N. and K. G. Mann, Activation of fluorescein labelled prothrombin. *J. biol. Chem.* 248, 3280-3287 (1973).
15. Butkowski, R. J., C. M. Heldebrant, S. P. Bajaj and G. L. Nelsestuen, [³H]-sialyl prothrombin: carbohydrate distribution during activation. *Fed. Proc.* 32, 318 (1973).
16. Butkowski, R. J., S. P. Bajaj and K. G. Mann, The activation of prothrombin IV; paravivo activation of [³H]-sialyl prothrombin. Submitted to *J. biol. Chem.* (1974).
17. Heldebrant, C. M., C. Noyes, H. S. Kingdon and K. G. Mann, The activation of prothrombin III, the partial amino acid sequences at the amino terminal of prothrombin and the intermediates of activation. *Biochem. Biophys. Res. Commun.* 54, 155-160 (1973).
18. Taswell, C., F. C. McDuffie and K. G. Mann, *Activation of prothrombin V, immunochemical relationships of the fragments of activation.* (In Preparation).
19. Hudson, B. G., C. M. Heldebrant and K. G. Mann, *Activation of prothrombin VI, The distribution of carbohydrate chain during activation.* (In Preparation).
20. Stenn, K. S. and E. R. Blout, Mechanism of prothrombin activation by an insoluble preparation of bovine factor Xa (thrombokinase). *Biochemistry* 11, 4502-4515 (1972).
21. Esmon, C. T., W. G. Owen and C. M. Jackson, The conversion of prothrombin to Thrombin, ll differentiation between thrombin and factor Xa catalyzed proteolyses, *J. biol. Chem.* 249, 606-611 (1974).
22. Stenflo, J. and P. O. Ganrot, Vitamin K and the biosynthesis of prothrombin I. Identification and purification of a dicoumarol-induced abnormal prothrombin from bovine plasma. *J. biol. Chem.* 247, 8160-8166 (1972).
23. Stenflo, J., Vitamin K and the biosynthesis of prothrombin II. Structural comparison of normal and dicoumarol-induced bovine prothrombin. *J. biol. Chem.* 247, 8167-8175 (1972).
24. Stenflo, J. and P. O. Ganrot, Binding of Ca⁺⁺ to normal and discoumarol-induced prothrombin. *Biochem. biophys. Res. Commun.* 50, 98-104 (1973).
25. Nelsestuen, G. L. and J. W. Suttie, The purification and properties of an abnormal prothrombin protein produced by dicoumarol-treated cows. A comparison to normal prothrombin. *J. biol. Chem.* 247, 8176-8182 (1972).

26. Bajaj, S. P., R. J. Butkowski, D. N. Fass and K. G. Mann, *Activation of Prothrombin – feed back regulation, abstracts*, 16th annual meeting American Society of Hematology, p. 61 (1973).
27. Mann, K. G., S. P. Bajaj, R. J. Butkowski, C. M. Heldebrant and D. N. Fass, *Intermediates of prothrombin activation*. Series Haematologica IV, 479 (1973).
28. Stark, G. R. and D. G. Smyth, The use of cyanate for the use of $NH_2$-terminal residues in proteins. *J. biol. Chem.* 238, 214-226 (1963).
29. Nelsestuen, G. L. and J. W. Suttie, The carbohydrate of bovine prothrombin. Partial structural determination demonstrating the presence of α-galactose residues. *J. biol. Chem.* 247, 6096-6102 (1972).

# THE CONVERSION OF PROTHROMBIN TO THROMBIN: THE FUNCTION OF THE PROPIECE OF PROTHROMBIN[1]

CRAIG M. JACKSON, CHARLES T. ESMON, SANFORD N. GITEL, WHYTE G. OWEN AND RUTH ANN HENRIKSEN

## INTRODUCTION

Prothrombin activation which under optimal conditions requires the pro-teolytic enzyme, Factor Xa, the paraenzyme, Factor Va, a negatively charged phospholipid surface, and $Ca^{2+}$ ions, has provided a fascinating system for investigation by scientists of virtually every persuasion. More-over, no process other than blood coagulation generally has depended so heavily upon the collective contributions of clinical, genetic, physical and biochemical investigators. Although the dependence of any current investi-gation on previous contributions and the evolutionary development of scientific ideas are both fully recognized, it seems most appropriate here to review only our recent work without attempting to place our observations in a historical context. That many of the ideas and approaches described here are derived from the work of earlier investigators is implicitly acknowledged and references to our sources can be found in the primary reports of this work (1-8).

Our investigation of bovine prothrombin activation was undertaken in an attempt to meet three principal objectives: 1) to account for the entire mass of the prothrombin molecule in the activation products; 2) to discover the function of the nonthrombin forming portions of the prothrombin molecule and 3) to determine the pathway by which prothrombin is converted to thrombin. During the early work on the third objective, a complication in accounting for the reaction kinetics arose which resulted in a fourth, sub-sidiary objective, viz. determining which of the two proteolytic enzymes present during prothrombin activation, factor Xa or thrombin, catalyzed the

1. This work was supported by grants from the United States Department of Health, Education and Welfare, National Institutes of Health, Heart and Lung Institute, Bethesda, Maryland 20014.

formation of each of the final activation products. The data which provided the solution to this problem were reported first, however, by Stenn and Blout (9).

PRODUCTS OF PROTHROMBIN ACTIVATION BY [XA, CA$^{2+}$] AND [XA, VA, PHOSPHOLIPID, CA$^{2+}$]

The stepwise cleavage of the prothrombin molecule and the enzymes responsible for each of the particular products are given in the chemical equations of figure 1[2]. It must be stated that these equations describe only

$$\text{PROTHROMBIN} \xrightarrow{\text{THROMBIN}} \text{INTERMEDIATE-1} + \text{FRAGMENT-1}$$

$$\text{INTERMEDIATE-1} \xrightarrow{\text{X}^a} \text{INTERMEDIATE-2} + \text{FRAGMENT-2}$$

$$\text{INTERMEDIATE-2} \xrightarrow{\text{X}^a} \text{THROMBIN}$$

*Fig.* 1. Precursor-product Relationships in the Proteolytic Cleavage of Prothrombin by Thrombin and Factor Xa. These chemical equations summarize only mass conservation, not cleavage as a function of time.

the conservation of mass in each of the written reactions, and do not define the activation mechanism in the usual sense, i.e. the stepwise activation

2. Intermediates are defined by us as partial proteolysis products which upon activation give rise to thrombin, i.e., contain the polypeptide sequence of thrombin. Activation fragments are nonthrombin-forming 'partial activation' or proteolysis products. The 'intermediates' and fragments are abbreviated: Intermediate 1 (I-1), Intermediate 2 ((I-2), Thrombin (T), Fragment 1 (F-1), Fragment 2 (F-2) and Fragment 1·2 (F-1·2). [Xa, Va, phospholipid, Ca$^{2+}$] or [Xa, etc.] are the abbreviations used to describe the various combinations of prothrombin activator components being employed in a particular experiment. In all cases phospholipid is an equimolar mixture of 1,2-dioleoyl-sn-glycero-3-phosphorylcholine and 1,2-dioleoyl-sn-glycero-3-phosphorylglycerol. iPr$_2$P-F is diisopropylphosphorofluoridate.

process as a function of time. This point is most clear when it is noted that the reaction of the first equation can only occur after some thrombin has been formed. The evidence upon which these equations are based is given below.

In order to facilitate presentation of the data which led to the equations of figure 1, all products of prothrombin activation obtained under the different conditions being investigated were separated by ion exchange chromatography on QAE Sephadex columns of identical dimension and with identical elution buffer conditions. A chromatogram of the starting bovine prothrombin and the relevant conditions are given in figure 2.

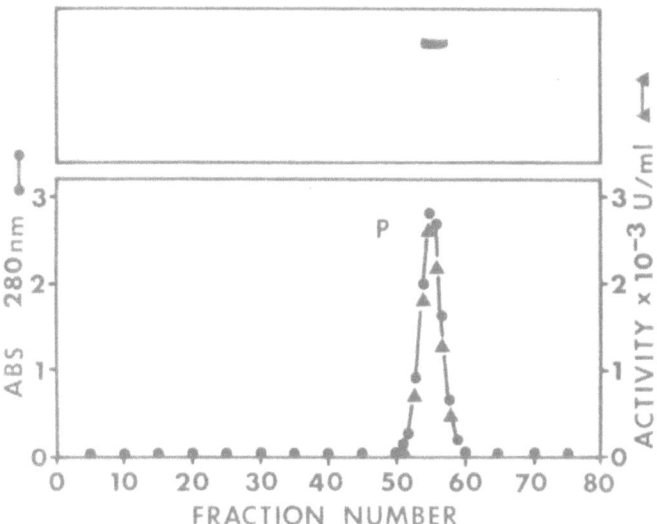

*Fig. 2.* Ion Exchange Chromatographic Behavior of Prothrombin. Column: 0.9 cm × 24 cm QAE Sephadex, Q50 overlaid with 1 cm of soybean trypsin inhibitor-Sepharose (3). Buffer: 0.02 M Tris, 0.10 M NaCl pH 7.5, Gradient: linear, 45 ml/chamber, 0.02 M Tris, 0.10 M NaCl to 0.02 M Tris, 0.60 M NaCl, pH 7.5, Flow rate: 6 ml/hr. Fraction vol: 1.0 ml. Sample 9 mg of bovine prothrombin, Sp Act 1240 NIH units/mg. in 3 ml of starting buffer. Activity (▲) is NIH units/ml of thrombin after activation. The sodium dodecyl sulfate electrophoresis gel is from the peak fraction.

The panel above the chromatogram shows the product of the peak column fraction as visualized by 'disc' acrylamide gel electrophoresis in the presence of sodium dodecyl sulfate. Activity[3] (▲) is thrombin activity in NIH units/

3. In all chromatograms ● is used for absorbance at 280 nm, ▲ is used for thrombin activity in a sample from a column fraction after incubation of the aliquot with [Xa, Va, phospholipid, Ca$^{2+}$] and ■ is used for the thrombin activity present in a column fraction prior to further activation.

ml after activation with [Xa, Va, phospholipid, $Ca^{2+}$]. The original report (3) should be consulted for complete experimental details for all activation reactions, chromatograms, and for the methods of preparation of the components employed here.

Incubation of prothrombin with thrombin (fig. 3) results in the formation

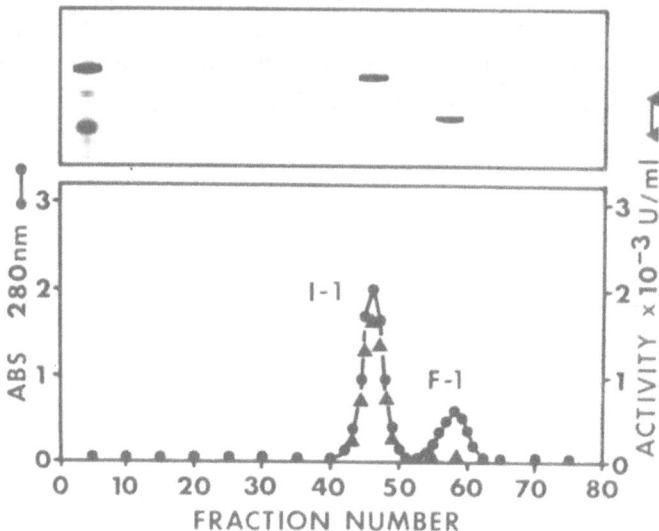

*Fig.* 3. The products of thrombin catalyzed proteolysis of prothrombin.

of the two products of equation 1 (fig. 1); viz. Intermediate 1 and Fragment 1. The first gel shown in Fig. 3 is from a sample of the reaction mixture prior to its application to the column. The doublet between the Intermediate 1 and Fragment 1 bands of this gel, is the added thrombin and an unidentified trace product. No thrombin activity other than that which was added was detectable after the incubation was terminated indicating that thrombin was not catalyzing its own formation from prothrombin.

Partial activation of Intermediate 1 with [Xa, $Ca^{2+}$] (fig. 4) results in formation of thrombin (■), Intermediate 2, a precursor of thrombin with chromatographic characteristics very similar to those of thrombin and Fragment 2. Further investigation demonstrated that Intermediate 2 was a single polypeptide chain protein with the same amino acid composition and molecular weight as thrombin, i.e. it is the direct precursor of thrombin in which the two polypeptide chains of thrombin are still linked by a peptide

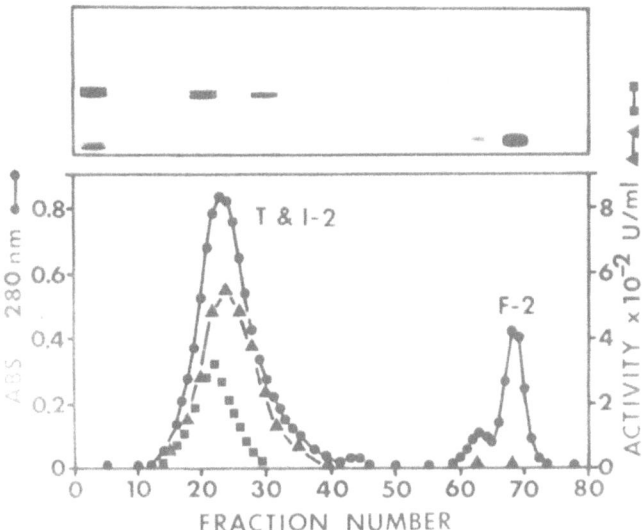

Fig. 4. The products of partial activation of Intermediate 1 with [Xa, Ca²⁺]. Gels contain from left to right: the reaction mixture prior to application to the column and aliquots from fraction 17, fraction 32, fraction 43, fraction 63 and fraction 68.

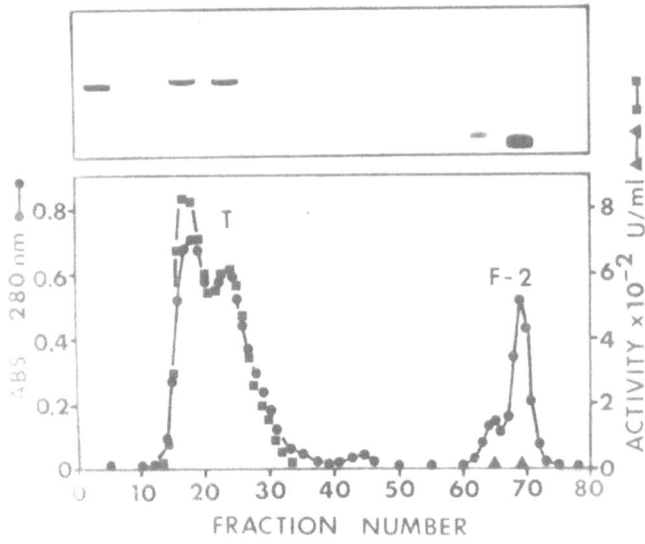

Fig. 5. Complete activation of Intermediate 1 with [Xa, Va, Phospholipid, Ca²⁺]. Gels are from left to right the activation mixture prior to chromatography and aliquots from fraction 14, fraction 25, fraction 65 and fraction 69. The double thrombin peak is an artifact caused primarily by the initial ionic strength of the sample applied to the column.

bond. Isolated Intermediate 2 was shown to be convertible to thrombin by [Xa, Ca²⁺] and by [Xa, Va, phospholipid, Ca²⁺]. These data collectively form the basis for equations 2 and 3 of figure 1. The complete conversion by [Xa, Va, phospholipid, Ca²⁺] of Intermediate 1 to thrombin and Fragment 2 (fig. 5) and prothrombin to thrombin plus Fragment 1 and Fragment 2 (fig. 6) was also demonstrated.

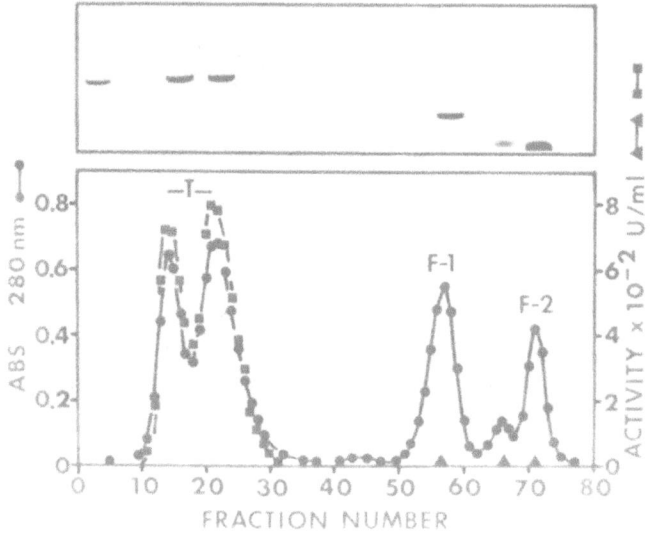

Fig. 6. Complete activation of prothrombin with [Xa, Va, Phospholipid, Ca²⁺]. Gels are from samples of: the final activation mixture, fraction 14, fraction 21, fraction 57, fraction 66 and fraction 71.

Confirmation of the relationships embodied in the chemical equations of figure 1 was obtained from the amino acid and carbohydrate compositions of prothrombin and its activation products, and from molecular weight determinations by sodium dodecyl sulfate gel electrophoresis and analytical ultracentrifugation (table 1). Composition comparisons of the products isolated from activations performed with [Xa, Ca²⁺] and [Xa, Va, phospholipid, Ca²⁺] indicated no chemical difference in the products as a consequence of inclusion of factor Va and phospholipid with [Xa, Ca²⁺].

Incubation of prothrombin, Intermediate 1 or Intermediate 2 with Va, phospholipid and Ca²⁺ *in the absence of Xa* resulted in neither thrombin formation nor proteolytic degradation as examined by sodium dodecyl sulfate gel electrophoresis demonstrating that the proteolytic cleavages of the activation process are due exclusively to factor Xa.

*Table* 1. Molecular weights of prothrombin and prothrombin activation products (Ref. 3).

| Component | Sedimentation Equilibrium | Molecular weight Sodium dodecyl sulfate Gel electrophoresis | Amino acid and Carbohydrate composition |
|---|---|---|---|
| Prothrombin | 74,000 ± 4,000 | 72,000 | 72,483 |
| Intermediate 1 | 49,700 ± 3,000 | 61,000[1] | 50,082 |
| Fragment 1 | 24,000 ± 1,000 | 17,500 − 25,000 | 22,371 |
| Intermediate 2 | | 38,000 | 36,961 |
| Fragment 2 | 12,900[2] | 11,000 | 12,843 |
| Thrombin | 37,000 ± 1,000 | 35,000[3] | 36,961 |

1. This discrepancy is reproducible and appears to be found in a number of laboratories.
2. Calculated from independent measurements of the sedimentation and diffusion coefficients.
3. B chain of thrombin only.

### DIFFERENTIATION BETWEEN THROMBIN AND FACTOR Xa CATALYZED PROTEOLYSIS OF PROTHROMBIN

Although it was shown above that thrombin *could* catalyze the formation of Intermediate 1 and Fragment 1, the question of what products are formed when thrombin action is prevented must also be asked. Activation in the presence of diisopropylphosphorofluoridate (iPr$_2$P-F) results in preferential inhibition of thrombin and thus this inhibitor was employed in experiments designed to differentiate between thrombin and Factor Xa catalyzed proteolysis.

Activation of prothrombin by [Xa, Va, phospholipid, Ca$^{2+}$] in the presence of iPr$_2$P-F (fig. 7) results in the formation of iPr$_2$P-thrombin and a previously undetected product with chromatographic characteristics similar to Fragment 2, but with a molecular weight by sodium dodecyl sulfate gel electrophoresis of 35,000. If both Factor Xa and iPr$_2$P-thrombin are removed prior to chromatography on QAE Sephadex, this new product, Fragment 1·2 can be isolated free of Fragment 2. Incubation of Fragment 1·2 with [Xa, Ca$^{2+}$] or [Xa, Va phospholipid, Ca$^{2+}$] is without effect, however, upon incubation with thrombin, Fragment 1·2 is cleaved to Fragments 1 and 2 (fig. 8). Amino acid analysis of Fragments 1 and 2 derived from Fragment 1·2 confirmed the identity of this product as the complete nonthrombin forming half or propiece of prothrombin.

On the basis of these latter observations and the data from which the equations of figure 1 are derived, a linear schematic diagram for the pro-

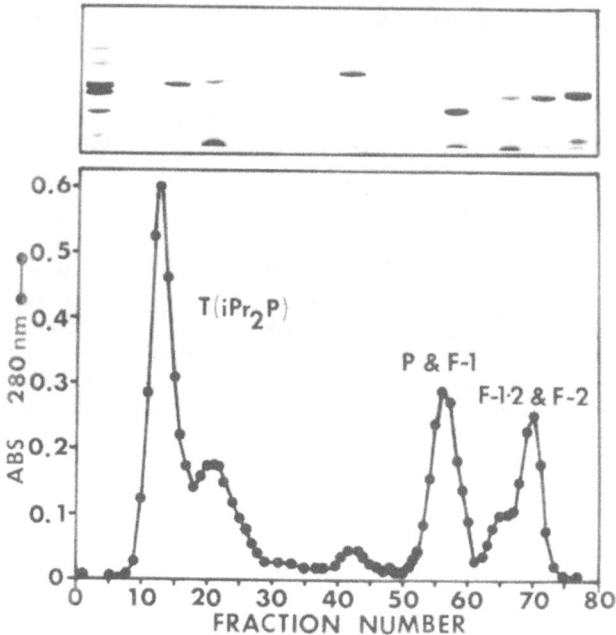

*Fig.* 7. Products of complete prothrombin activation when thrombin catalyzed proteolysis is prevented by iPr₂P-F. Gels are from left to right: the activation mixture prior to chromatography, and aliquots taken from fractions 12, 21, 42, 55, 65, 68, 71.

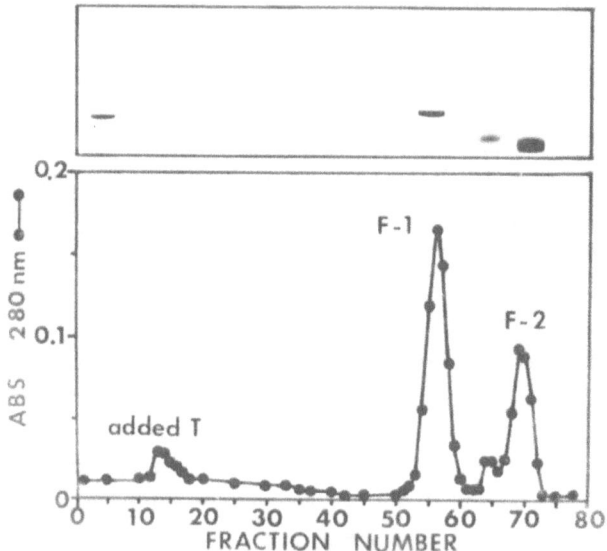

*Fig.* 8. Cleavage of Fragment 1·2 by thrombin to yield Fragment 1 and Fragment 2. Gels are from the reaction mixture, fraction 55, fraction 64 and fraction 69.

thrombin molecule can be constructed (fig. 9). Furthermore, if the peptide bonds which are cleaved in prothrombin are numbered beginning from the amino terminal end, a simple mnemonic results which simplifies both the

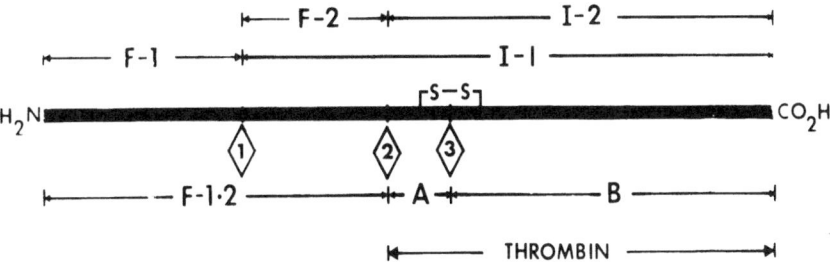

*Fig.* 9. A Schematic Diagram for the Linear Structure of the Prothrombin Molecule. The lengths of the line segments are proportional to the number of amino acid residues in each Intermediate or Fragment region.

nomenclature and structural representation of the steps of prothrombin proteolysis. Specifically, equation 1 (fig. 1) is the cleavage of bond $\langle 1 \rangle$ ; equation 2, bond $\langle 2 \rangle$ and equation 3, bond $\langle 3 \rangle$ and, except for equation 3, the intermediate and fragment numbers are the same as the bond number which leads to their formation in the mass conservation scheme.

### THE FUNCTION OF THE PROPIECE OF PROTHROMBIN: INTERACTION OF THE FRAGMENT 1 REGION WITH PHOSPHOLIPID AND CALCIUM

The first clue to the function of the Fragment 1 portion of the propiece came from the observation that activation of Intermediate 1 was not stimulated by the addition of phospholipid to $[Xa, Ca^{2+}]$ whereas prothrombin activation can be increased greater than 50 fold by appropriate phospholipid (fig. 10 and 11). As Intermediate 1 is prothrombin from which Fragment 1 has been cleaved by the action of thrombin (fig. 9), the hypothesis that Fragment 1 contained the structural features of prothrombin responsible for the known lipid binding ability of prothrombin was immediately tested. Qualitative evidence demonstrating that Fragment 1 binds to phospholipid in the presence of $Ca^{2+}$ whereas Intermediate 1 does not was obtained and has been reported elsewhere (1).

Quantitation of the Fragment $1$-$Ca^{2+}$-phospholipid interaction provides considerably greater insight into the mechanism of Fragment 1 function in prothrombin activation than the qualitative results. The technique of

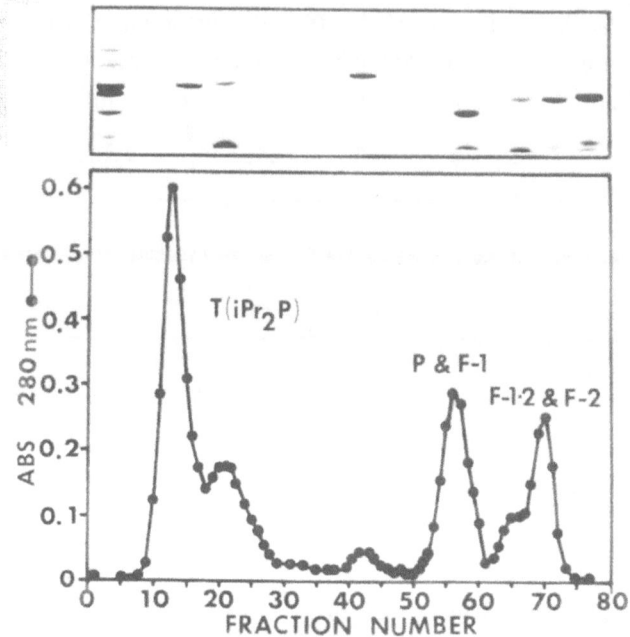

*Fig.* 7. Products of complete prothrombin activation when thrombin catalyzed proteolysis is prevented by iPr₂P-F. Gels are from left to right: the activation mixture prior to chromatography, and aliquots taken from fractions 12, 21, 42, 55, 65, 68, 71.

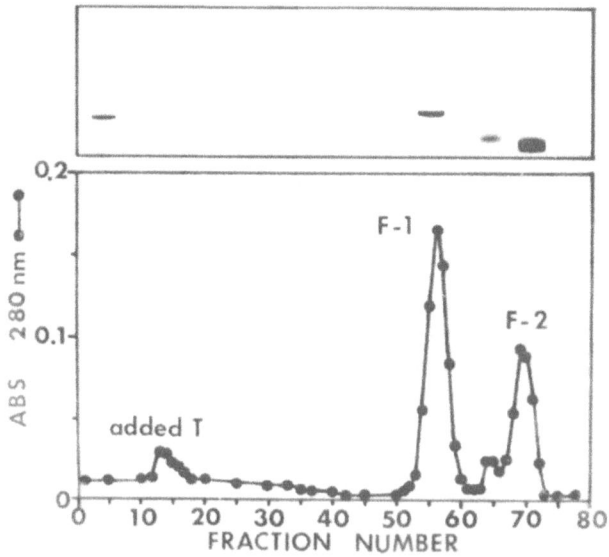

*Fig.* 8. Cleavage of Fragment 1·2 by thrombin to yield Fragment 1 and Fragment 2. Gels are from the reaction mixture, fraction 55, fraction 64 and fraction 69.

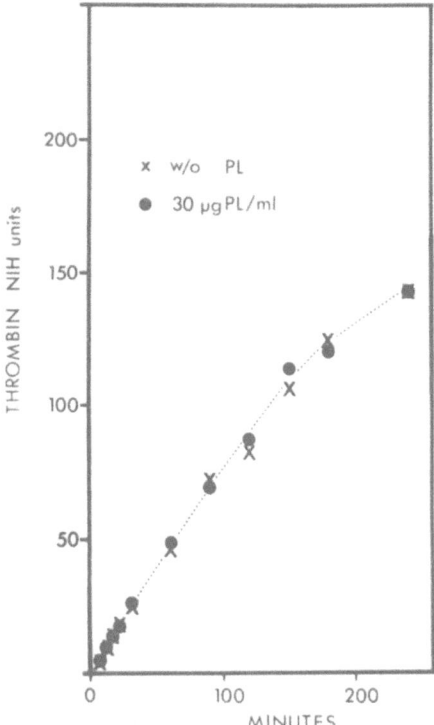

*Fig.* 11. Failure of phospholipid to accelerate the activation of Intermediate 1 by [Xa, Ca²⁺]. Intermediate 1 (0.3 mg/ml), 0.02 M Tris HCl, 0.10 M NaCl, pH 7.5, 0.010 M CaCl₂.

and Fragment 1 binding to vesicles composed of 1,2-dioleoyl sn-glyero-3-phosphorylcholine (PC) and 1,2-dioleoyl-sn-glycero-3-phosphorylglycerol (PG) in equimolar mixture by the 'Hummel-Dreyer' column technique are given in figure 12.

The average number of protein molecules bound/vesicle is calculated from the peak by employing $^{14}C$ labelled phospholipid to correct for lipid loss on the column, and from the trough, which represents the protein bound to the lipid added to the column. Similar measurements of the number of prothrombin or Fragment 1 molecules bound/phospholipid vesicle as a function of protein and $Ca^{2+}$ concentration indicate that both the number of sites on the surface of a vesicle and the binding affinity are indistinguishable for prothrombin and Fragment 1.

Isotherms for Fragment 1 and prothrombin binding to PC/PG vesicles are shown in figure 13 for 1.0 mM to 9.0 mM $Ca^{2+}$. From such isotherms

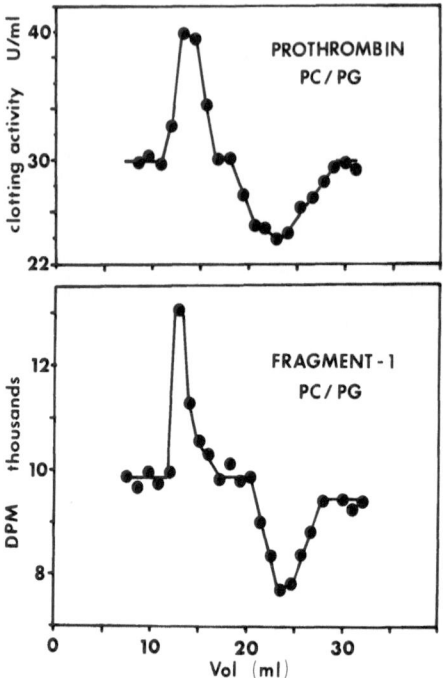

*Fig.* 12. Protein binding to phospholipid surfaces. Quantitative binding of prothrombin and Fragment 1 to phospholipid vesicles. Top: Prothrombin binding to 0.10 μMol (added to column) of single compartment vesicles made from an equimolar mixture of PC and PG Column: Biogel A 1.5, 0.9 × 45 cm equilibrated with 0.05 M Tris HCl, 0.10 M NaCl, pH 7.5, 2 mM CaCl₂, and prothrombin, 0.32 μM at 23°C. Ordinate: thrombin activity after activation, NIH units/ml. Bottom: Fragment 1 binding to 0.095 μMol of single compartment vesicles, as in the prothrombin experiment above. Column: Biogel A 1.5, 0.9 × 30 cm equilibrated with 0.05 M Tris HCl, 0.10 M NaCl, 2 mM CaCl₂, ³H Fragment 1, 0.7 μM at 23°C.

it can be deduced that 38 ± 5 Fragment 1 or prothrombin molecules bind to each lipid vesicle. Furthermore, a detailed analysis of these equilibrium binding data employing the equations for linked functions derived by Wyman (14) indicates that each protein molecule is bound to the phospholipid via 20 ± 2 Ca²⁺ ions, figure 14. A detailed discussion of the analysis of these data, including protein-phospholipid stoichiometry and affinity will be presented elsewhere (8). The relationship of Ca²⁺ in the lipid-protein complex to the Ca²⁺ bound by prothrombin and Fragment 1 in the absence of phospholipid is discussed below.

The binding of Fragment 1 to phospholipid suggests that this fragment

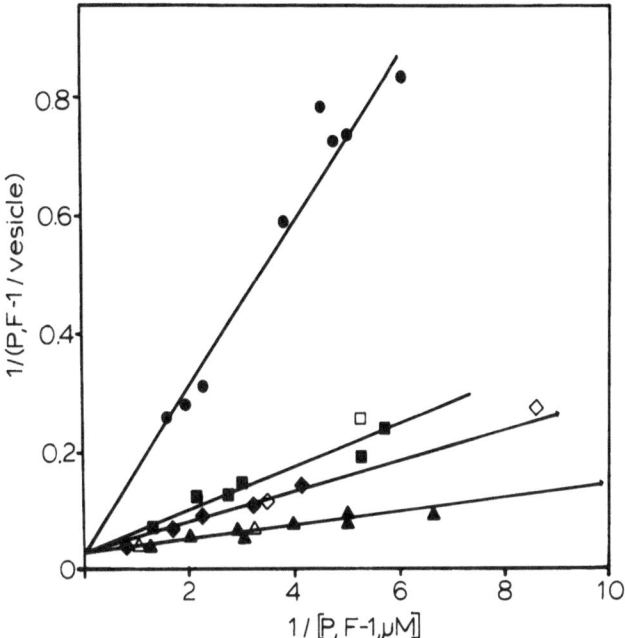

*Fig.* 13. Isotherms for Fragment 1 and prothrombin binding to single compartment vesicles containing PC and PG in equimolar ratio. Graph – the reciprocal of the concentration of prothrombin or Fragment 1 in equilibrium with bound protein versus the reciprocal of the average number of protein molecules bound to each vesicle. The solid lines are calculated for 38 protein sites/vesicle for all $Ca^{2+}$ concentrations. Individual curves are for different $Ca^{2+}$ concentrations: ● 0.5 mM, □ ■ 1.0 mM, ◇ ◆ 1.8 mM and △ ▲ 9.0 mM. Closed symbols are from data points obtained from $^3$H labelled Fragment 1, open symbols are from data points obtained from prothrombin.

should inhibit prothrombin activation by [Xa, phospholipid, $Ca^{2+}$] by competing with prothrombin for the phospholipid surface. The occurrence of such inhibition has been reported by us previously (15). Moreover, the equal affinity of Fragment 1 and prothrombin for phospholipid (fig. 13) leads to a very simple quantitative prediction about the effect of Fragment 1 on the rate of prothrombin activation by [Xa, phospholipid, $Ca^{2+}$].

38 PROTHROMBIN + 38 (20 $Ca^{2+}$) + PHOSPHOLIPID VESICLE $\rightleftharpoons$ $\left[\text{PROTHROMBIN } (Ca^{2+})_{20}\right]_{38}$ PHOSPHOLIPID VESICLE

LIPID-PROTEIN COMPLEX

*Fig.* 14. Stoichiometry of Prothrombin and Fragment 1 binding to vesicles containing Phosphatidylcholine and Phosphatidylglycerol; calculated from the data of Fig. 13.

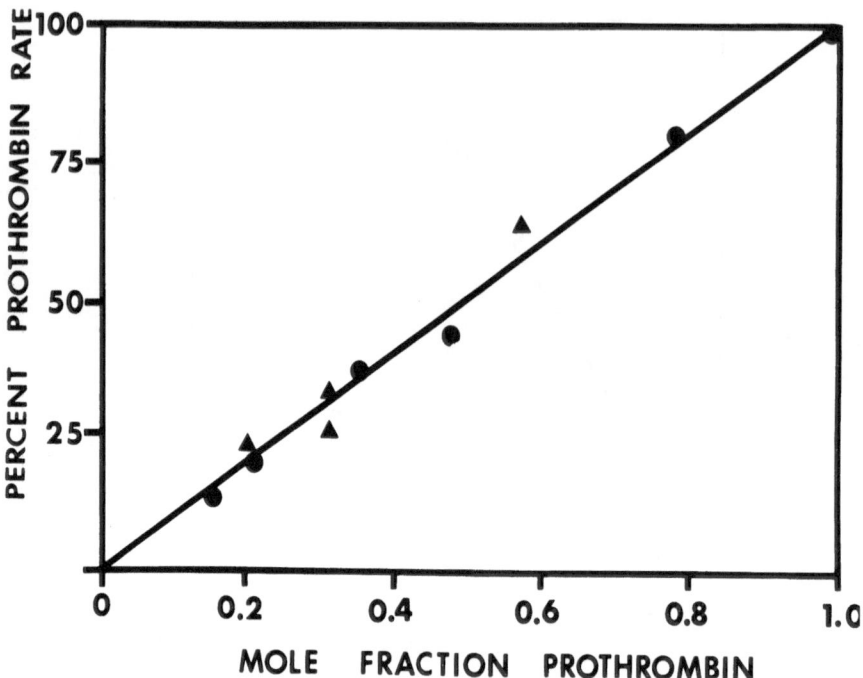

*Fig.* 15. Fragment 1 inhibition of prothrombin activation by [Xa, Phospholipid, Ca²⁺].
Prothrombin concentrations: ▲, 0.13 mg/ml, and ●, 0.26 mg/ml.

Specifically, the initial rate of thrombin formation in mixtures of Fragment 1 and prothrombin should be directly proportional to the mole fraction of prothrombin. Figure 15 shows that this is in fact so, confirming by an independent technique the equal affinity of these proteins for phospholipid which was demonstrated in the binding experiments.

As prothrombin and Fragment 1 binding to phospholipid are $Ca^{2+}$ mediated, consideration of the relationship between $Ca^{2+}$ binding to these proteins in free solution and in the presence of phospholipid provides some insight into the probable nature this protein-$Ca^{2+}$-lipid interaction. In agreement with previous reports (16, 17), prothrombin and Fragment 1 have been found by us to bind a total of $10 \pm 1$ $Ca^{2+}$ ions in free solution. This number which is one half the number reported above (fig. 14) for the protein-phospholipid-$Ca^{2+}$ complex, is most easily interpreted if the protein-lipid interaction is envisioned as occurring via $Ca^{2+}$ bridges between ligands on the protein and the phosphoryl moieties of the negatively charged phosphatidylglycerol molecules in the lipid bilayer. In solution, $Ca^{2+}$ binding to the protein is envisioned as occurring via 2 ligands on the protein, in the presence of lipid the protein is proposed to contribute only a single ligand to each bound $Ca^{2+}$ ion. Determination of the apparent $Ca^{2+}$-protein dissociation constants yields values not inconsistent with carboxylate mediated $Ca^{2+}$ binding to the protein and likewise, direct measurement of the number of free carboxylate groups on Fragment 1 indicates that there are a sufficient number of such groups to account for the $Ca^{2+}$-protein-lipid interaction[4].

Although much less is known about factor Xa binding to phospholipid via $Ca^{2+}$, a considerable amount of recent evidence suggests that the light chain of Factor Xa functions in a fashion analogous to Fragment 1 (15, 18, 19).

## THE FUNCTION OF THE PROPIECE OF PROTHROMBIN: PARTICIPATION OF THE FRAGMENT 2 REGION IN FACTOR Va CATALYSIS OF PROTHROMBIN ACTIVATION

The first evidence that the Fragment 2 region is involved in the activation process was the observation that Intermediate 1 activation is accelerated by [Xa, Va, $Ca^{2+}$] and [Xa, Va, phospholipid, $Ca^{2+}$] (15)[5]. At first glance, acceleration by the latter combination of components, i.e. [Xa, Va, phospholipid, $Ca^{2+}$] was puzzling in view of the absence of any effect of phospholipid on Intermediate 1 activation in the absence of Factor Va, viz. by [Xa, phospholipid, $Ca^{2+}$] (see above). However, the demonstration that Factor Va could function as a substrate binding protein (2) suggested that if the region of the substrate which specifically interacts with Factor Va were present in both prothrombin and Intermediate 1, such a result might be quite simply explained.

Systematic experiments to determine if the Fragment 2 region was functioning specifically in conjunction with Factor Va were carried out by comparing the activation by [Xa, Va, $Ca^{2+}$] of substrates which contain a

---

4. Detailed interpretation of $Ca^{2+}$ binding to the proteins and to the phospholipid residues is not yet possible as large corrections for electrostatic effects must be made to obtain intrinsic binding constants for comparison with small carboxylate containing molecules and simple phosphodiesters. A further complication exists also as the $Ca^{2+}$-protein binding is probably dependent upon the particular buffer ions used in the experiments, e.g., Tris or HEPES and the univalent cation of the supporting electrolyte, i.e., $Na^+$ and $K^+$ (17).

5. Intermediate 1 and Prethrombin (Ser) are now known to be the same molecular species. Work by Seegers and coworkers demonstrated at least 6 years ago that in the presence of sufficient Factor V prethrombin could be rapidly converted to thrombin (20).

Fragment 2 region, i.e. prothrombin and Intermediate 1 with Intermediate 2, the substrate which contains no part of the propiece. As an additional control on the Factor Va dependence, activation of each of the substrates by [Xa, Ca²⁺] was investigated also, i.e. without Factor Va being present in the mixture. Figure 16A shows the formation of thrombin from Intermediate 1 and Intermediate 2 by [Xa, Ca²⁺] as a function of time; figure 16B shows the result of the addition of Factor Va to such mixtures, i.e. thrombin formation from the same substrates by [Xa, Va, Ca²⁺].

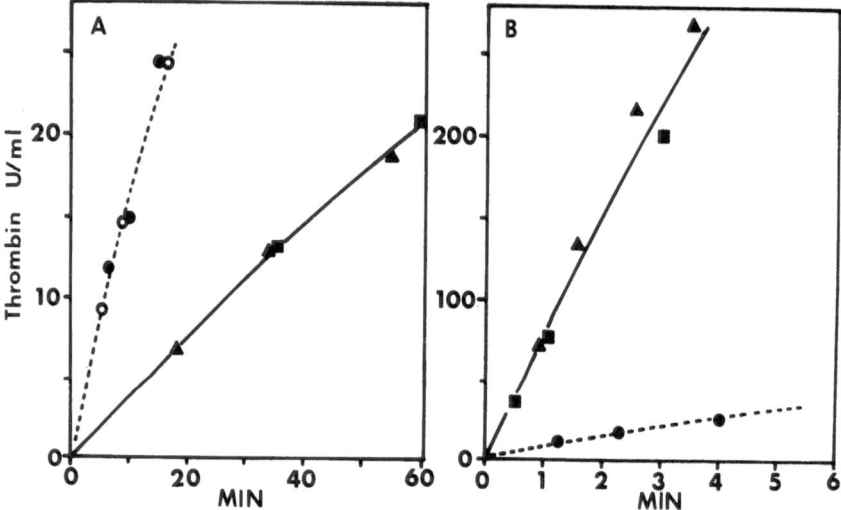

*Fig.* 16. Reversal of the relative rate of activation of Intermediate 1 and Intermediate 2 by factor Va. A. A comparison of the activation of prothrombin, Intermediate 1 and Intermediate 2 by [Xa, Ca²⁺]. Solution composition, 0.02 M Tris HCl, 0.10 M NaCl, pH 7.5. Equimolar concentrations (5.4 μM) of prothrombin (0.39 mg/ml), Intermediate 1 (0.27 mg/ml) or Intermediate 2 (0.21 mg/ml) were incubated with [Xa, 3.3 μg/ml; Ca²⁺, 10 mM final conc.]. Phospholipid is *absent* from all reaction mixtures. In one experiment, Fragment 2 (0.02 mg/ml) was added to Intermediate 2 in order to assess the effect of Fragment 2 on the Xa catalyzed activation of Intermediate 2. B. The effect of factor Va: a comparison of the activation of prothrombin, Intermediate 1 and Intermediate 2 by [Xa, Va, Ca²⁺]. All reactant concentrations are the same as in A, except that Va is present at a final concentration of 12.5 units/ml. (Note that the scales on both abscissa and ordinate are different in A and B). Prothrombin, ▲ – ▲; Intermediate 1, ■ – ■; Intermediate 2, ●--- ●; and Intermediate 2 plus Fragment 2, ○--- ○.

Two striking features are seen from these experiments. First, a large increase in the rate of thrombin formation occurs upon addition of Factor Va to Intermediate 1 or prothrombin activation mixtures and second, whereas Intermediate 2 is activated more rapidly by [Xa, Ca²⁺] than Intermediate 1 or prothrombin, the relative rates of activation are reversed when [Xa, Va, Ca$^{2+}$] is the activator and Intermediate 1 or prothrombin are activated more rapidly than Intermediate 2. A comparison of the actual rates of activation of Intermediate 1 or prothrombin by [Xa, Va, Ca$^{2+}$] with the rate of activation of these substrates by [Xa, Ca$^{2+}$] indicates that this process is accelerated 200 fold by Factor Va. It should also be noted here that the rate of activation of prothrombin and Intermediate 1 are the same with these activators, i.e. in the absence of phospholipid there is no effect of the Fragment 1 region on the activation rate.

The dramatic effect of the presence of the Fragment 2 region in the substrate for activation by [Xa, Va, Ca$^{2+}$] immediately prompted us to ask if covalent attachment of Fragment 2 and Intermediate 2 was necessary or

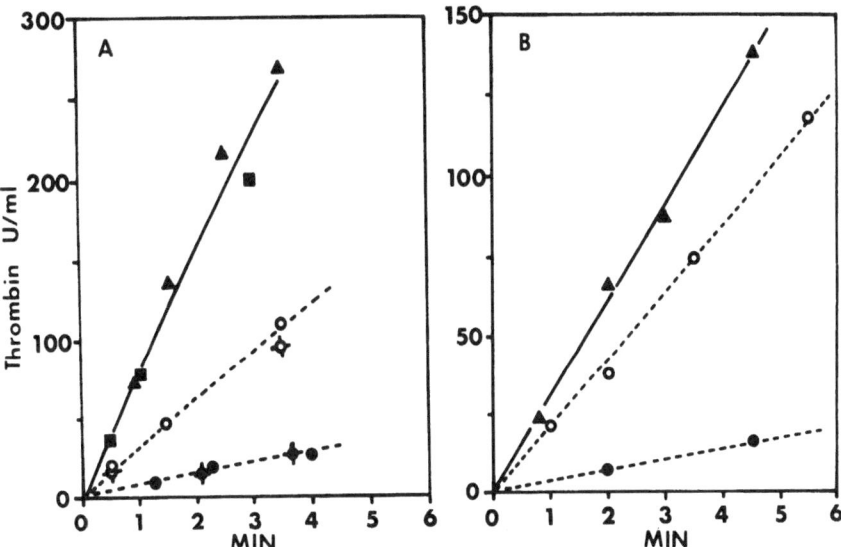

*Fig.* 17. Acceleration of the activation of Intermediate 2 by Fragment 2 in the presence of factor Va. A. Intermediate 2 (0.21 mg/ml) was incubated with [Xa, 3.3 µg/ml; Va, 12.5 units/ml; Ca$^{2+}$, 10 mM final conc.] in the presence and absence of Fragment 2 (0.018 mg/ml). Prothrombin and Intermediate 1 activation curves obtained with the same molar concentration as Intermediate 2 are shown for comparison. In one pair of control experiments Fragment 1 (0.03 mg/ml) was added to activation mixtures consisting of [Xa, Va Ca$^{2+}$] and Intermediate 2 alone and Intermediate 2 plus Fragment 2. B. Intermediate 2 (0.08 mg/ml) was incubated with [Xa, Va, Ca$^{2+}$] at the same concentrations as employed in A but in the presence and absence of Fragment 2 (0.018 mg/ml). The activation of prothrombin (0.15 mg/ml) at the same molar concentration as Intermediate 2 was examined for comparison. Prothrombin, ▲ – ▲; Intermediate 2, ●--- ●; Intermediate 2 plus Fragment 2, ○--- ○; Intermediate 2 plus Fragment 1, ◗--- ◗; and Intermediate 2 plus Fragment 2 and Fragment 1, ⬡--- ⬡.

if a mixture of Fragment 2 with Intermediate 2 could also be rapidly activated by [Xa, Va, Ca²⁺]. Addition of Fragment 2 to Intermediate 2 was
found to restore the rapid activation observed for Intermediate 1 and
prothrombin demonstrating that covalent attachment is in fact unnecessary
for this effect (figure 17). The dependence of Intermediate 2 activation rate on
Fragment 2 or Fragment 1·2 concentration is shown in figure 18. As predicted from the indistinguishable activation rates found for Intermediate 1
and prothrombin, Fragment 2 and Fragment 1·2 are identical in their
ability to accelerate Intermediate 2 activation.

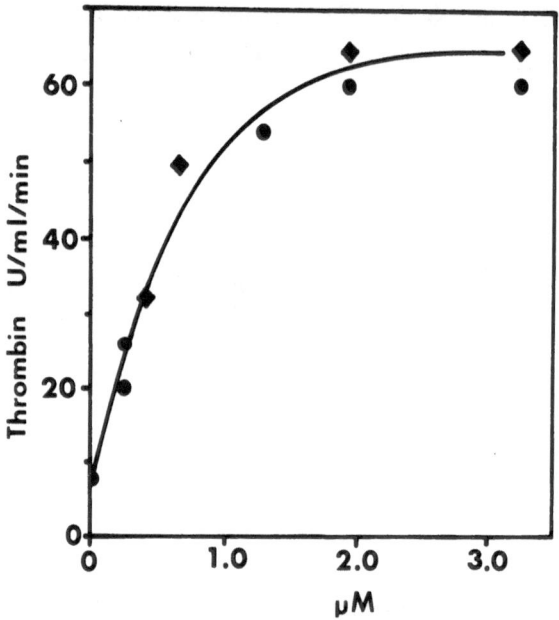

*Fig.* 18. Intermediate 2 activation by [Xa, Va, Ca²⁺]: a comparison of the effects of Fragment 2 and Fragment 1·2. Intermediate 2 (70 μg/ml) was incubated with [Xa, 14 μg/ml;
Va, 32 units/ml; Ca²⁺, 10 mM final conc.] and either Fragment 2 or Fragment 1·2 at the
final concentration shown on the absicca of the figure. The initial rate of thrombin formation was determined from plots of the concentration of thrombin versus time. Intermediate
2 plus Fragment 2, ●; Intermediate 2 plus Fragment 1·2◆ .

The maximum extent of stimulation of Intermediate 2 activation occurs
with equimolar Intermediate 2 and Fragment 2 or 1·2 suggesting that 1 to 1
recombination of the Intermediate 2 and either Fragment 2 or Fragment 1·2
may be occurring to form a product with properties indistinguishable from
Intermediate 1 or prothrombin respectively. Electrophoresis of mixtures of

Intermediate 2 and Fragment 2 or Fragment 1·2 (fig. 19) demonstrates that such reassociation does in fact occur and thus the ability of the noncovalently linked Fragment 2 or 1·2 to restore dramatic Factor Va acceleration to Intermediate 2 activation appears to have a simple explanation[6]. In contrast, Fragment 1 is without either stimulatory or inhibitory effect on the Factor Va related acceleration nor does Fragment 1 recombine with Intermediate 1 to form a species electrophoretically like prothrombin.

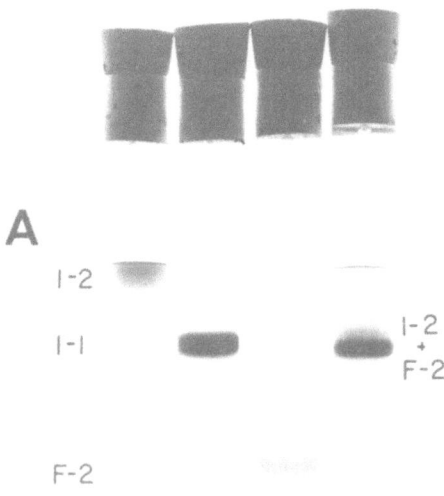

*Fig.* 19A. Noncovalent interaction between Intermediate 2 and Fragment 2. Acrylamide gel electrophoresis at pH 7.5 was performed as described by Williams and Reisfeld (22), except that stacking gels were not used. Samples (50 µl each in 0.1 M NaCl, 0.02 M Tris-HCl, pH 7.5 and containing 5% glycerol) were layered under the upper buffer, directly over the gel. Electrophoresis was carried out at 3 ma per column and at room temperature, with the gel completely immersed in the lower buffer. Samples are, from left to right, Intermediate 2, 13 µg; Intermediate 1, 18 µg; Fragment 2, 4 µg; Intermediate 2, 13 µg + Fragment 2, 4 µg.

6. The noncovalent association between Fragment 1·2 or Fragment 2 and Intermediate 2 is reflected in the chromatographic behavior of Intermediate 2 and thrombin on QAE Sephadex. In figure 4 Intermediate 2 activity can be seen to lag thrombin, consistent with preferential interaction between Fragment 2 and Intermediate 2. Such interactions may also contribute to the double peaking found for thrombin on QAE Sephadex.

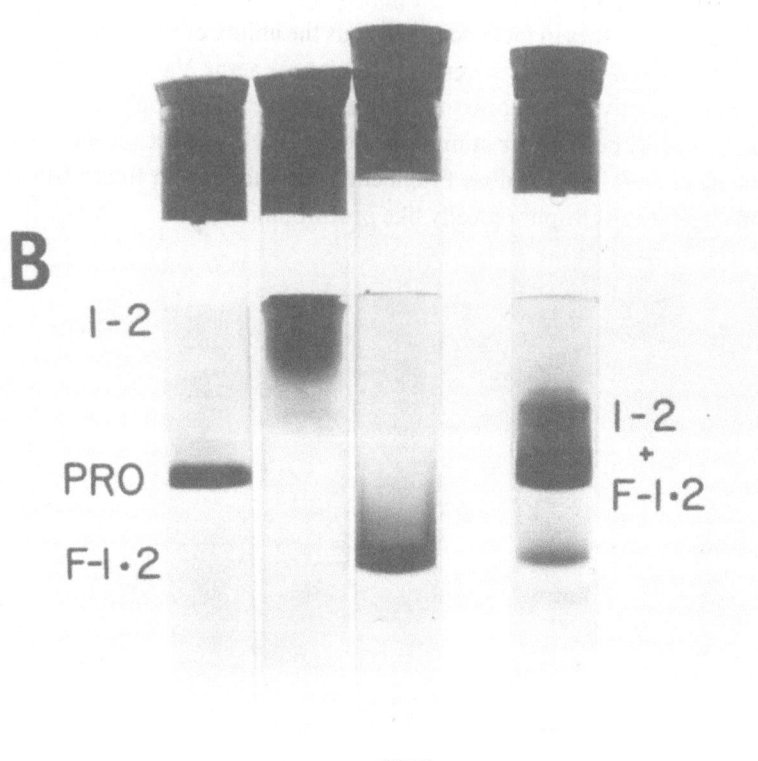

B. Noncovalent interaction between Intermediate 2 and Fragment 1·2. Acrylamide gel electrophoresis at pH 7.5 was performed as described above. Samples (50 μl each in 0.1 M NaCl, 0.02 M Tris-HCl, pH 7.4 containing 5 percent glycerol) were layered under the upper buffer, directly onto the gel. Electrophoresis was run at 3 ma per tube and at room temperature. The samples are from left to right: Prothrombin, 20 μg, Intermediate 2, 15 μg. Fragment 1·2, 15 μg, and Intermediate 2, 15 μg plus Fragment 1·2, 15 μg. The two components seen in the gel on the far right which are not identified by samples in the other gels are nearest to the top, 'Intermediate 1', i.e. (Intermediate 2 plus Fragment 2), and nearest the bottom, a trace of Fragment 1. These products are the consequence of trace thrombin contamination in the Intermediate 2.

On the basis of the organization of the Fragments and Intermediates in the linear sequence of the prothrombin polypeptide chain and the function of the Fragment 1 region in interaction with phospholipid and $Ca^{2+}$, and the Fragment 2 region with Factor Va, the following more specific schematic model for prothrombin can be drawn (fig. 20A). This particular representation also permits easy comparison of prothrombin with Factor X (figure 20B). The data which form the basis for this comparison are discussed elsewhere (15, 18, 19).

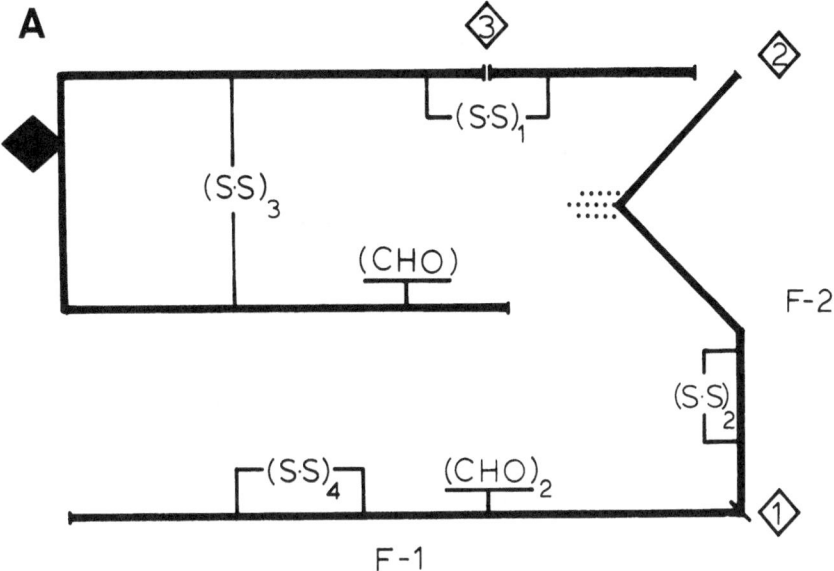

*Fig.* 20. Schematic structural comparison of prothrombin and Factor X. A. Prothrombin: the diamonds, ◇ represent the peptide bonds which are cleaved by thrombin; ①, and Factor Xa; ② and ③, the symbol, ◆, represents the active serine of the catalytic site and ... represents the noncovalent interaction between Intermediate 2 and the Fragment 2 region.

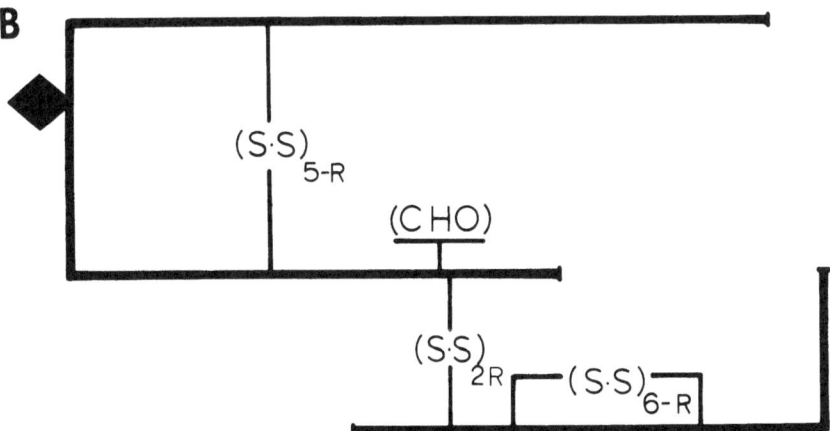

B. Bovine Factor X: The bottom polypeptide chain, which is the light chain, commences with N terminal alanine and is both the principal $Ca^{2+}$ binding chain and responsible for Factor Xa binding to phospholipid. The symbol, ◆, in the heavy chain represents the active site serine.

A MECHANISM FOR PROTHROMBIN ACTIVATION

Experiments carried out to elucidate the mechanism(s) of prothrombin activation are based on the structural information about the prothrombin molecule summarized in figure 9, and the functional properties of the Fragment 1 and Fragment 2 regions described above. Clearly, with this information in hand, each proposal for a mechanism must specifically take into account the two polypeptide chain structure of thrombin, i.e. the requirement for cleavage of at least 2 peptide bonds in prothrombin and the fact that thrombin itself catalyzes one proteolytic cleavage in prothrombin. As thrombin does not catalyze its own formation, but only the reaction leading to Intermediate 1 and Fragment 1 (fig. 1, equation 1) or cleavage of Fragment 1·2 to Fragments 1 and 2 (fig. 8), the principal focus of the mechanism investigation is on the Factor Xa catalyzed cleavages. The two peptide bonds which are cleaved by Factor Xa are designated ⟨2⟩ and ⟨3⟩ (fig. 9) and thus the problem of mechanism elucidation is reduced to determining the order of cleavage of these two peptide bonds. The two alternative mechanisms are designated Pathway II (bond ⟨2⟩ cleaved first) and Pathway III (bond ⟨3⟩ cleaved first). The chemical equations which define these pathways are given in figure 21. Pathway I, which can only exist after sufficient thrombin has been formed to catalyze the production of Intermediate 1, is shown also. The detailed kinetic evidence which shows that Pathway I is not competitive with the major pathway even under conditions in which it can be operating is given below.

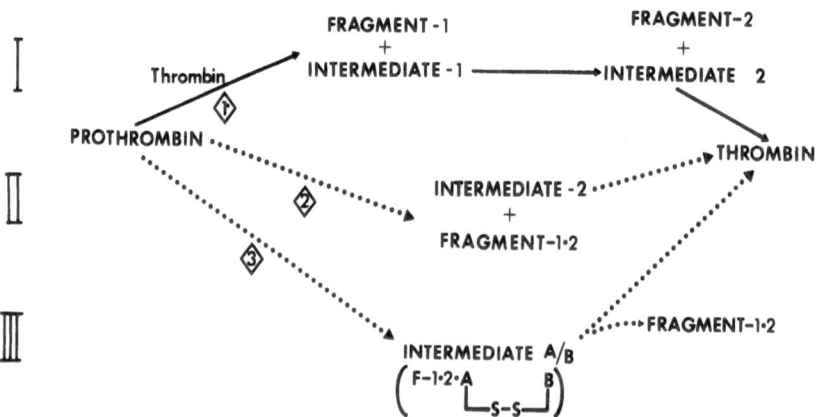

*Fig.* 21. Three possible pathways for prothrombin activation.

Experimentally, the task of determining the mechanism(s) of thrombin formation lies in showing that the following conditions or situations occur.

1) If Pathway II exists it must be possible to demonstrate that Intermediate 2 is formed *directly* from prothrombin; or, likewise if Pathway III exists, Intermediate A/B must be shown to be formed or its existence required from kinetic considerations. It should be recalled that Intermediate 2 already exists but, as it can arise from Intermediate 1 (fig. 4) what is crucial for Pathway II is that its direct formation from prothrombin be demonstrated.

2) The rate of formation of the particular activation intermediate (Intermediate 2 or Intermediate A/B) must be increased upon addition of the accessory components, i.e. phospholipid and Factor Va to [Xa, Ca$^{2+}$] if the 'basic protease only' pathway is to operate for the complete prothrombin activator.

3) The rate of conversion of the activation intermediate to thrombin must not be slower than prothrombin conversion to thrombin with any specific prothrombin activator mixture, e.g. [Xa, Ca$^{2+}$] or [Xa, phospholipid, Ca$^{2+}$].

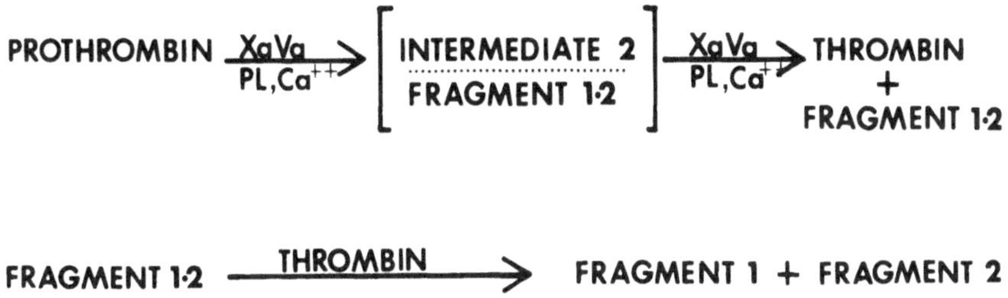

$$\text{PROTHROMBIN} \xrightarrow[\text{PL,Ca}^{++}]{\text{Xa Va}} \left[ \begin{array}{c} \text{INTERMEDIATE 2} \\ \hline \text{FRAGMENT 1·2} \end{array} \right] \xrightarrow[\text{PL,Ca}^{++}]{\text{Xa Va}} \begin{array}{c} \text{THROMBIN} \\ + \\ \text{FRAGMENT 1·2} \end{array}$$

$$\text{FRAGMENT 1·2} \xrightarrow{\text{THROMBIN}} \text{FRAGMENT 1 + FRAGMENT 2}$$

*Fig.* 22. A mechanism for prothrombin activation.

The only mechanism found which meets all three criteria (fig. 22) is Pathway II with the added restriction that the activation intermediate consist of both Intermediate 2 and Fragment 1 · 2.

The direct formation of Intermediate 2 from prothrombin by [Xa, Ca$^{2+}$], [Xa, phospholipid, Ca$^{2+}$] and [Xa, Va, Ca$^{2+}$] was investigated by sodium dodecyl sulfate gel electrophoresis monitoring of the activation time course. The results of one such experiment on prothrombin activation by [Xa, Ca$^{2+}$] in the presence of iPr$_2$P-F are shown in figure 23. As neither Intermediate 1 nor Fragment 1 are observed in this reaction mixture, the Intermediate 2 which is seen in the gels must be arising directly from prothrombin and the first criterion is therefore fulfilled. The same situation is found for [Xa,

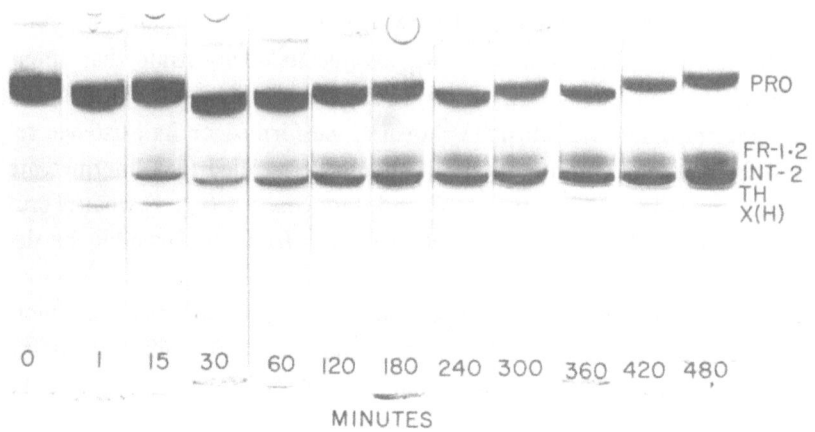

*Fig.* 23. Time course of prothrombin activation by [Xa, Ca$^{2+}$] in the presence of iPr$_2$P-F. Prothrombin (0.23 mg/ml) was activated by [Xa, 5 μg/ml, CaCl$_2$, 0.01 M] at room temperature, in the presence of iPr$_2$P-F (0.01 M), in 0.02 M Tris-HCl, 0.10 M NaCl, pH 7.5. At the times indicated in the figure, 100 μl aliquots were removed from the reaction mixture and added to 10 μl of 10% sodium dodecyl sulfate, 0.05% ethylenediaminetetraacetic acid at 70°. In samples for electrophoresis after disulfide reduction, 10 μl of βmercaptoethanol were added to the protein-sodium dodecyl sulfate mixture. Each gel contains 23 μg of protein. X(H) is the heavy chain of Factor Xa.

phospholipid, Ca$^{2+}$] and [Xa, Va, Ca$^{2+}$] and thus Pathway II is demonstrated to exist for these three activator combinations. Activation of $^3$H labeled prothrombin in the presence and absence of iPr$_2$P-F confirms the qualitative conclusions derived from figure 23, and also permits quantitation of the products. By comparison of tritiated prothrombin activation reactions carried out with [Xa, Ca$^{2+}$] and [Xa, phospholipid, Ca$^{2+}$], the requirement of condition 2 above was shown to be met also.

A representative radiolabel distribution from prothrombin activation by [Xa, phospholipid, Ca$^{2+}$] in the presence of iPr$_2$P-F is shown in figure 24. After conversion of the radiolabel distribution to mols of products it can be concluded: 1) that in the presence of iPr$_2$P-F, Intermediate 2 and Fragment 1·2 are formed at the same rate; 2) that Intermediate 2 and Fragment 1·2 formation is accelerated by phospholipid; and 3) that from reactions carried out in the absence of iPr$_2$P-F (data not shown here (5, 7) these data are not in some way dependent upon iPr$_2$P-F. No clear evidence for Intermediate A/B could be found in any of the experiments and thus Pathway III, if it exists at all, must be a minor pathway. The more extensive data and their analysis upon which these conclusions are based are found in references 5 through 7.

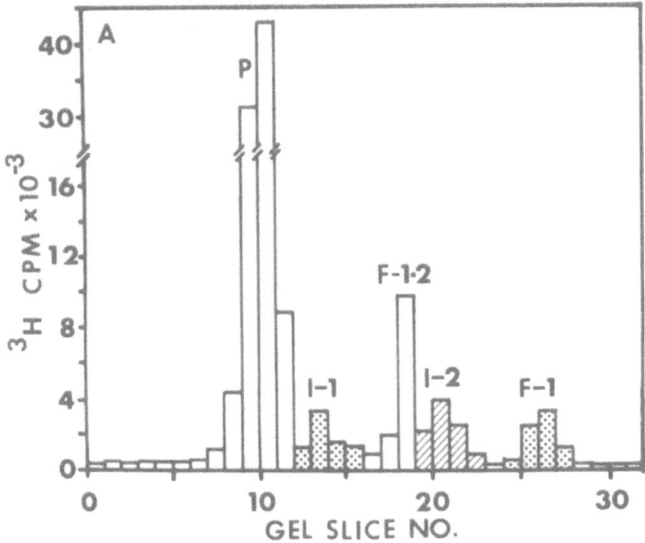

*Fig.* 24. Quantitation of prothrombin activation products. Tritiated prothrombin (0.125 mg/ml) was activated in the presence of iPr$_2$P-F by [Xa, 5 µg/ml, phospholipid, 20 µg/ml CaCl$_2$, p.010 M]. Reaction products were separated by sodium dodecyl sulfate gel electrophoresis, the gels sliced and the distribution of radioactivity determined by liquid scintillation counting.

A. Distribution of radioactive products after activation for 1 min in the presence of iPr$_2$P-F. Disulfide bridges were reduced prior to electrophoresis.

The requirement that the activation intermediate be comprised of both Fragment 1·2 and Intermediate 2 was discovered from experiments required to ensure fulfillment of criterion 3. Although when [Xa, Ca$^{2+}$] is employed to activate isolated Intermediate, condition 3 is readily met (see fig. 16), upon addition of phospholipid to the activator, Intermediate 2 activation becomes slow relative to prothrombin and thus Intermediate 2 alone cannot be the intermediate in the [Xa, phospholipid, Ca$^{2+}$] catalyzed activation. However, the noncovalent association between Fragment 1·2 and Intermediate 2 (fig. 19) suggested that 'reconstituted prothrombin' might also be a structure which could satisfy the kinetic requirements. Such 'reconstitution' was found to satisfy criterion 3 and consequently with Intermediate 2 and Fragment 1·2 together, Pathway II was demonstrated to be a satisfactory mechanism (fig. 25). Similarly, condition 3 is met with [Xa, Va, phospholipid, Ca$^{2+}$] as the activator only when Fragment 1·2 and Intermediate 2 are both present. On this basis, Pathway II appears also to be an acceptable mechanism for prothrombin activation with the complete prothrombin activator. It is important to note that whereas Fragment 1·2 is sufficient in meeting the kinetic requirement for thrombin formation from Intermediate 2, Fragment 1 plus Fragment 2 *are not* able to do so (fig. 25).

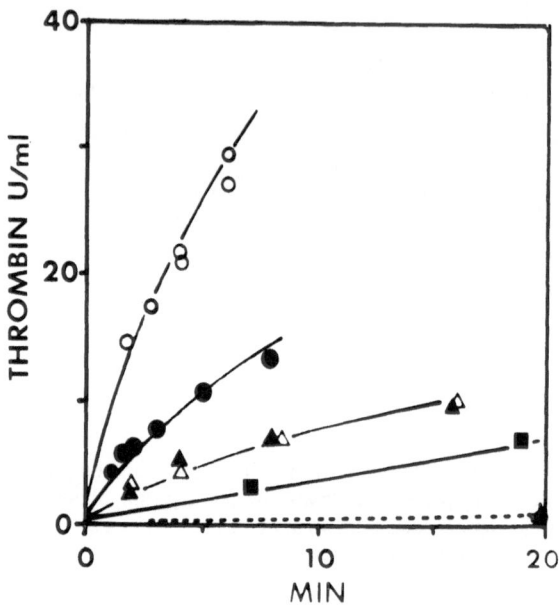

*Fig*. 25. A requirement for Fragment 1·2 for rapid activation of Intermediate 2 by [Xa, phospholipid, Ca$^{2+}$]. Intermediate 2 (0.066 mg/ml) was activated by [Xa, 2.3 μg/ml, phospholipid, 33 μg/ml, CaCl$_2$, 0.01 M] in the presence and absence of equimolar Fragment 1·2 (0.062 mg/ml). Activation was carried out in 0.02 M Tris-HCl, pH 7.4, 0.1 M NaCl, at room temperature. For comparison, the following were also activated by this same activator under identical conditions: Prothrombin, (0.134 mg/ml), and Intermediate 2 (0.066 mg/ml) plus Fragment 1 (0.04 mg/ml) and Fragment 2 (0.022 mg/ml). In order to establish a reference activation curve in the absence of phospholipid, prothrombin (0.134 mg/ml) and Intermediate 2 were activated by [Xa, 2.3 μg/ml, CaCl$_2$, 0.01 M] also.
Prothrombin, [Xa, phospholipid, Ca$^{2+}$] ● — ●
Intermediate 2, [Xa, phospholipid, Ca$^{2+}$] ▲ — ▲
Intermediate 2 plus Fragment 1 and Fragment 2, [Xa, phospholipid, Ca$^{2+}$] △ — △
Intermediate 2 plus Fragment 1·2, [Xa, phospholipid, Ca$^{2+}$] ○ — ○
Prothrombin, [Xa, Ca$^{2+}$] ● --- ●
Intermediate 2, [Xa, Ca$^{2+}$] ■ — ■

Although Pathway I (fig. 21) exists, it can be shown to be quantitatively unimportant in the initial thrombin forming process when [Xa, phospholipid, Ca$^{2+}$] is the activator from the following experiment. If thrombin formation from 1) prothrombin, 2) prothrombin at twice the concentration of 1) and 3) prothrombin and Intermediate 1 at equimolar concentration and together equal to the substrate concentration of reaction 2) is compared, the ability of Intermediate 1 to compete for the enzyme will be measured by how nearly the rate of thrombin formation in 3) approaches the rate found in 2) (fig. 26).

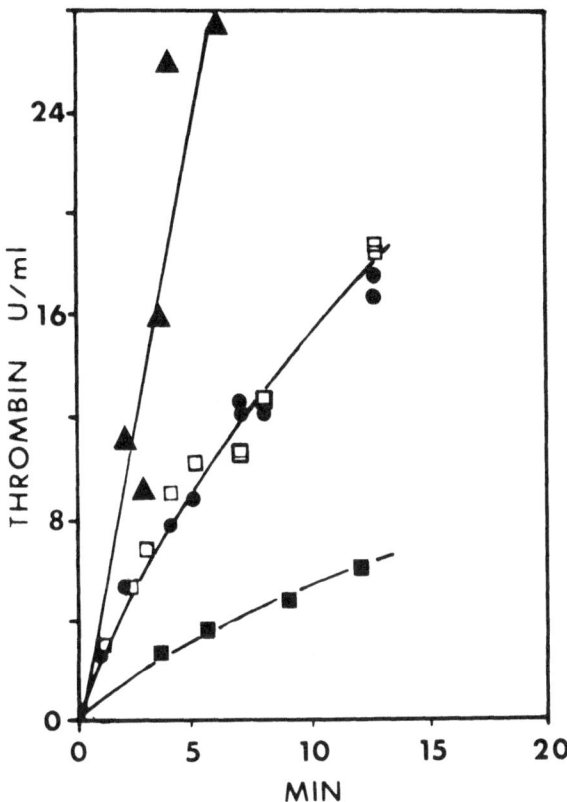

*Fig.* 26. Activation of prothrombin by [Xa, phospholipid, $Ca^{2+}$] in the presence of Intermediate 1 and Fragment 1. Solutions of prothrombin at 0.32 mg/ml and 0.65 mg/ml were activated by [Xa, 3 μg/ml, phospholipid, 20 μg/ml, $CaCl_2$, 0.010 M] in 0.02 M Tris-HCl, pH 7.4, 0.10 M NaCl at room temperature. In a set of parallel experiments, prothrombin (0.32 mg/ml) prothrombin (0.32 mg/ml) plus Intermediate 1 (0.22 mg/ml) and prothrombin (0.32 mg/ml) plus Intermediate 1 (0.22 mg/ml) and Fragment 1 (0.11 mg/ml) were also activated by the same activation mixture. Thrombin formation was determined as a function of time by bioassay.

Prothrombin (0.65 mg/ml) ▲—▲
Prothrombin (0.32 mg/ml) ●—●
Intermediate 1 plus prothrombin □—□
Intermediate 1 plus Fragment 1 plus prothrombin ■—■

From these data Intermediate 1 is seen to contribute nothing to the net rate of thrombin formation and furthermore, when Fragment 1 is added in an attempt to 'reconstitute' prothrombin from these two polypeptides, the reaction is inhibited, as predicted from figure 15. The addition of Factor Va markedly reduces the disparity between prothrombin and Intermediate 1 as competing substrates, as anticipated from the experiments on Factor Va and the Fragment 2 region, however, except under special limiting circumstances, Intermediate 1 never becomes an equally competitive substrate.

Several features of prothrombin activation emerge from these studies. First, the entire prothrombin molecule has been shown to participate obligatorily in the activation process. The propiece (Fragment 1·2) participates by interaction via the Fragment 1 region with $Ca^{2+}$ and phospholipid and via the Fragment 2 region with Factor Va. Second, in addition to these interactions, Fragment 1·2 noncovalently attaches Intermediate 2 to both the lipid and Factor Va during Factor Xa catalyzed cleavage of the peptide bond (bond 3) which generates active thrombin. These specific observa-

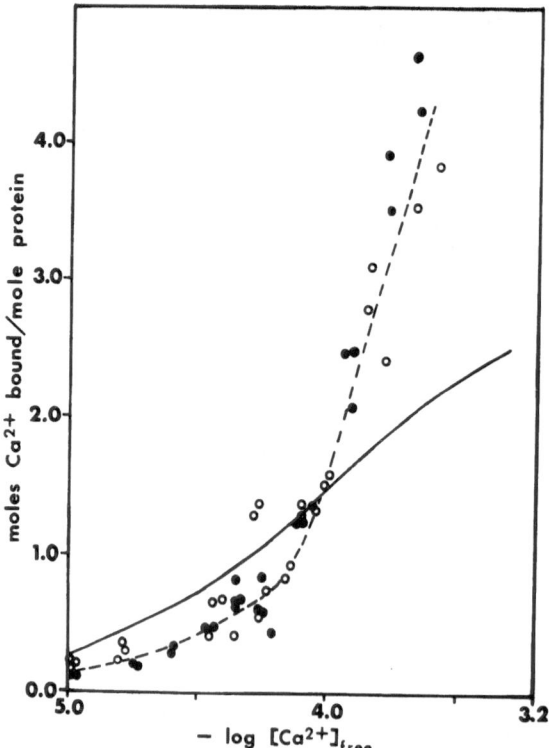

*Fig. 27.* Binding of Ca++ to prothrombin and Factor X.

tions, coupled with the previously demonstrated interaction between Factor V and Factor Xa (21) suggest that both protein-protein and protein-$Ca^{2+}$-lipid interactions within the prothrombin activator result in a system which localizes thrombin formation. The physiological significance of local thrombin formation for hemostasis seems obvious. The availability of a molecular mechanism which can account for this phenomenon suggests a myriad of experiments which should provide insight into both local hemostasic mechanisms and what may in part by viewed as delocalized *in vivo* thrombin formation, thrombosis.

In agreement with Stenflo (23) we also observe positively cooperative binding of $Ca^{2+}$ to prothrombin at low $Ca^{2+}$ concentration. Studies carried out by R. A. Henriksen in my laboratory also demonstrate similar $Ca^{2+}$ binding to bovine Factor X. As there are approximately twice as many total sites on Factor X as on prothrombin, the figure 27 most clearly illustrates the extreme similarity in $Ca^{2+}$ binding of these two vitamin K dependent proteins. Open circles ○, are Factor X data, the closed circles ●, are for Prothrombin. Within error, the binding of $Ca^{2+}$ by these proteins is indistinguishable. The solid line is the theoretical curve for $Ca^{2+}$ binding to *3* identical, noninteracting sites with k-diss of $10^{-4}M$.

## REFERENCES

1. Gitel, S. N., W. G. Owen, C. T. Esmon and C. M. Jackson, *Proc. Nat. acad. Sci.* 70, 1344 (1973).
2. Esmon, C. T., W. G. Owen, D. L. Duiguid and C. M. Jackson, *Biochim. biophys. Acta* 310, 289 (1973).
3. Owen, W. G., C. T. Esmon and C. M. Jackson, *J. biol. Chem.* 249, 594 (1974).
4. Esmon, C. T., W. G. Owen and C. M. Jackson, *J. biol. Chem.* 249, 606 (1974).
5. Esmon, C. T. and C. M. Jackson, *J. biol. Chem.* 249, 7782 (1974).
6. Esmon, C. T. and C. M. Jackson, *J. biol. Chem.* 249, 7791 (1974).
7. Esmon, C. T., W. G. Owen and C. M. Jackson, *J. biol. Chem.* 249, 7798 (1974).
8. Gitel, S. N., F. A. Dombrose and C. M. Jackson, *J. biol. Chem.* Manuscript in preparation.
9. Stenn, K. S. and E. R. Blout, *Biochemistry* 11, 4502-4515 (1972).
10. Hummel, J. P. and W. J. Dreyer, *Biochim. biophys. Acta* 63, 530-532 (1962).
11. Johnson, S. M., A. D. Bangham, M. W. Hill and E. D. Korn, *Biochim. biophys. Acta* 233, 820-826 (1971).
12. Huang, C. H., *Biochemistry* 8, 344 (1969).
13. Van Lenten, L. and G. Ashwell, *J. biol. Chem.* 246, 1889-1894 (1971).
14. Wyman, J., In Anson, M. L. and J. T. Edsall, *Adv. in protein chem.* 4, 436-443 (1948).
15. Jackson, C. M., W. G. Owen, S. N. Gitel and C. T. Esmon, *In physiology and biochemistry of prothrombin conversion, thrombosis et diath. haemorrh.* Supplement 57 p. 293 E. F. Mammen, G. F. Anderson and M. I. Barnhart, eds., In press.

16. Stenflo, J. and P. O. Ganrot, *Biochem. biophys. Res. Commun.* 50, 98-104 (1973).
17. Benson, B. J., W. Kisiel and D. J. Hanahan, *Biochim. biophys. Acta.* 329, 81-87 (1973).
18. Jackson, C. M., *Biochemistry* 11, 4873 (1972).
19. Henriksen, R. A., S. N. Gitel and C. M. Jackson, Manuscript in preparation.
20. Baker, W. J. and W. H. Seegers, *Thrombos. Diathes. haemorrh.* 17, 205-213 (1967).
21. Papahadjopoulos, D. P. and D. J. Hanahan, *Biochim. biophys. Acta.* 90, 436-439 (1964).
22. Williams, D. E. and R. A. Reisfeld, *Ann. N.Y. Acad. Sci.* 121, 373-381 (1964).
23. Stenflo, J. and Ganrot, P. O., *Biochem. Biophys. Res. Comm.* 50, 98-104 (1973).

# DISCREPANCIES BETWEEN THE ONE- AND TWO-STAGE PROTHROMBIN ESTIMATIONS IN PURIFIED PROTHROMBIN PREPARATIONS

H. C. HEMKER AND A. D. MULLER

Recently, Kisiel and Hanahan (1) reported a method to purify prothrombin. In the purified product a discrepancy was observed between the one-stage and the two-stage determination. The same phenomenon has been observed by other investigators (2). We tried to find the cause of this discrepancy and we think that in the light of the results reported by Stenflo (3) (this volume, ref. 3) we can offer a hypothesis to explain it.

In previous work we investigated the kinetic mechanism at the basis of the one-stage and the two-stage prothrombin determinations (4-6).

All prothrombin determinations are based upon thrombin generation. Thrombin generation in the absence of antithrombins has a time course as depicted in figure 1. The initial velocity of thrombin generation ($\alpha$) levels off to approach zero when all prothrombin has been converted into thrombin. The amount of thrombin then formed ($\beta$) of course reflects the amount of prothrombin originally present.

In a one-stage test $\alpha$ is measured, in a two-stage test one determines $\beta$. In both tests normal plasma is used as a standard. $\alpha$ and $\beta$ are interdependent. When this interdependancy in a preparation is the same as it is in normal plasma by definition no differences will be found between the one and the two-stage determination. When on the other hand a certain type of prothrombin is converted at a slower rate than normal prothrombin (d in fig. 1) but eventually produces the same final amount of thrombin ($\sim 50$ U/ml in fig. 1) one will estimate a low level in the one-stage and a normal one in the two-stage. This is what is actually observed with PIVKA-II (7). We determined the thrombin generation curve of four types of preparation: a) A euglobulin precipitate from normal plasma; b) a preparation of prothrombin prepared according to a method developed in our laboratory using the selective effect of Cd-ions upon the adsorbtion of prothrombin onto $Al(OH)_3$ (8, 9); c) a preparation of prothrombin prepared according to Kisiel

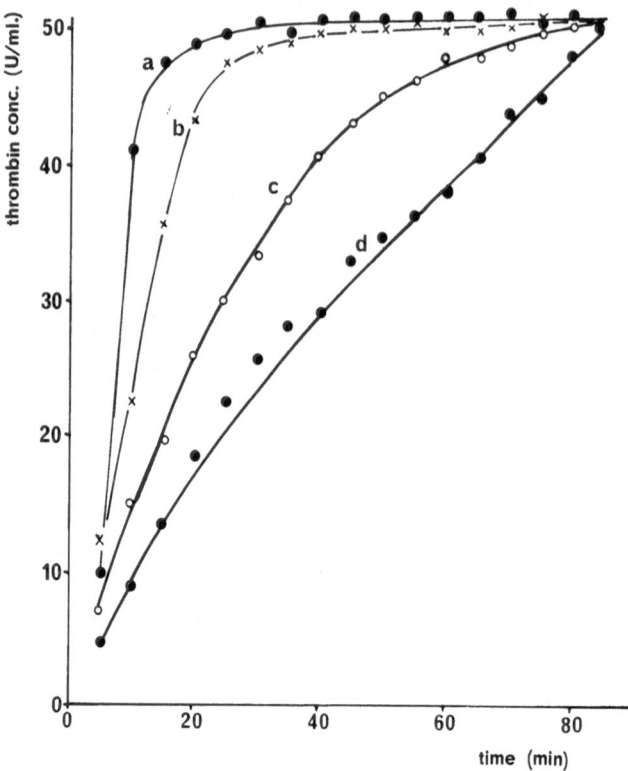

*Fig.* 1. Time course of thrombin generation. At zero time a fixed high amount of pro-thrombinase is added to a prothrombin preparation. The incubation is done at 37°C. At 2 min. intervals 0.1 ml aliquots of the incubation mixture are assayed for their thrombin content.

a : normal plasma (euglobulin preparation)
b : prothrombin preparation prepared according to ref. 8.
c : prothrombin preparation prepared according to ref. 1.
d : plasma from patients under deep oral anticoagulation.

and Hanahan and d) a euglobulin preparation from plasma of a deeply anticoagulated patient. Care was taken to add a fixed high amount of prothrombinase at zero time.

One would like to do this type of experiments with native prothrombin, but untreated plasma cannot be used because of the antithrombin 3 present in it. We therefore used a euglobulin precipitate, i.e. a preparation where the prothrombin went through only one purification step *viz.* acid precipitation. We adjusted the dilutions of the different preparations so that eventually the same amount of thrombin was formed.

The initial rates of thrombin formation differed considerably. The amount of prothrombinase as well as all other conditions being the same with the four preparations, the differences must be due to the properties of the prothrombin present.

We observe that the kinetic properties of the purified preparations lie between those of normal prothrombin and PIVKA-II. We can safely assume that PIVKA-II owes its aberrant activity to the absence of $\gamma$-carboxy glutamyl residues necessary for normal function (3). Hypothetically the slow conversion of the purified prothrombins may be caused by a loss of $\gamma$-carboxy glutamyl groups during preparation. Kisiel and Hanahans prothrombin generates thrombin at a rather slow pace. During preparation it is subjected to preparative electrophoresis in addition to a chromatographic procedure whereas in our procedure we can proceed with one column chromatography only. We conclude that a discrepancy between the one- and the two-stage determination in a prothrombin preparation is indicative of a reduced specific velocity of thrombin generation, possibly because of loss of $\gamma$-carboxy glutamyl groups.

*Table* 1. Comparison of different prothrombins in different tests.

|  | A | B | C | D | E |
|---|---|---|---|---|---|
| one-stage | 100 | 100 | 100 | 100 | 21 |
| two-stage | 72 | 60 | 97 | 100 | 43 |
| initial velocity | 1,2 | – | 2,7 | 3,4 | 0,8 |

The activities are expressed in % of normal plasma, the initial velocity as U of thrombin per minute.

A : prothrombin prepared according to Kisiel and Hanahan as estimated in our laboratory

B : the same, calculated from the author's results (1)

C : prothrombin prepared according to Devilee (8), (9)

D : normal plasma

E : plasma from a patient receiving dicoumarol.

REFERENCES

1. Kisiel, W. and D. J. Hanahan, *Biochem. biophys. Acta* 304, 103-113 (1973).
2. Josso, F., *Personal communication*.
3. Stenflo, J., P. Farmlund, W. Egen and P. Roapstorf, *Proc. nat. Acad. Sci.* 71 2730-2733 (1974).
4. Hemker, H. C., A. C. W. Swart and A. J. M. Alink, *Thrombos. Diathes. haemorrh.* 27, 205-211 (1972).

5. Hemker, H. C., P. W. Hemker, K. van der Torren, P. P. Devilee, W. Th. Hermens and E. A. Loeliger, *Thrombos. Diathes. haemorrh.* 25, 545-554 (1971).
6. Hemker, H. C. and P. W. Hemker, *Proc. roy. Soc. B* 173, 411-420 (1969).
7. Hemker, H. C., A. D. Muller and E. A. Loeliger, *Thrombos. Diathes. haemorrh.* 23, 633-637 (1970).
8. Devilee, P. P., B. M. Bas and H. C. Hemker, *Biochom. bioph. Acta* 379, 172-179 (1975).
9. Devilee, P. P., J. S. de Graaf and J. M. van der Voort-Beelen, B. M. Bas. *This volume* p. 93-98.

# PREPARATION OF PURE PROTHROMBIN BY THE Cd++ METHOD

P. P. DEVILEE, J. S. DE GRAAF, J. M. VAN DER VOORT-BEELEN AND
B. M. BAS

In the presence of cadmium ions $Al(OH)_3$ shows a tendency to adsorb less of prothrombin than of the factors VII, IX, and X (fig. 1 and 2). This property can be used to purify prothrombin in a procedure employing column chromatography only once (ref. 1).

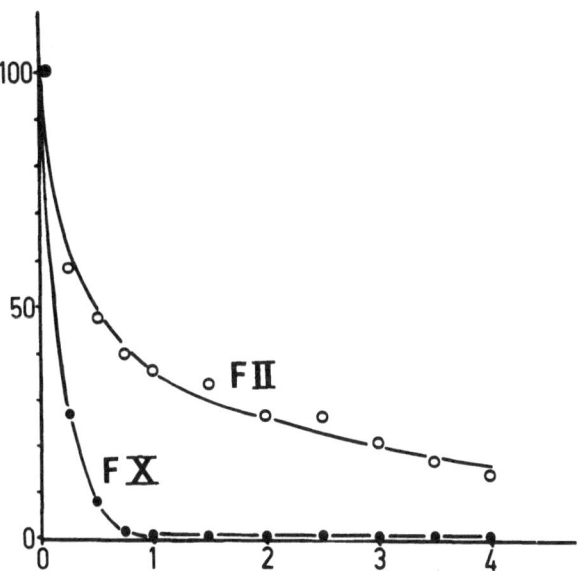

Fig. 1. Influence of $Cd^{++}$ on the adsorption of coagulation factors onto Al $(OH)_3$.
$CdSO_4$ was added to normal plasma to the final concentration indicated. 2% (w/v) of Al $(OH)_4$ was added, incubated for 10 min and separated by centrifugation. The concentration of coagulation factors in the supernatant was determined.
Abcissa: Concentration $Cd^{++}$ in mM.
Ordinate: % coagulation factor left in supernatant.
The values for the factors VII and IX were O at $Cd^{++}$ concentrations < 1.4 mM and differed less than 5% from those for factor X, at higher concentrations; they are not represented.

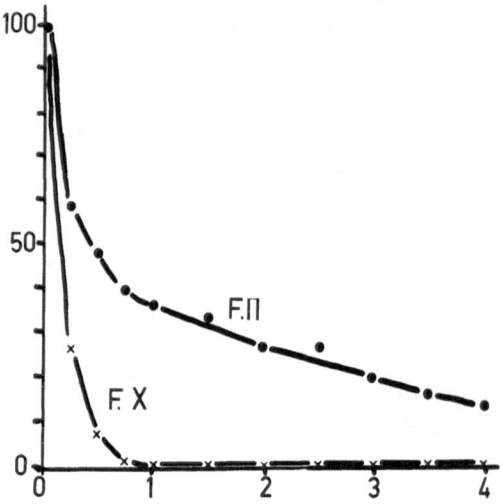

*Fig.* 2. Adsorption of the coagulation factors II, and X onto Al(OH)$_3$ in the presence of CdSO$_4$ (1 mM). To normal plasma 1/80 volume of CdSO$_4$ 0.1 M was added and 1/5 volume of a mixture of a 20% (w/v) suspension of Al(OH)$_3$ and water to obtain the desired concentration of Al(OH)$_3$.
Abcissa: concentration Al(OH)$_3$ in % w/v.
Ordinate: % coagulation factor left in supernatant.
Further details as in the legend to fig. 1.

## PURIFICATION PROCEDURE

The entire procedure is carried out in the cold room at 4°C and in cooled centrifuges at the same temperature. To the plasma are added successively 1/100 volume of a 0.1 M CdSO$_4$ solution and 1/15 volume of Al(OH)$_3$ in the form of a 20% (w/v) moist gel. The mixture is stirred for 10 min, after which the Al(OH)$_3$ is removed by centrifugation. All sedimentations of inorganic material are effected by centrifugation for 15 min at 6,000 g. The supernatant plasma contains 1 mM CdSO$_4$, ~ 50% of the original factor II and less than 0.5% of factors VII, IX, and X (supernatant a, table 1). The Cd$^{++}$ in the supernatant is precipitated by adding 3 g solid Na-oxalate per 100 ml of the preparation. The precipitated Cd-oxalate is removed by centrifugation.

The factor II remaining in the supernatant (supernatant b, table 1) can then be adsorbed onto Al(OH)$_3$ as described above. The resulting Al(OH)$_3$ sediment is washed first with 1/5 plasma volume 0.1 M EDTA (pH 8.0) and then with 1/5 plasma volume 0.15 M NaCl. The proteins adsorbed are eluted with 1/20 volume 0.25 M K-Na phosphate buffer (pH 8.0). Centrifugation

*Table* 1. Purification of human plasma factor II.

| Fraction | Vol. (ml) | Act. (U/ml) | Prot. conc. (mg/ml) | Spec. act. (U/mg) | Recovery (%) | Purification (fold) |
|---|---|---|---|---|---|---|
| plasma | 500 | 0.83 | 68.8 | 0.0121 | 100 | 1.00 |
| Supernatant a | 535 | 0.44 | 67.0 | 0.0066 | 57 | 0.54 |
| Supernatant b | 535 | 0.42 | 67.0 | 0.0063 | 54 | 0.52 |
| Al (OH)$_3$ eluant | 25 | 5.98 | 5.90 | 1.014 | 36 | 84 |
| Sephadex A-50 | 44 | 2.26 | 0.25 | 9.04 | 24 | 749 |

leaves factor II and other proteins in the supernatant. The eluate is dialysed overnight against 0.1 M NaCl in 0.01 M K-Na-phosphate buffer pH 6.8. The material is then applied to a 9 × 1 cm column containing DEAE Sephadex A-50 previously equilibrated with 0.1 M NaCl in 0.01 M K-Na-phosphate buffer pH 6.8. After 30 ml of the same buffer have flown through, a linear gradient of 100 ml of this buffer and 100 ml of the same buffer containing 0.6 M NaCl is applied.

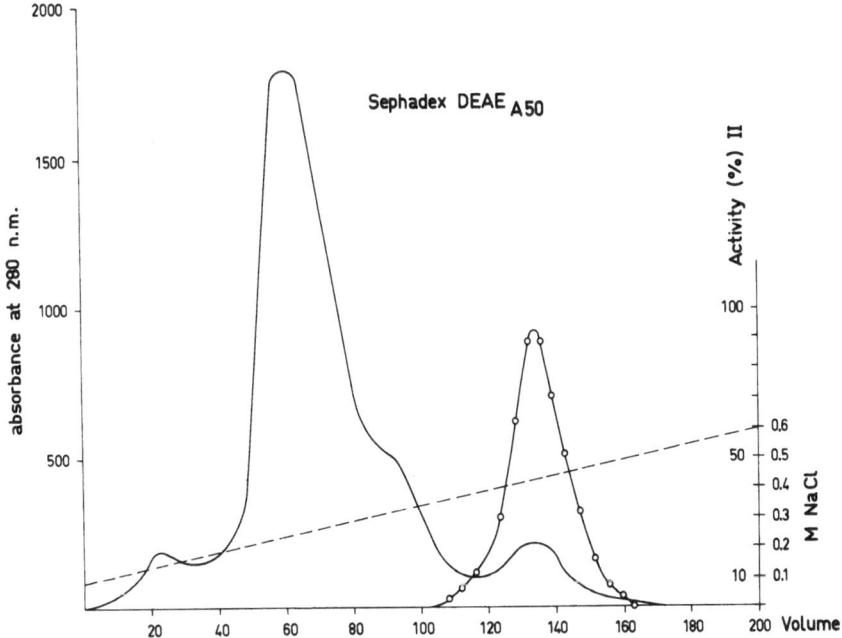

*Fig.* 3. Chromatography of human factor II.
Drawn line: adsorbance at 280 nm
Dashed line: NaCl concentration in the eluant (M)
○ — ○ : factor II activity (one-stage determination).

A typical elution pattern is shown in figure 3. Prothrombin elutes as a single peak at about 0.51 M NaCl. The fractions containing more than 30% of the original factor II activity are pooled. The mean purification and yield obtained in 12 of these procedures are shown in table 1.

PROPERTIES OF THE PURIFIED MATERIAL

The preparation never contained detectable amounts of factors VII, IX, or X. (In our assay systems (2) this means that for a factor II activity of 1 U/ml, less than 0.0025 U/ml of the factors VII, X, or IX are present). The isolated protein shows a single band on polyacrylamide-gel electrophoresis (fig. 4). An antibody raised against this preparation showed one precipita-

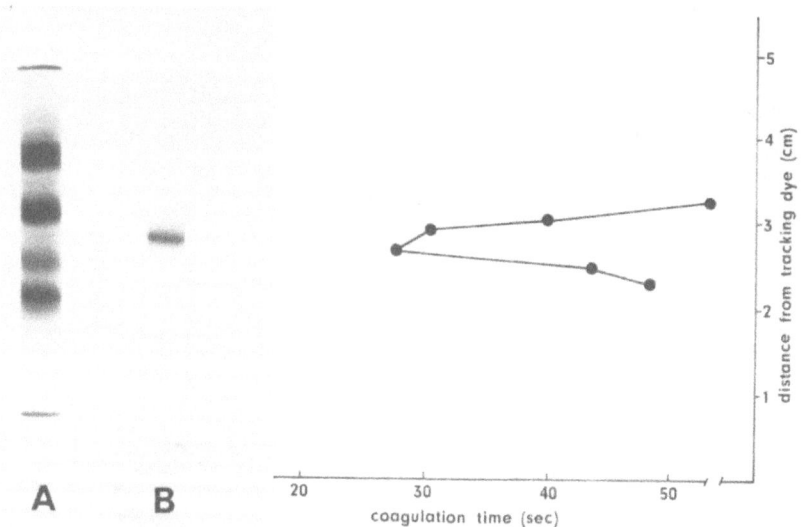

*Fig.* 4. Polyacrylamide gel electrophoresis of human factor II.
A: sample before chromatography
B: sample after chromatography.
The graph gives the coagulation times in a factor II estimation as found with fragmented 2 mm segments of a gel obtained under the same conditions as B.

tion arc with normal human plasma (fig. 5). There was a reaction of complete identity between the prothrombin prepared according to the method described here; the prothrombin found in normal plasma, and the prothrombin prepared according to Kisiel and Hanahan (3).

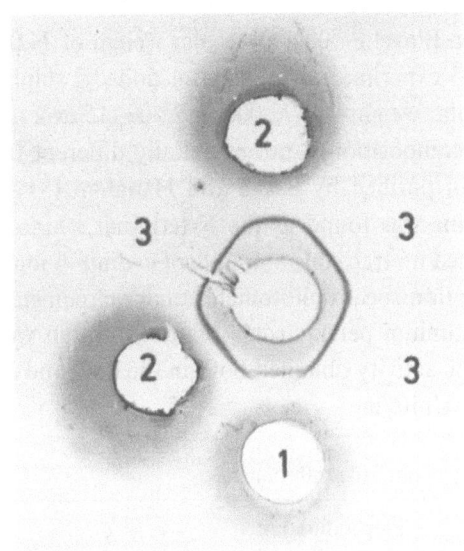

*Fig.* 5. Immuno diffusion pattern with an antibody against prothrombin.
The centre well contains the antibody. The other wells contain human serum (1), human plasma (2) and purified prothrombin (3). Two types of the latter are tested, upper wells: preparation as described in this article; lower well: preparation according to Kisiel and Hanahan.

*Table* 2. Amino acid composition of human factor II.

| Amino acid | Lanchantin (4) | Hanahan (3) | Devilee (1) |
|---|---|---|---|
| lysine | 4.81 | 5.19 | 4.85 |
| histidine | 1.78 | 1.91 | 1.98 |
| arginine | 7.94 | 8.34 | 8.18 |
| aspartic acid | 9.14 | 9.85 | 9.89 |
| threonine | 5.52 | 4.90 | 5.21 |
| serine | 4.67 | 4.36 | 4.25 |
| glutamic acid | 12.72 | 13.17 | 13.36 |
| proline | 4.28 | 4.28 | 4.50 |
| glycine | 3.52 | 3.83 | 3.75 |
| alanine | 3.48 | 3.75 | 3.61 |
| cystine (half) | 3.35 | 2.51 | 3.84 |
| valine | 4.15 | 4.53 | 4.53 |
| methionine | 1.30 | 1.29 | 1.38 |
| isoleucine | 3.42 | 3.30 | 3.18 |
| leucine | 6.11 | 6.52 | 6.48 |
| tyrosine | 4.90 | 4.31 | 4.95 |
| phenylalanine | 4.42 | 5.07 | 3.80 |
| tryptophan* | 5.34 | 3.28 | 3.09 |
| totals | 90.85 | 90.39 | 90.83 |

* Determined according to Scoffone (5).

By gelfiltration on Biogel P-100 a molecular weight of 74,000 $\pm$ 2,000 was found (means of 15 experiments) by sodium dodecyl sulphate gel electrophoresis the molecular weight was 72,000 $\pm$ 2,500 (15 experiments).

The amino acid composition is not essentially different from that of the human prothrombin purified by Kisiel and Hanahan (3) and Lanchantin (4) (table 2). Alanine was found as the N-terminal amino acid. The final preparation contained no traceable amounts of cadmium ions when assessed in an atomic adsorption spectrophotometer under circumstances where less than one ion of cadmium per molecule of prothrombin would have been detected. The specific activity obtained both in the one- and in the two-stage determination was 9 Units/mg.

*Table* 3. Specific activity of purified prothrombin.

| Method | Preparation | | |
|---|---|---|---|
| | A | B | C |
| one-stage | 9.04 | 5.34 | 6.52 |
| two-stage | 9.06 | 9.34 | 11.32 |
| staphylocoagulase | 9.07 | 9.02 | – |
| Echis carinata | 9.01 | 8.98 | – |

The figures give specific activities in Units per mg.
A: preparation as described in this article (means of 12 experiments).
B: preparation according to Kisiel and Hanahan (means of 2 batches).
C: data from Kisiel and Hanahan recalculated for the use of Units as defined in this article. Due to a different method for the two-stage assay, the figures for this assay in the columns B and C are not directly comparable.

### REFERENCES

1. Devilee, P. P., H. C. Hemker and B. M. Bas, *Biochem. biophys. Acta* 379, 172-179 (1975).
2. Hemker, H. C., A. C. W. Swart and A. J. M. Alink, *Thrombos. Diathes. haemorrh.* 27, 205-211 (1972).
3. Kisiel, W. and D. J. Hanahan, *Biochem. biophys. Acta* 304, 103-113 (1973).
4. Lanchantin, G. F., D. W. Hart, J. A. Friedman, N. V. Saavedra and J. W. Mekl, *J. biol. Chem.* 243, 5479-5485 (1968).
5. Scoffone, E., A. Fontana and R. Rocchi, *Biochemistry* 7, 971 (1968).

# STAPHYLOCOAGULASE

B. M. BAS AND A. D. MULLER

Staphylocoagulase is a protein secreted by certain strains of Staphylococcus Aureus. Upon interaction of Staphylococcus Aureus with prothrombin, a thrombin-like activity arises. In order to study the interaction underlying this effect, we had to purify staphylocoagulase as existing methods (1-9) proved insufficient.

## Materials used

Brain heart infusion was obtained from DIFCO. Sephadex G-100 and DEAE Sephadex A-100 were from Farmacia Fine Chemicals. The DEAE cellulose used for step 2 was Batch D 8382 from Sigma. For the chromatography, microgranular DEAE cellulose DE 32 from Whatman was used; for ultrafiltration, a Diaflow apparatus with membrane XM-50.

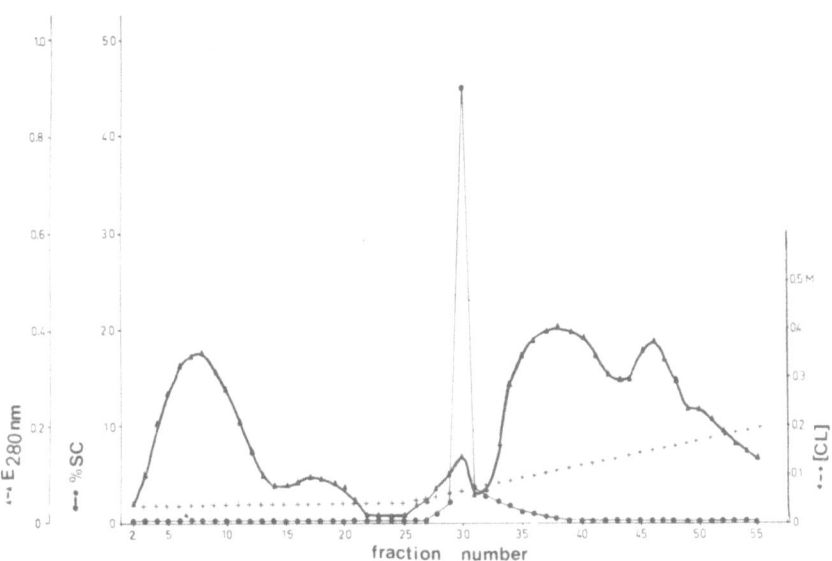

*Fig.* 1. DEAE cellulose chromatography of staphylocoagulase.

*Method*

A modification of the method of Soulier was followed (7). A glass tube in a waterbath was provided with

0.1 ml rabbit plasma diluted 1:20

0.1 ml bovine fibrinogen 4 mg/ml

0.2 ml veronal acetate buffer (pH 7.35)

0.1 ml sample containing staphylocoagulase,

and the clotting time was recorded.

When the activity was to be assessed in slices of a polyacrylamide gel, each 2-mm slice was fragmented in 0.2 ml buffer after which 0.2 ml of a mixture of equal parts of diluted rabbit plasma and bovine fibrinogen solution were added. One crude preparation of staphylocoagulase (obtained after the acid preparation step to be described below) was considered to contain 100 arbitrary units per ml.

Coagulation times obtained with dilutions of this preparation were used to construct a reference curve. This curve was a hyperbola, since the plot of coagulation times against the inverse of the concentration of staphylocoagulase was a straight line. The standard preparation was frozen at $-70°C$ in small portions and remained stable for more than two years. This approach is preferable to basing the definition of a unit on a coagulation time (7) because variations in rabbit plasma or fibrinogen will not influence the unit defined.

PROCEDURE

*Preparation of the starting material*

A strain of Staphylococcus aureus (originally strain 104 of Tager (7)) kindly provided by Professor Soulier, was stored at $-70°C$ in broth. Every two months the strain was cultured on a blood-agar plate and inoculated in 50 ml of fresh broth. After 24 hours at $37°C$ the culture was frozen and kept for another two months. For mass culture, the broth was used to inoculate 1% glucose blood agar. After 24 hours at $37°C$, three tubes of blood agar were mixed into 100 ml brain heart infusion (Difco). This infusion was kept at $37°C$ for 48 to 72 hours in 1-litre Roux flasks, after which the material from 30 flasks was pooled and centrifuged for 30 minutes at $7,000 \times g$. The supernatant was then filtered through a G-5 glass filter.

*Step 1. Isoelectric precipitation*
Under rigorous stirring, 3 N HCl was added to the preparation to obtain pH 4.5. The material was then allowed to stand for 18 hours at 0°C. The precipitate was collected by centrifugation (20 min at 5,000 × g, 4°C) and washed twice in 1/10 vol 0.15 M Na acetate (pH 3.8) before being dissolved in 1/20 vol 0.05 M Tris-HCl (pH 7.35) containing 0.10 M NaCl. The activity of this preparation was tested; if a 1:10 dilution gave coagulation times longer than 40 seconds, the material was discarded.

*Step 2. DEAE cellulose adsorption*
To the preparation was added one half its volume of a DEAE-cellulose slurry (75 mg/ml in 0.015 M Tris-HCl, pH 7.35). After being stirred for 10 min at room temperature, the cellulose was separated on a G-2 sintered glass filter. The cellulose cake was then washed repeatedly with 20 ml of a Tris-HCl buffer 0.05 M (pH 7.35) containing 0.15 M NaCl. The coagulation time was determined after each washing. Washing was stopped when coagulation times longer than 60 seconds were obtained, usually after 9-12 washings. The washing fluids were pooled and concentrated by ultrafiltration using a Diaflow apparatus with a XM-50 membrane.

*Step 3. Lipid extraction*
A 100-ml aliquot of the preparation (0°C) was added slowly to a mixture of 100 ml ethanol and 100 ml diethylether at −10°C. After 30 min of incubation 2.5 ml water was added. A two-phase system results. The ethanol-water layer (about 240 ml) was separated from the ether layer and to this phase 160 ml of a saturated solution of ammonium sulfate was added. This again results in a two-phase system. The lower (aqueous) phase, which contains the staphylocoagulase in the form of a fine precipitate, was collected by centrifugation for 10 min at −10°C and 2,000 g. The precipitate was suspended in 100 ml n-pentane at −10°C and again collected by centrifugation and freezedried. The dry powder was extracted by 20-min of stirring at room temperature with 20 ml Tris buffer (pH 7.35) 0.15 M NaCl. This procedure was repeated 2 to 4 times until the coagulation time of the supernatant exceeded 60 seconds.

*Step 4. DEAE cellulose chromatography*
The preparation was diluted five times with a 0.02 M borate buffer (pH 5.5) and applied to a 2.5 × 10 cm column of DEAE cellulose equilibrated with the same buffer containing 0.03 M NaCl. When 280-mμ adsorbing material

*Table 1.* Purification of staphylocoagulase*

| Procedure | Vol. ml | Activity U/ml | Protein** mg/ml | Spec. act. U/mg | Yield % | Purification x |
|---|---|---|---|---|---|---|
| filtered broth | 20,000 | 17 | 15.4 | 1.1 | 100 | 1 |
| isoelectric ppt | 1,000 | 110 | 8.7 | 12.6 | 32 | 11 |
| DEAE cell. ads. | 4,000 | 24.5 | .650 | 37.7 | 29 | 34 |
| ultrafiltration | 200 | 479 | .742 | 661 | 20 | 600 |
| lipid extraction | 120 | 532 | .325 | 1640 | 18 | 1490 |
| chromatography | 20 | 2360 | .060 | 39300 | 14 | 35700 |

\* Values represent the means of 10 purification procedures. The highest specific activity observed was 41,800 U/mg, the lowest 35,200.

\*\* Estimated according to ref. 10.

no longer appeared in the eluant, a linear gradient of 0.03-0.25 M NaCl in the same buffer was applied (2 × 100 ml). The staphylocoagulase elutes as a sharp peak shortly afterward, at about 0.07 M NaCl (fig. 2).

The means of the data from ten purification procedures are given in table 1.

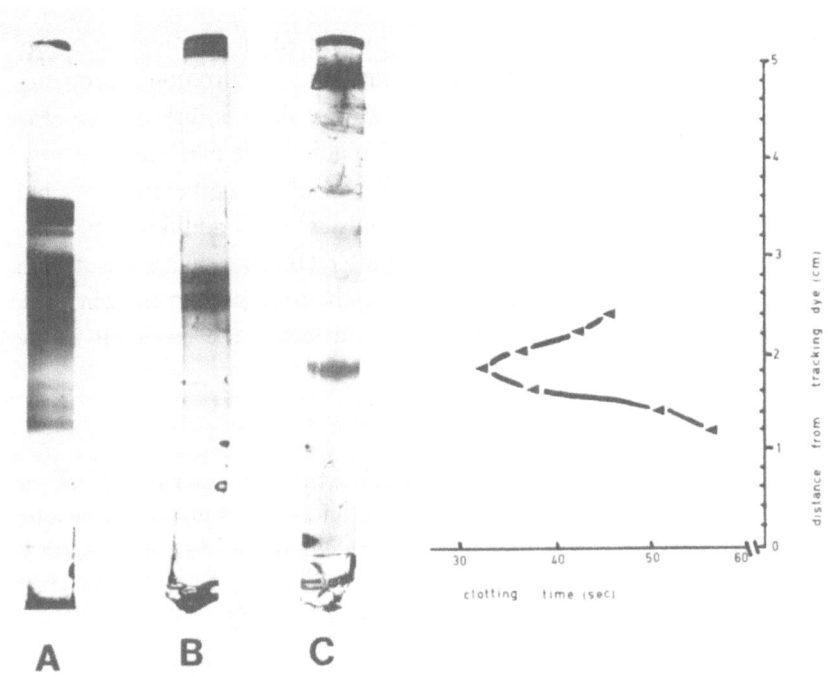

*Fig.* 2. Polyacrylamide gel electrophoresis of different preparations.
A. After DEAE cellulose adsorption and elution (step 2).
B. After lipid extraction (step 3).
C. After DEAE cellulose chromatography (step 4).
The graph gives the coagulation times obtained with fragmented 2 mm segments of an unstained gel prepared under the same conditions as gel C.


## VARIATIONS OF THE METHOD

### Isoelectric precipitation
Usually, isoelectric precipitation is done at pH 3.8 (7); in our hands this gave a 7-fold purification at a 36% yield. We preferred the higher purification (11 times) at a slightly lower yield (32%), obtained at pH 4.5.

*DEAE cellulose adsorption*
DEAE cellulose concentrations between 10 and 500 mg/ml were tested
systematically. All activity adsorbed at 40 mg/ml or higher. The lowest concentration of NaCl in 0.05 M Tris HCl pH 7.35 at which complete elution
was observed was 0.15 M.

*Lipid extraction*
An extensive series of separation methods was tried on the preparation obtained by DEAE cellulose adsorption, including gelfiltration, chromatography on P-, SE-, TEAE-, CM-, and DEAE-celluloses, preparative electrophoresis etc. None of them resulted in an acceptable purification.

The results were more promising after alcohol-ether extraction, but
successful chromatography was possible only after an additional pentane
extraction. Lipid analysis of the material after DEAE cellulose adsorption
showed 43 μg phospholipid and 628 μg triglyceride per mg protein (11).
After lipid extraction no phospholipid was detected and less than 20 μg
triglyceride was found.

*Chromatography*
Chromatography of the material after lipid extraction was carried out on
DEAE-, TEAE-, CM-, P-, SE- and exteola-cellulose c.q. Sephadex in various
buffers and at various pH values. Under the conditions described, DEAE
cellulose (Whatman DE 32, microgranular) appeared to be the material of
choice, combining good purification with reasonable yield.

The polyacrylamide electrophoresis pattern at various steps of the purification are shown in figure 2.


PROPERTIES OF THE PURIFIED STAPHYLOCOAGULASE

*Molecular weight*
Gel filtration on P-150 acrylamide gel columns with the use of yeast alcohol
dehydrogenase (molecular weight: 126,000), bovine serum albumin (molecular weight: 70,000), ovalbumin (molecular weight: 43,000), lactic dehydrogenase (molecular weight: 36,000), and chymotrypsinogen (molecular
weight: 25,700) as reference molecules gave a molecular weight of 62,000 ±
3,000 as the mean of ten separate estimations, calculated according to
Andrews (13). The molecular weight as estimated with the aid of SDS
electrophoresis was 60,000 ± 2,300 (15 estimations), with both methods

we obtained a calculated molecular weight of 61,000 ± 2,300 (12). Reduction does not change the behaviour in SDS polyacrylamide electrophoresis.

*Isoelectric points*
Upon isoelectric focusing the staphylocoagulase activity eluted in a single peak in fractions with a pH of 4.51 to 4.55.

*Chemical composition*
The amino acid composition is shown in table 2. The N-terminal amino acid is aspartic acid. Carbohydrate staining of the polyacrylamide gels of the purified product was negative.

*Table* 2. Amino acid composition of staphylocoagulase.

| Aminoacid | a | b |
|---|---|---|
| lysine | 9.10 | 43 |
| histidine | 1.89 | 8 |
| arginine | 4.01 | 16 |
| aspartic acid | 13.18 | 70 |
| threonine | 4.74 | 29 |
| serine | 3.71 | 26 |
| glutamic acid | 17.58 | 83 |
| proline | 2.82 | 18 |
| glycine | 3.38 | 36 |
| alanine | 5.09 | 44 |
| cystine (half) | 1.64 | 10 |
| valine | 6.96 | 43 |
| methionine | 1.57 | 7 |
| isoleucine | 6.42 | 35 |
| leucine | 7.70 | 42 |
| tyrosine | 3.99 | 15 |
| phenylalanine | 4.53 | 19 |
| tryptophan* | 0.60 | 2 |

Column a: g. aminoacid/100 g protein
    b: nearest integer to mol aminoacid/mol protein.

* Determined according to Scoffone et al. (14).

*Purity*
We could detect only one N-terminal amino acid. Cochromatography showed that Dns-amino acids in a concentration of 1/20 of the Dns-asp found were readily detectable. Individual contaminants therefore were probably less than 5% of the main protein. An unstained gel showed staphylo-

coagulase-activity at the same position as the main protein. When the optical density of the stained gel was scanned the total of the parasitic bands amounted to less than 16% of the main protein. The purification obtained was more than seven times higher than the highest we found reported in the literature. (14).

## REFERENCES

1. Blobel, H., D. T. Berman and J. Simon, *J. Bact.* 79, 807-815 (1960).
2. Duthie, E. S. and G. Haughton, *Biochem. J.* 70, 125-134 (1958).
3. Jackerts, D., *Ztschr. Hyg.* 142, 213-218 (1956).
4. Jeljaszewicz, J., *Acta microbiol. Pol.* 7, 17-34 (1958).
5. Murray, M. and P. Ghodes, *Biochem. biophys. Acta* 40, 518-522 (1960).
6. Siwecka, M. and J. Jeljaszewicz, *Zentralblatt Bakt.* 208, 385-394 (1968).
7. Soulier, J. P., S. Lewi, A. M. Panty and O. Prou-Wartelle, *Rev. franc. etud. clin. biol.* 12, 544-588 (1967).
8. Tager, M., *Yale J. Biol. Med.* 20, 487-501 (1948).
9. Zolli, Z. and C. L. San Clemente, *J. Bact*, 86, 527-535 (1963).
10. Lowry, O. H., N. J. Rosebrough, A. L. Farr and R. J. Randall, *J. biol. Chem.* 193, 265-275 (1951).
11. Bligh, E. G. and W. Dyer, *Canad. J. Biochem.* 37, 911-917 (1959).
12. Hemker, H. C., A. D. Muller and B. M. Bas, *Biochem. biophys. Acta,* 379, 180-188 (1975).
13. Andrews, P., *Biochem. J.* 91, 222-233 (1964).
14. Scoffone, E., A. Fontana and R. Rocchi, *Biochemistry* 7, 971 (1968).

# THE INTERACTION BETWEEN PROTHROMBIN
# AND STAPHYLOCOAGULASE

B. M. BAS, A. D. MULLER, J. S. DE GRAAF AND H. C. HEMKER

*Introduction*

Thrombin is a two-chain serine protease (39,000 daltons), derived from prothrombin (a single-chain protein of about 73,000 daltons) by limited proteolysis (1-5). Staphylocoagulase produces a thrombin-like activity in prothrombin. This activity we call coagulase-thrombin (6, 7).

Coagulase-thrombin can be distinguished from normal thrombin in that it is not inhibited by heparin and soybean trypsin inhibitor (8); also its chromatographic behaviour on DEAE-cellulose is different (9).

Soulier found that purified coagulase-thrombin is inhibited by antibodies against prothrombin as well as by antibodies against staphylocoagulase (9). Muller and Hemker showed that the molecular weight of coagulase-thrombin equals the sum of the molecular weights of staphylocoagulase and prothrombin (10). The purpose of this study was to determine whether staphylocoagulase induces activity in prothrombin by limited proteolysis or by a stoichiometric reaction.

EXPERIMENTS

*Generation of activity*

The addition of purified staphylocoagulase to purified prothrombin (11, 13) leads to the generation of a product that has both TAMe[1]-esterase activity and the ability to clot fibrinogen.

The amount of esterase activity that evolves is a function of both the quantity of staphylocoagulase and the quantity of prothrombin present. Figure 1 shows that after two minutes the activity in the mixture is maximal and stable. Figure 2 shows that for each concentration of staphylocoagulase

---

1. TAMe = tosyl arginine methylester.

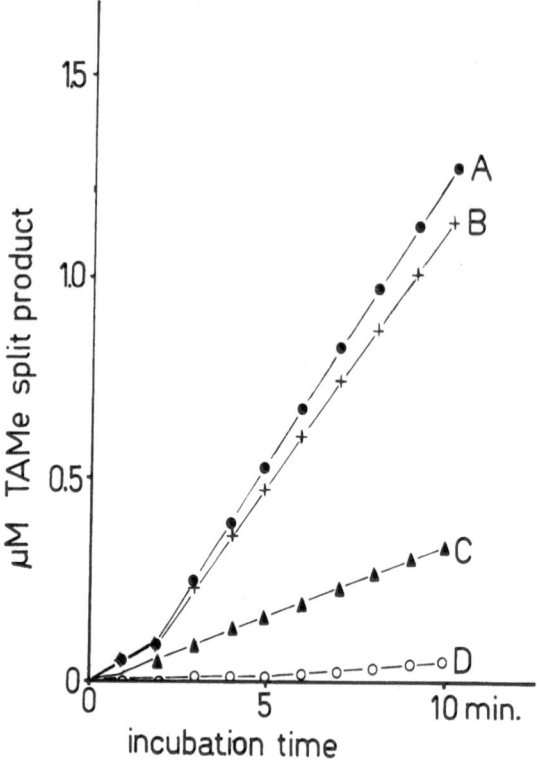

Fig. 1. TAMe hydrolysis by coagulase-thrombin.
The amount of ester hydrolysed is given as a function of time. Reaction mixture C: 0.10 ml
staphylocoagulase (2 mg/ml) and 0.10 ml prothrombin (10 mg/ml); 4.8 ml TAMe 5 mM
(pH 7.35) in 0.1 M NaCl. In the other mixtures prothrombin or staphylocoagulase solutions were (partially) replaced by 0.1 M NaCl so as to obtain the concentrations indicated
below. No observable esterase activity developed when no prothrombin was added.
Final concentrations: A: staphylocoagulase 40 μg/ml; prothrombin  50 μg/ml
                      B: staphylocoagulase 40 μg/ml; prothrombin 200 μg/ml
                      C: staphylocoagulase 10 μg/ml; prothrombin 200 μg/ml
                      D: staphylocoagulase  0 μg/ml; prothrombin 200 μg/ml.

there is a lowest concentration of prothrombin that gives maximal activity.
Any further increase in prothrombin concentration will not raise the
esterase activity further. The same phenomenon can be observed with the
coagulation times: for each concentration of staphylocoagulase there is a
lowest concentration of prothrombin that will cause maximal coagulation
activity, i.e. a minimal coagulation time (fig. 3).

   This type of experiment indicates the minimal concentration of prothrombin that will just cause optimal activity in a given amount of staphylocoagulase (and vice versa). The pairs of concentrations thus found are plotted in

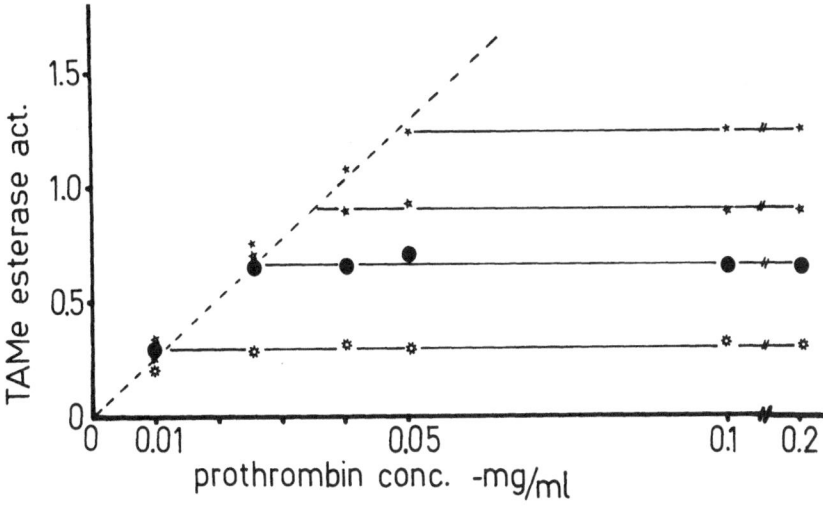

*Fig.* 2. Esterase activity in μM/min in mixtures of prothrombin and staphylocoagulase. The esterase activity was determined with varying amounts of prothrombin as indicated on the abcissa and the following amounts of staphylocoagulase:

✿ : 10 μg/ml
● : 20 μg/ml
☆ : 30 μg/ml
★ : 40 μg/ml.

fig. 4. Optimal esterase activity coincided with optimal coagulation activity (fig. 2 and 3).

*Estimation of the molecular weight*

Preparations of prothrombin, staphylocoagulase, coagulase-thrombin and normal thrombin were subjected to gelfiltration on various types of material. Crude preparations of staphylocoagulase digested Sephadex to some extent, and the behaviour of prothrombin on Sephadex was also anomalous. We therefore changed to polyacrylamide gels. Biogel P-150 showed the most appropriate fractionation range. The molecular weight was determined from the partition coefficient *de modo* Andrews (14). Dextran blue (molecular weight: > 150,000) was used to estimate the void volume; alcohol dehydrogenase (molecular weight: 126,000), bovine serum albumin (molecular weight: 70,000), ovalbumin (molecular weight: 43,000), lactate dehydrogenase (molecular weight: 36,000), and chymotrypsin (molecular weight: 25,700) were used as reference substances. Prothrombin, staphylocoagulase and thrombin were run separately five times each. Coagulase-thrombin was obtained in three ways: i.e. using:

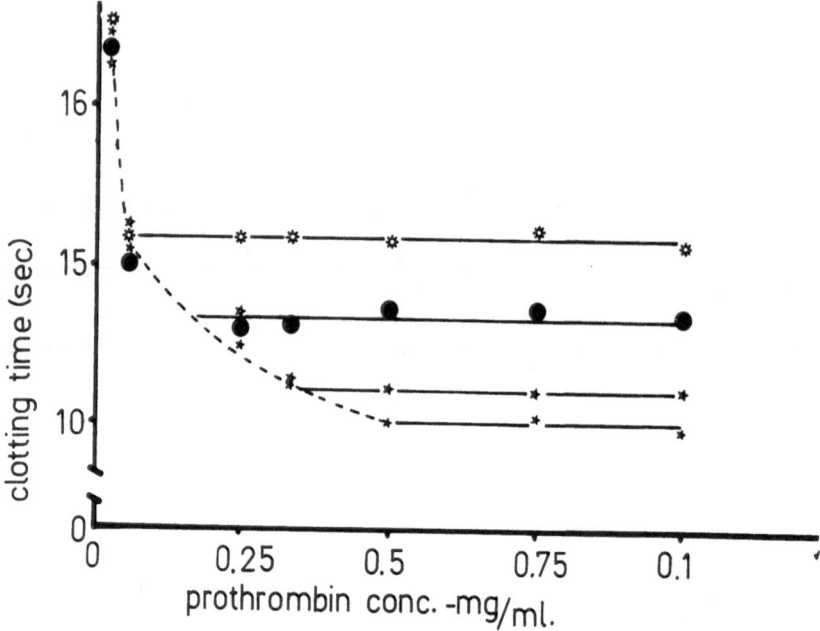

*Fig.* 3. Clotting activity in mixtures of prothrombin and staphylocoagulase.
The coagulation activity was determined with varying amounts of prothrombin, as indicated on the abcissa, and the following amounts of staphylocoagulase:
✿ : 10 µg/ml
● : 20 µg/ml
☆ : 30 µg/ml
★ : 40 µg/ml.

a. roughly equimolar amounts of staphylocoagulase and prothrombin;
b. an excess of prothrombin; or
c. an excess of staphylocoagulase.

In case a) a peak of coagulase-thrombin activity was obtained, followed in-
cidentally by a very small peak of either prothrombin or staphylocoagulase.
In case b) the peak of coagulase-thrombin was followed by a peak of prothrombin and in case c) by a peak of staphylocoagulase. The positions of
these peaks were used to calculate partition coefficients. Each type of experiment was repeated five times. Essentially the same results were found at pH
values of 6, 6.5, 7.35, 7.5 and 8 in both the absence and presence of 0.15 M
NaCl.

For staphylocoagulase, a molecular weight of 61,000 was found; for
thrombin this value was 37,000, for prothrombin 74,000, and for coagulase-
thrombin 135,000.

Molecular-weight determinations were also carried out by means of

Table 1. Amino acid composition of staphylocoagulase, prothrombin, and coagulase-thrombin.

| Amino acid | Staphylocoagulase M = 61,000 | | Prothrombin M = 74,000 | | Coagulase-thrombin M = 135,000 | | Calculated difference | |
|---|---|---|---|---|---|---|---|---|
| | a | b | a | b | a | b | c | d |
| Lysine | 9.10 | 43 | 4.85 | 28 | 5.54 | 58 | 71 | +13 |
| histidine | 1.89 | 8 | 1.98 | 11 | 2.15 | 21 | 19 | − 2 |
| arginine | 4.01 | 16 | 8.18 | 39 | 7.56 | 65 | 55 | −10 |
| aspartic acid | 13.18 | 70 | 9.89 | 64 | 10.99 | 129 | 134 | + 5 |
| threonine | 4.74 | 29 | 5.21 | 38 | 5.49 | 73 | 67 | − 6 |
| serine | 3.71 | 26 | 4.25 | 36 | 4.68 | 73 | 62 | −11 |
| glut. acid | 17.58 | 83 | 13.36 | 77 | 13.92 | 145 | 160 | +15 |
| proline | 2.82 | 18 | 4.50 | 34 | 3.83 | 53 | 52 | − 1 |
| glycine | 3.38 | 36 | 3.75 | 49 | 4.76 | 113 | 85 | −28 |
| alanine | 5.09 | 44 | 3.61 | 38 | 5.17 | 98 | 82 | −16 |
| cystine | 1.64 | 10 | 3.84 | 28 | 2.58 | 34 | 38 | + 4 |
| valine | 6.96 | 43 | 4.53 | 34 | 5.97 | 81 | 77 | − 4 |
| methionine | 1.51 | 7 | 1.38 | 8 | 1.52 | 16 | 15 | − 1 |
| isoleucine | 6.42 | 35 | 3.18 | 21 | 4.28 | 51 | 56 | + 5 |
| leucine | 7.70 | 42 | 6.48 | 42 | 6.88 | 82 | 84 | + 2 |
| tyrosin | 3.99 | 15 | 4.95 | 22 | 3.72 | 31 | 37 | + 6 |
| phenylalanine | 4.53 | 19 | 3.80 | 19 | 3.81 | 35 | 38 | + 3 |
| tryptophan | .60 | 2 | 3.09 | 12 | 1.83 | 13 | 14 | + 1 |
| totals | 98.85 | 546 | 90.83 | 600 | 94.68 | 1171 | 1146 | +54 / −79 |

Column a :  g amino acid/100 g protein.
Column b :  nearest integer to mol amino acid/mol protein.
Column c :  calculated amino acid composition assuming that one molecule of coagulase-thrombin consists of one molecule of prothrombin and one molecule of staphylocoagulase.
Column d :  difference between preceding columns b and c.

polyacrylamide gel electrophoresis in buffers contaning sodium dodecyl sulfate (12). Chymotrypsinogen, lactate dehydrogenase, ovalbumin, bovine serum albumin, and β-galactosidase were used as reference molecules. The means of 10 experiments were for thrombin 39,000, for prothrombin 72,000, for staphylocoagulase 60,000 and for coagulase-thrombin 125,000.

### N-terminal amino acid analysis
N-terminal amino acid analysis was carried out by labeling with dansyl-chloride. For prothrombin, a N-terminal alanine was confirmed (5) as well as N-terminal threonine and isoleucine for thrombin (5). Staphylocoagulase has a N-terminal aspartic acid (12). In coagulase-thrombin the only N-terminals detectable were alanine and aspartic acid. No trace of either threonine or isoleucine could be demonstrated.

### Amino acid analysis
Table 1 shows the results of the amino acid analysis of staphylocoagulase (from ref. 12), our preparation of prothrombin, and coagulase-thrombin. Coagulase-thrombin was obtained by mixing equimolar amounts of prothrombin and staphylocoagulase and separating the product (molecular weight: 135,000) by gelfiltration on Biogel P-150. The values represent the means of three experiments.

### Immuno precipitation
Antibodies were prepared in rabbits against a coagulase-thrombin preparation. These antibodies show single precipitation lines against prothrombin and staphylocoagulase. Against coagulase-thrombin a double line was observed, one continuous with the precipitation line of prothrombin, another continuous with that of staphylocoagulase. Against normal thrombin no precipitation line was found (fig. 5).

### DISCUSSION

A thrombin-like activity can be induced in a prothrombin preparation by the addition of staphylocoagulase. The data in figure 1 are incompatible with the assumption that in this system staphylocoagulase acts as an enzyme that converts prothrombin into thrombin. The amounts of both staphylocoagulase and prothrombin determine the final amount of esterase activity, whereas the velocity of generation of this activity is not influenced by changes in the concentration of staphylocoagulase. From figure 2 and 3 it can be seen that at each concentration of staphylocoagulase there is a smallest concentration of prothrombin that causes optimal activity. Optimal activity is found when prothrombin and staphylocoagulase are present in equimolar amounts (fig. 4).

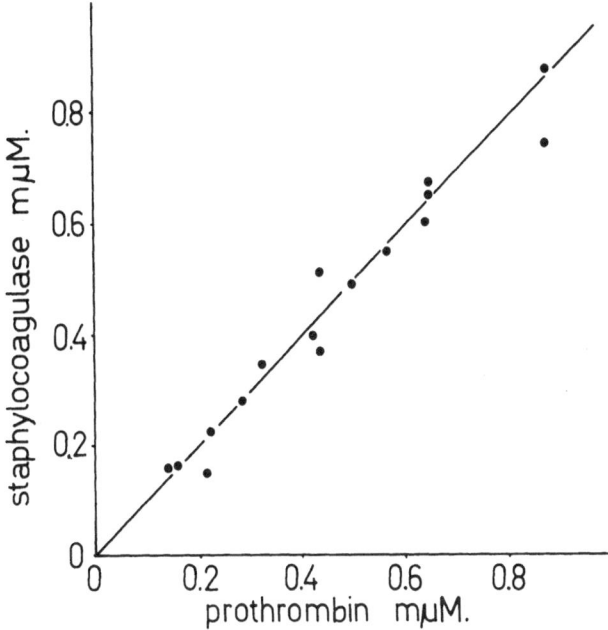

Fig. 4. Ratio of prothrombin to staphylocoagulase at optimal activity.
Molar concentrations calculated for a molecular weight of prothrombin of 73,000 daltons and staphylocoagulase 61,000 daltons.

The active product (coagulase-thrombin) can be separated from the components by gel filtration. The molecular weight calculated from the results of these experiments, is 135,000. This value can be interpreted as the sum of the molecular weights of the constituent proteins (prothrombin: 74,000; staphylocoagulase: 61,000).

Essentially the same results are found when the molecular weights are estimated on the basis of SDS gel electrophoresis, which gives a molecular weight of 125,000 for coagulase-thrombin, 72,000 for prothrombin, and 60,000 for staphylocoagulase.

Within the limits of the experimental error, the amino acid composition of thrombin-coagulase is equal to the sum of the amino acid compositions of staphylocoagulase and prothrombin. It therefore seems that one molecule of thrombin-coagulase results from the reaction between one molecule of pro-thrombin and one molecule of staphylocoagulase.

As for all of the other serine-protease zymogens, the generation of throm-bin activity from prothrombin under physiological circumstances is due to limited proteolysis (1-5). Trypsin and a fraction from Echis carinata venom induce activity in prothrombin in a comparable way (15, 16).

It is conceivable that staphylocoagulase splits covalent bonds in prothrom-bin but forms an extraordinarily stable enzymeproduct complex. The mole-cular weight determinations and the determinations of the amino acid com-position suggest that a peptide with a molecular weight of maximally 14,000 daltons or about 130 amino acid residues could split off during this process (on the assumption of a 10% error in the molecular weight determinations).

Neither in the gel filtration elution pattern nor in the SDS gel electropho-resis patterns were we able to demonstrate polypeptides smaller than 50,000 daltons. This does not, however, preclude the possibility that covalent bonds in prothrombin are split by staphylocoagulase, all the products remaining attached to the staphylocoagulase. Nevertheless, the finding that the N-terminal amino acids in coagulase-thrombin consist of alanine and aspartic acid make it unlikely that proteolysis underlies the generation of thrombin-like activity. Unless prothrombin is split so as to render another N-terminal alanine or aspartic acid, no new N-terminal and hence no form of proteolysis can be demonstrated. The N-terminals threonin and isoleucine, that are typical for thrombin, could not be found in coagulase-thrombin.

Figure 5 shows that antibodies directed against coagulase-thrombin preci-pitate with prothrombin and staphylocoagulase, but not with thrombin. The fact that with coagulase-thrombin two precipitation lines are obtained, one continuous with prothrombin, the other with staphylocoagulase, can be explained by assuming that coagulase-thrombin dissociates under the ex-perimental conditions. This is slightly puzzling as under a variety of other experimental procedures (gel filtration, column chromatography, SDS polyacrylamide gel electrophoresis) we did not obtain separation. Alterna-tively, one can imagine that immunisation against coagulase-thrombin gives rise to two populations of antibodies recognising the antigenic determinants of the prothrombin and the coagulase part separately. The problem is under further investigation. Anyhow, the pattern is compatible with the con-cept of thrombin-coagulase consisting as a complex of prothrombin and staphylocoagulase but not having antigenic determinants in common with thrombin.

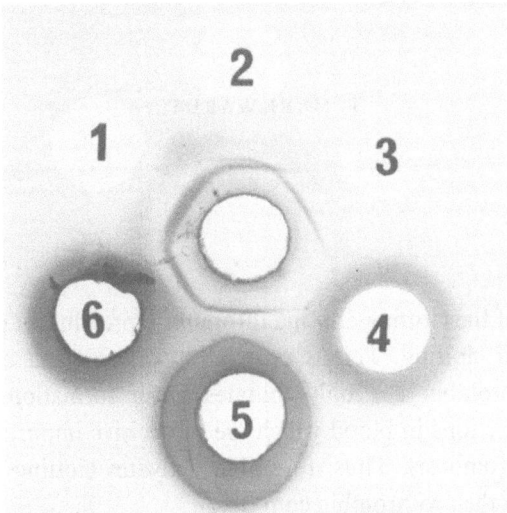

*Fig. 5.* Double immunodiffusion of an antibody against coagulase-thrombin.
The centre well contains the antibody, the other wells contain: 1. prothrombin; 2. coagulase-thrombin; 3. staphylocoagulase; 4. thrombin; 5. normal serum; 6. normal plasma.

We conclude that apart from limited proteolysis there is a fundamentally
different way to obtain thrombin activity from a prothrombin molecule, viz.
by a stoichiometric interaction with one molecule of staphylocoagulase.

### REFERENCES

1. Mann, K. G., C. M. Heldebrant and D. N. Fass, *J. biol. Chem.* 246, 6106-6114 (1971).
2. Heldebrant, C. M. and K. G. Mann, *J. biol. Chem.* 248, 3642-3652 (1973).
3. Owen, W. G., C. T. Esmon and C. M. Jackson, *J. biol. Chem.* 249, 594-605 (1974).
4. Jesty, J. and M. P. Esnouf, *Biochem. J.* 131, 791-799 (1973).
5. Magnusson, S., In *The enzymes* (P. D. Boyer, ed.) 3rd. ed. Vol. 3 277-321, Acad. Press.
6. Tager, M., *Yale J. Biol. Med.* 20, 487-501 (1948).
7. Tager, M., *J. exp. Med.* 104, 675-686 (1956).
8. Drummond, M. C. and M. Tager, *J. Bact.* 83, 975-980 (1962).
9. Soulier, J. P., O. Prou-Wartelle and L. Hallé, *Thrombos. Diathes. haemorrh.* 17, 321-331 (1967).
10. Muller, A. D. and H. C. Hemker, *Abstracts 6th FEBS Meeting*, Madrid. no. 834 (1968).
11. Devilee, P. P., J. S. de Graaf and J. M. v. d. Voort-Beelen and B. M. Bas, *This issue.* p. 93-98.
12. Bas, B. M., A. D. Muller and H. C. Hemker, *Biochem. biophys. Acta* 379, 164-171 (1975).
13. Devilee, P. P., H. C. Hemker and B. M. Bas, *Biochem. biophys. Acta* 379, 172-179 (1975).
14. Andrews, T., *Biochem. J.* 91, 222-233 (1964).
15. Engel, A. M. and B. Alexander, *Biochem. biophys. Acta* 320, 687-700 (1973).
16. Schieck, A., F. Kornalik and E. Habermann, Naunyn-Schmiedebergs *Arch. Pharm.* 264, 259 (1969).

# INHIBITION OF THROMBIN

F. MARKWARDT

The inhibition of the clotting enzyme thrombin represents an effective interference in blood clotting. This is especially evident when one takes into
account that thrombin not only initiates fibrin formation but also induces further reactions in blood which are of decisive importance in hemostasis and in thrombosis. Thus, thrombin activates clotting factors which
are necessary for the prothrombin conversion.

As known, the fibrin-stabilizing factor XIII (plasma transglutaminase) is
activated by thrombin too. Furthermore, thrombin causes a drastic change
in the permeability of the platelet membrane followed by biochemical and
morphological changes in blood platelets, whereby the initial phase of
thrombus formation is triggered. Therefore, the use of a thrombin inhibitor
as an anticoagulant is not only based on its inhibitory effect on the thrombin-
fibrinogen reaction but also on its inhibitory influence on the other thrombin-catalyzed reactions involved in hemostasis and thrombosis.

To elucidate the mechanism of action of thrombin inhibitors the knowledge of the biochemistry of the clotting enzyme, and especially the findings
of the past several years on the structure of its active center are of special
importance (8, 11, 13, 44). As an enzyme, thrombin exhibits distinct speci-
ficities for proteolysis of large substrates and for esterolytic hydrolysis of
small substrates. The reaction of the enzyme (E) with the substrate (S)
comprises the formation of an adsorptive complex (E·S) and a covalent
intermediate, the acyl enzyme (E - S'), liberating the first product $P_1$ and $P_2$
is the finally released other product.

$$E + S \underset{k_{-1}}{\overset{k_1}{\rightleftarrows}} E \cdot S \xrightarrow{k_2} E - S' + P_1 \xrightarrow{k_3} E + P_2$$

Thrombin is a serine proteinase (10). That means, a proteolytic enzyme
which displays its catalytic activity with the aid of an especially reactive

serine residue, the β-hydroxyl group of which forms a covalent bond with the substrate molecule. They are cleaving polypeptide chains only in such bonds in which the carboxyl group of the basic amino acids lysine or arginine participate. This specificity of the enzymes is achieved by the characteristics in structure of their substrate binding centers which in these proteinases are built according to the same principle. They consist of a hydrophobic slit formed by apolar side chains of amino acids and a dissociated side chain-situated carboxyl group of an aspartic acid residue at the bottom.

The substrate most widely studied has been the protein fibrinogen, which can polymerize into a gel or clot after partial proteolysis by thrombin. A first approximation to illustrate the fit of fibrinogen to the surface of the enzyme is given in figure 1. The fibrinopeptide moiety of the fibrinogen

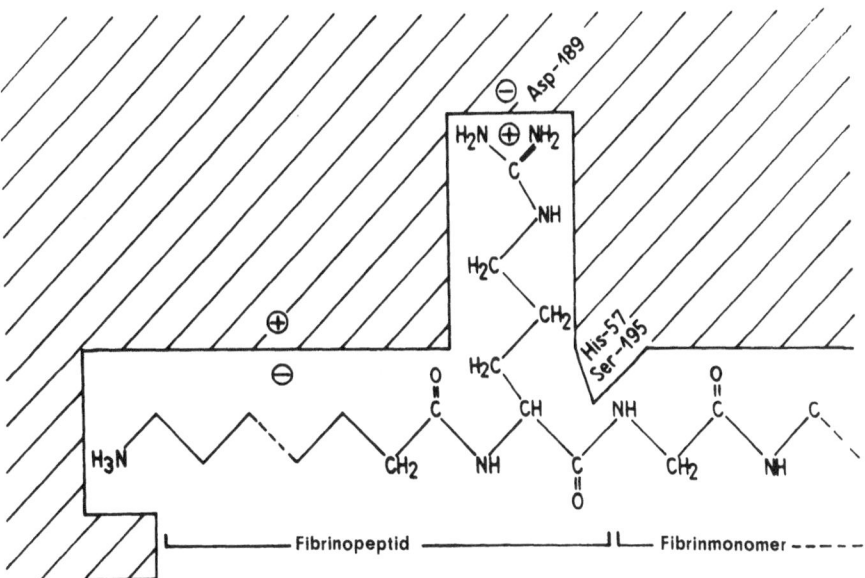

*Fig.* 1. Illustration of the fit of fibrinogen to thrombin.

molecule is bound to positively charged areas by its polyanionic character and the basic guanidium ion of the arginyl residue of fibrinogen reacts with the complementary anionic part in the depth of the active site (E·S). In this case the fibrinogen molecule is brought into a position which allows a splitting of specific Arg-Gly peptide bonds in fibrinogen forming the acyl enzyme fibrinopeptidyl thrombin (E — S') and releasing fibrin monomer $(P_1)$. This is followed by liberation of fibrinopeptides and the enzyme is ready for reaction with the next fibrinogen molecule $(E + P_2)$.

ANTITHROMBIN III AND HEPARIN

Physiologically, the most important thrombin inhibitor in blood plasma is antithrombin III (AT III) which inactivates the enzyme in a time- and temperature-dependent reaction (26). Table 1 shows the most relevant data of

*Table* 1. Antithrombin in human plasma.

| | |
|---|---|
| Molecular weight: | 65000 |
| Peptide content: | 85% |
| Carbohydrate content: | 13.4% |
| Concentration in plasma: | 388 mg/l = 6.0 μMol |
| Molar ratio of 'potential' thrombin (E) to antithrombin (A): | 1 : 4.5 |

$$E + A \underset{k_{-1}}{\overset{k_1}{\rightleftharpoons}} E \cdot A \xrightarrow{k_2} E - A' \xrightarrow{k_3} E + P$$

AT III (41). Although the thrombin-antithrombin reaction is of decisive importance for the regulation of the blood clotting process, its mechanism has not yet been finally clarified. So far, investigations of the kinetics of this reaction indicate that it is comparable to an enzyme-substrate reaction (34, 43).

$$E + A \underset{k_{-1}}{\overset{k_1}{\rightleftharpoons}} E \cdot A \xrightarrow{k_2} E - A' \xrightarrow{k_3} E + P_2$$

According to this scheme, the formation of a thrombin-antithrombin complex $(E \cdot A)$ would be followed by the acylation of the enzyme. In contrast to normal enzyme-substrate reactions, however, a very slow deacylation follows ($k_3 \approx 0$), resulting in a very stable acyl enzyme (E—A') and a long-term but not permanent inhibition of the enzyme. The influence of synthetic thrombin inhibitors on the thrombin-antithrombin reaction supports the assumption that it proceeds like an enzyme-substrate reaction (24). This is in agreement with the fact that the formation of a reversible complex with competitive inhibitors and irreversible acylation of the active center hinder the reaction of thrombin with antithrombin. One might therefore come to the assumption that AT III cannot react with thrombin if the active site of the latter is blocked in any way which interferes with its enzymatic activity.

From the physiological point of view the slow progressive reaction of thrombin with AT III seems to be useful, since by this way thrombin is inactivated after fulfilling its function. However, AT III does not cause a marked inhibition of coagulation, since fibrinogen conversion proceeds more rapidly than the reaction of thrombin with AT III.

The inactivation of thrombin by AT III follows the kinetics of a second order rate reaction, when the acidic polysaccharide heparin is added the reaction is increased and AT III produces a powerful inhibition of thrombin (fig. 2). Since heparin is not consumed during the reaction, it seems to act as a catalyzer of the AT III reaction.

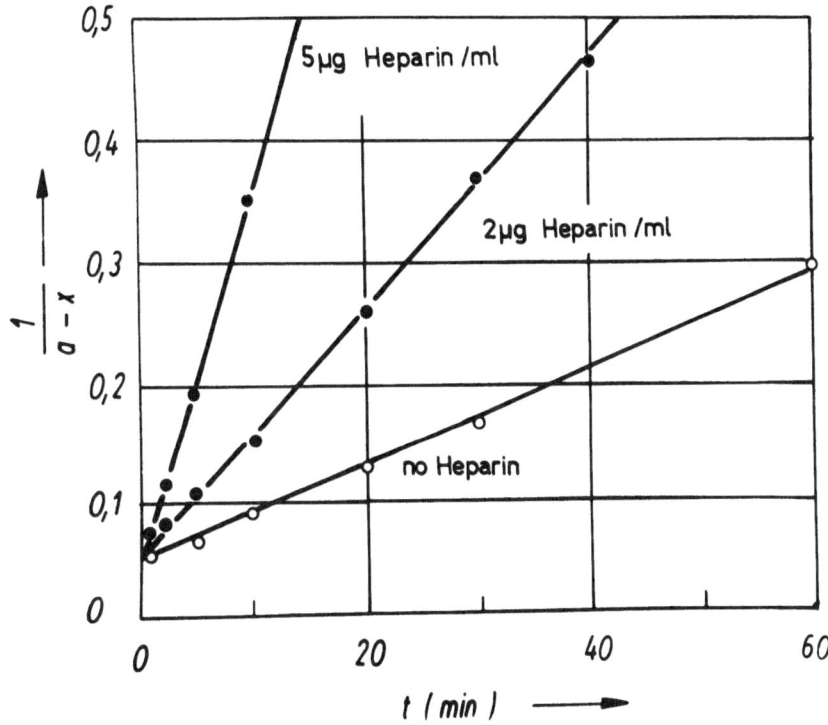

*Fig.* 2. Influence of heparin on the rate of the thrombin-antithrombin reaction at pH 7.8 and 35°C.
a = initial concentration: thrombin 20 NIH-U/ml, antithrombin 20 AT-U/ml
x = amount of thrombin inactivated in the time t
t = reaction time in minutes.

This action of heparin as an accelerator of the inactivation of thrombin by AT III is of therapeutic importance, because a distinct inhibition of coagulation can be obtained with small amounts of heparin, and similar effects can be demonstrated in plasma.

Concerning the role of AT III in the case of the anticoagulant effect of heparin we could prove for the first time that AT III is identical to the heparin cofactor, as was previously assumed by several workers (34). By other investigators it was also concluded that the plasmatic cofactor of heparin is identical to the main thrombin inhibitor of plasma, AT III (1, 2, 3, 5).

## THROMBIN INHIBITORS FROM BLOOD SUCKING ANIMALS

Blood sucking animals contain substances with anticoagulant properties (9, 20, 28, 31). During leeching, the blood sucker secretes anticoagulants into the wound in order to keep the blood from clotting. The analysis of these substances revealed that most of them are specific proteins with strong thrombin-neutralizing potencies. They inhibit blood coagulation by blocking the end product of the first stage of clotting, thrombin, and thereby prevent the conversion of fibrinogen to fibrin.

Among these antithrombins hirudin from Hirudo medicinalis is the best characterized so far (21). It was first isolated in 1955 and identified as a polypeptide (table 2) (14, 16, 30, 35).

*Table* 2. Hirudin (H).

| | |
|---|---|
| Molecular weight: | $9060 \pm 190$ |
| Amino acid composition: | Asp 10, Glu 13, Cys 6, Ser 4, Gly 10, Thr 4, Ala 1, Val 4, Leu 4, Ileu 2, Pro 3, Phe 2, Tyr 2, His 2, Lys 4 |
| Amino acid sequence from the C-terminal end: | Ala – Gly – Ser – Glu – Leu |
| Isoelectric point: | 3.8 |
| Specific activity: | $10\,400 \pm 600$ AT U/mg |

$$E + H \overset{K_I}{\rightleftarrows} E \cdot H \quad (K_I = 0.8 \cdot 10^{-10}\ M)$$

Hirudin is a specific inhibitor of thrombin (15). For its effect it does not require the presence of other coagulation factors or plasma constituents. This acidic polypeptide forms an extremely tight stoichiometric complex which can be identified by means of electrophoresis and chromatography.

$$E + H \underset{k_{-1}}{\overset{k_1}{\rightleftarrows}} E \cdot H$$

The inactive thrombin-hirudin complex $(E \cdot H)$ is only poorly dissociable $(Km = 0.8 \cdot 10^{-10}$, pH 7.4, 20°C), so that for all practical purposes the complex can be regarded as nondissociable $(k_{-1} \approx 0)$.

When thrombin reacts with hirudin, which leads to the immediate inactivation of the enzymatic activity of thrombin, the active surface of the enzyme is occupied by hirudin. To further elucidate the mode of action of hirudin, its reaction with chemically modified forms of thrombin was studied (33). The binding sites for hirudin were found in the cationic groups of the active surface of the enzyme which binds the fibrinopeptide portion of the fibrinogen substrate. Acetylation of these groups, as in esterase thrombin, blocks the binding of hirudin and thrombin.

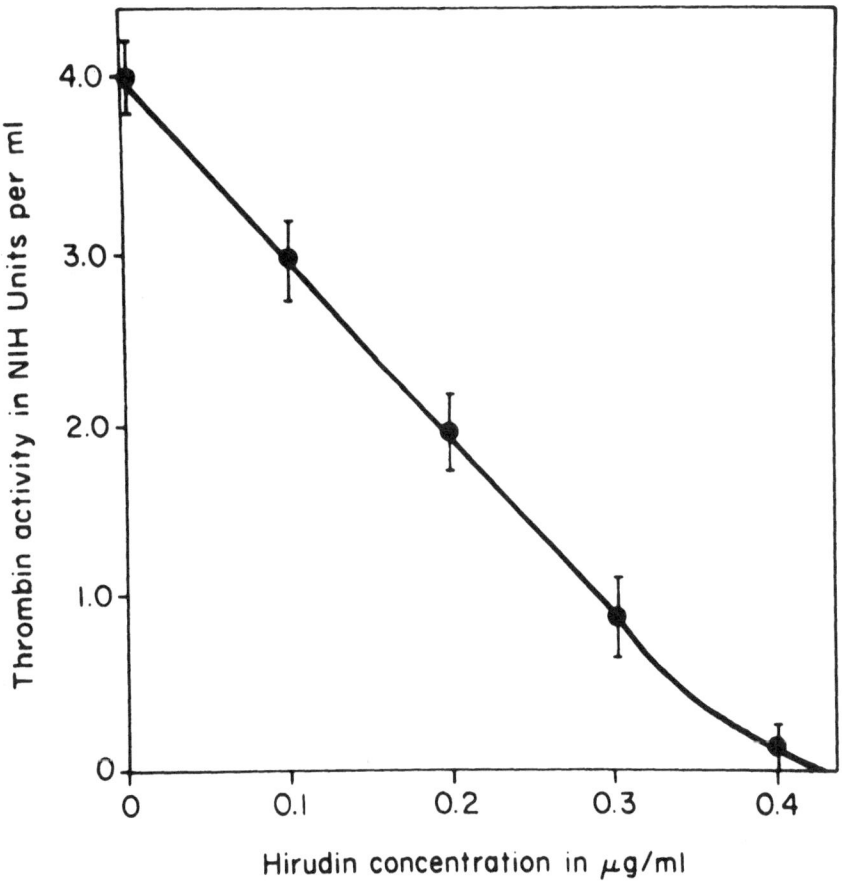

*Fig.* 3. Inhibition of clotting activity of thrombin by hirudin.

Based on the specific, rapid and stoichiometric reaction between hirudin and thrombin, hirudin activity can be quantitatively determined by titration with a standardized thrombin solution (fig. 3). The hirudin activity is expressed in antithrombin units (AT-U), whereby one AT-U is the amount of hirudin which neutralizes one NIH unit of thrombin. One AT-U corresponds to 0.1 μg of pure hirudin (21).

After knowing that thrombin activity is neutralized by hirudin, hirudin can be employed for the determination of thrombin activity by titrating a thrombin solution of unknown activity against a known concentration of hirudin. The determination of thrombin and those reactions which are closely related to formation and action of thrombin can be easily handled in a rather simple procedure. The practical application of this procedure has revealed certain advantages over other techniques (17, 19).

## LOW MOLECULAR WEIGHT THROMBIN INHIBITORS

With the introduction of the directly and indirectly acting antithrombins of the hirudin and heparin type, the search for new anticoagulant compounds has continued since both still have certain disadvantages. In the past several years low molecular weight inhibitors of thrombin have received increasing attention, because such substances could find potential use as oral, rapidly acting anticoagulants.

Biochemical studies of serine proteinases led us to the development of several types of synthetic thrombin inhibitors (22). Corresponding to their mechanism of action the inhibitors (1) will be divided into competitive, reversible, and temporary or irreversible inhibitors.

$$E + I \underset{k_{-1}}{\overset{k_1}{\rightleftharpoons}} E \cdot I \overset{k_2}{\longrightarrow} E - I' + P_1 \overset{k_3}{\longrightarrow} E + P_2$$

competitive inhibitors : $k_2 = 0$

irreversible inhibitors : $k_3 = 0$

temporary inhibitors : $k_3 < k_2$

The competitive inhibitors are assumed to be fixed at the active center of the enzyme on account of their structural relationship to the basic amino acids arginine and lysine. In this way, a displacement of the substrate is brought about which results in a competitive inhibition of the enzyme. This effectiveness of the inhibitors can be determined from their $K_i$ value.

Table 3. Low molecular weight inhibitors of thrombin (E) Competitive Inhibitors (I) (Benzamidine derivatives)

$E + I \rightleftarrows E \cdot I$

| R | $K_i$ [mM]* | $I_{50}$ [mM]** |
|---|---|---|
| — H | 0.22 | 1.0 |
| — $NH_2$ | 0.08 | 0.9 |
| — NHCO—⟨⟩ | 0.1 | 0.35 |
| — $NHSO_2$—⟨⟩ | 0.06 | 0.15 |
| — CONH—⟨⟩ | 0.12 | 0.4 |
| — CONH—⟨Cl⟩—Cl | 0.04 | 0.08 |
| — $CONHCH_2$—⟨⟩ | 0.14 | 0.6 |
| — $CH_2$—CO—COOH | 0.008 | 0.008 |

\* Hydrolysis of synthetic substrates (BANI).
\*\* Thrombin induced coagulation of fibrinogen.

Especially aromatic amidino compounds are found to be competitive inhibitors of thrombin (table 3). We suppose that the basic amidino groups of the inhibitors react with an anionic aspartic acid residue in the depth of the active site of the enzyme. The aromatic parts of the inhibitor molecules can be assumed to fit to the enzyme by hydrophobic bonds. Substituents at the aromatic ring system may influence the strength of the hydrophobic bond, and thus vary the inhibitor activity (27, 36, 37, 38).

*Table* 4. Low molecular weight inhibitors of thrombin (E) irreversible inhibitors (1).
$E + I \rightleftarrows E \cdot I \rightarrow E - I' + P_1$

| Compound | $k_2$ $[M^{-1} \cdot s^{-1}]$ |
|---|---|
| (CH₃)₂CH—O, O / P / (CH₃)₂CH—O F <br> Diisopropylfluorophosphate (DFP) | 1.3 |
| ⬡—CH₂—SO₂F <br> Phenylmethylsulfonyl fluoride (PMSF) | 2.0 |
| H₂N—CH₂—⬡—SO₂F <br> 4-Aminomethylbenzenesulfonyl fluoride (AMBSF) | 3.4 |
| HN C—⬡—SO₂F / H₂N <br> 4-Amidinobenzenesulfonyl fluoride (ABSF) | 15.0 |

Active-site-directed irreversible inhibitors are equipped with chemical groups that bind specifically to one of the amino acids at the active site of the enzyme, usually to either histidine or serine (table 4). The reaction sequence involves the initial formation of a reversible enzyme-inhibitor complex which is converted in the irreversible complex. In previous investigations it was shown that competitive inhibitors after combining with chemically reactive groups may be converted in inhibitors which form a stable covalent bond with the enzyme. Starting from the competitive inhibitors benzylamine and benzamidine, we studied the thrombin inactivating action of derivatives of these compounds with a reactive fluorosulfonyl moiety at the aromatic ring (39, 45).

These compounds, aminomethyl and amidinofluorosulfonylbenzenes possessed the highest rate of inactivation. The inhibitory effect of both the compounds on thrombin surpassed that of diisopropylfluorophosphate (DFP) and phenylmethylsulfonylfluoride (PMSF) which are commonly used as irreversible inhibitors of serine proteinases (6, 7, 12, 42).

Temporary inhibitors are defined as compounds that can enter into a more or less permanent bond with the enzyme and, as a consequence, can reduce its activity. Several esters of the amidino and guanidino benzoic acid, especially the nitrophenyl esters, react with thrombin like a substrate by acylation of the serine residue of the active center and by simultaneous release of the alcoholic component (4). However, the rate of deacylation is slower than the rate of acylation. Therefore, a temporary inhibition of the enzyme results (29). Furthermore, amidinophenyl esters of benzoic and other aromatic carboxylic acids also react with the enzyme like a substrate and the inactivation is caused by temporary acylation of the active center of thrombin (32, 40) (table 5).

*Table 5.* Low molecular weight inhibitors of thrombin (E) Temporary inhibitors (1).
$E + I \rightleftarrows E \cdot I \rightarrow E - I' + P_1 \rightarrow E + P_2$

| Compound | $k_2 \cdot 10^{-3} \ [M^{-1} \cdot s^{-1}]$ |
|---|---|
| Phenyl 4'-amidinobenzoate | 0.04 |
| 4-Nitrophenyl 4'-amidinobenzoate | 0.06 |
| 4-Amidinophenyl benzoate | 5.5 |
| Phenyl 4'-guanidinobenzoate | 10.0 |
| 4-Nitrophenyl 4'-guanidinobenzoate | 13.0 |

As shown, these inhibitors can serve as chemical probes into the configuration and reactivity of the active site of the thrombin molecule. With the advent of synthetic thrombin inhibitors, however, the question naturally arises whether any of those agents could serve a useful role as anticoagulants in vivo. In the case of spontaneous activation of the enzyme inhibitors are required to interfere with the immediately starting reaction with the permanently present substrate. Only such inhibitors are effective the reaction rate of which equals or surpasses that of the enzyme-substrate reaction. The ideal inhibitor should possess a very low $K_i$ value for entering into the initial reversible complex with thrombin and should then be able to establish rapid covalent bonding to the enzyme molecule. All the known rapidly acting temporary inhibitors, such as phenylguanidino benzoate, are ester compounds which are hydrolyzed and inactivated in the blood by nonspecific esterases. The irreversible inhibitors, such as amidinobenzene sulfonylfluoride, which can enter into a permanent covalent bond with the enzyme require minutes or even hours to achieve a significant inactivation of thrombin, while a few seconds would be the tolerable upper limit.

Investigating the different types of inhibitors with a possible anticoagulant effect in the blood, it could be shown that competitive inhibitors, especially aromatic amidino compounds, such as amidinophenylpyruvic acid (APPA), were most suitable for the chemical control of thrombin activity in the blood, if their inhibitory effect was sufficient. For in vivo investigations APPA is proved to be the most useful compound. Already at this time, this inhibitor can serve as a pharmacological model for compounds of this nature and allows an estimate for the potential therapeutic effect of this class of drugs.

These findings are of fundamental importance since so far no anticoagulant with a similar mode of action has been studied in vivo. The differences to the known anticoagulants are apparent since the protease inhibitors are synthetic, low molecular weight compounds with a direct action and can be administered orally.

*Antithrombotic Action*

To estimate the possible therapeutic use of the natural macromolecular and the synthetic low molecular inhibitors thrombin time of blood samples was studied in man after application of hirudin and APPA (23).

Since the polypeptide hirudin is destroyed by the influence of proteolytic enzymes only parenteral application is possible. Intravenously injected hirudin disappears from the blood relatively fast. The half life of hirudin amounts to 15 min (fig. 4). In the 24-hours-urine 70-80% of the injected hirudin are excreted in unchanged form.

Following the injection of APPA the blood level drops sharply initially corresponding to the distribution between intra- and extravascular compartments. The average half life was 100 min (fig. 5). The absorption of APPA following oral administration was 30%. 40% of APPA were recovered in an unaltered form in the 24-hours-urine.

It is evident that the inhibitors display their antithrombin effect in the

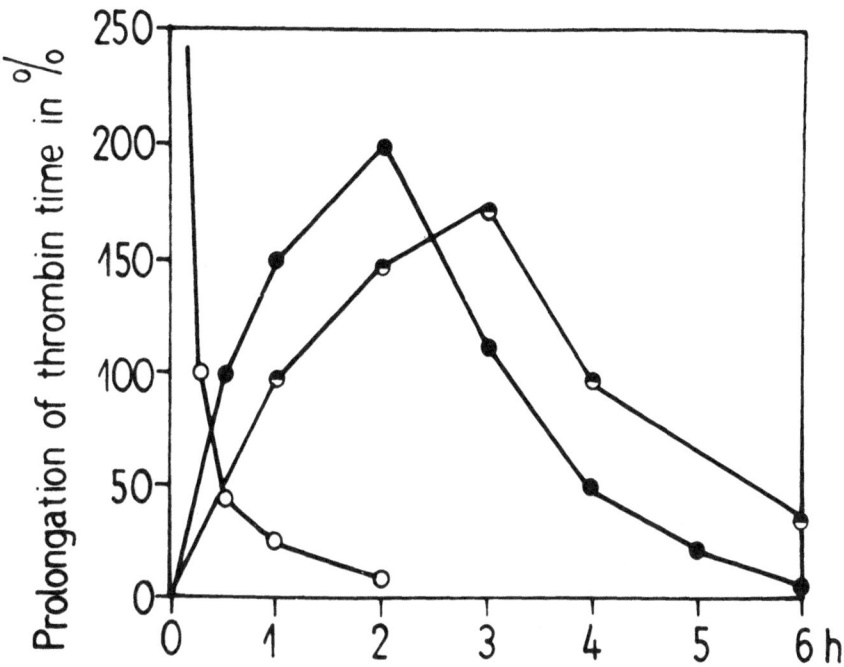

*Fig.* 4. Prolongation of thrombin time after injection of hirudin, 0.01 mg/kg in man.
( ○ ) i. v.; ( ● ) i.m.; ( ◓ ) s. c.

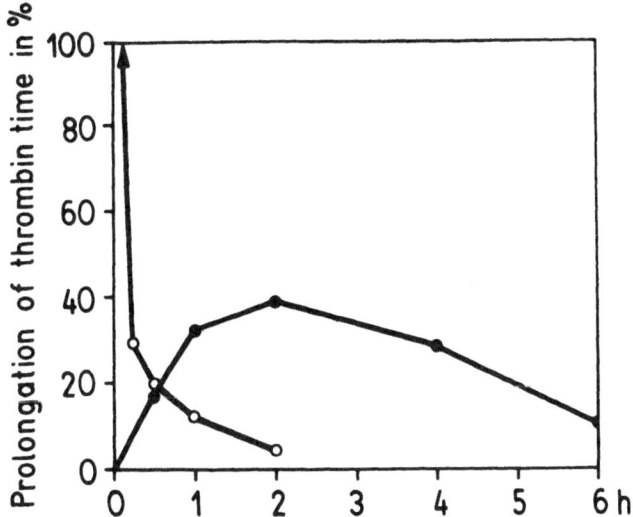

*Fig.* 5. Prolongation of thrombin time after application of APPA in man
( ○ ) 1 mg/kg i. v.; ( ● ) 10 mg/kg per os.

128        F. MARKWARDT

*Table* 6. The effect of thrombin inhibitors on lethal thrombin doses ($LD_{100}$ = 900 NIH. U/kg i.v. over 30 sec.).

| Number of animals n | Inhibitor dose per kg i.v.* | Number of dead animals after thrombin injection | | p |
|---|---|---|---|---|
| | | n | % | |
| 44 | – | 44 | 100 | – |
| 40 | 10 mg heparin | 4 | 10 | <0.001 |
| 32 | 2 mg hirudin | 4 | 12 | <0.001 |
| 46 | 10 mg APPA | 4 | 9 | <0.001 |

* 5 min before thrombin injection.

streaming blood too. The antithrombotic action of the thrombin inhibitors in vivo was demonstrated by preventing thrombus formation (18, 25). In experimental animals lethal effects caused by thrombin infusion (table 6), the incidence of experimental thrombosis (table 7) and endotoxin-induced disseminated intravascular coagulation (table 8), as it is observed in the Sanarelli-Shwartzman phenomenon, were prevented by administration of hirudin, APPA and heparin.

*Table* 7. The effect of thrombin inhibitors on the formation of clotting thrombi in rats. (Produced in an exposed segment of jugular vein by injection contact activated human serum followed by stasis).

| Number of animals n | Inhibitor dose per kg i.v.* | Animals with thrombi | | p |
|---|---|---|---|---|
| | | n | % | |
| 18 | – | 16 | 89 | – |
| 15 | 2 mg heparin | 1 | 6 | <0.01 |
| 10 | 0,5 mg hirudin | 1 | 10 | <0.01 |
| 12 | 10 mg APPA | 2 | 13 | <0.01 |

* 5 min prior to the injection of serum.

The inhibition of the clotting enzyme thrombin represents an effective influence on blood clotting. Accordingly, intrinsic plasmatic inhibitors (AT III and heparin), specific inhibitors obtained from blood sucking animals (hirudin), and synthetic low molecular weight inhibitors of serine proteinases (APPA) are therapeutically relevant substances.

*Table 8.* Influence of thrombin inhibitors on the localized Sanarelli-Shwartzman phenomenon (SSP) in rabbits. (Produced by injections of endotoxin: 0.1 mg intracutaneously and after 24 h 0.2 mg intravenously).

| Number of animals n | Inhibitor dose per kg i.v.* | Animals with SSP** | | |
|---|---|---|---|---|
| | | n | % | p |
| 30 | – | 29 | 96 | – |
| 20 | 8 mg hirudin | 1 | 5 | <0.001 |
| 16 | 20 mg heparin | 4 | 25 | <0.01 |
| 13 | 20 mg APPA | 4 | 30 | <0.01 |

\* Given after the 2nd injection of endotoxin over a period of 5 h.
\*\* 4-6 h after the 2nd injection of endotoxin.

## REFERENCES

1. Abildgaard, U., Binding of thrombin to antithrombin III. *Scand. J. clin. Lab. Invest.* 24, 23 (1969).
2. Abildgaard, U., Thrombin inhibiting action of heparin. *Folia haemat.* 98, 408 (1972).
3. Burstein, M. and A. Guinand, Héparine et consommation de l'antithrombine. *Arch. int. Pharmacodyn.* 54, 435 (1956).
4. Chase, T. Jr. and E. Shaw, Comparison of the esterase activities of trypsin, plasmin and thrombin on guanidinobenzoate esters: titration of the enzymes. *Biochem.* 3, 2212 (1969).
5. Gerendas, M., Die Thrombininaktivierung als Enzymprozeß. *Thrombos. Diathes. haemorrh. (Stuttg.)* 4, 56 (1960).
6. Gladner, J. A. and K. Laki, The inhibition of thrombin by diisopropyl-phosphorofluoridate. *Arch. Biochem.* 62, 501 (1956).
7. Glover, G. and E. Shaw, Purification of thrombin and affinity labeling of an active center histidine. *J. biol. Chem.* 246, 4594 (1971).
8. Hartley, B. S., Homologies in serine proteinases. *Phil. Trans. Roy. Soc.* B 257, 77 (1970).
9. Hellmann, K. and R. J. Hawkins, An antithrombin (maculatin) and plasminogen activator extractable from the blood sucking hemipteran Eutrioma maculatus. *Brit. J. Haemat.* 12, 376 (1966).
10. Laki, K., J. A. Gladner, J. E. Folk and D. R. Kominz, The mode of action of thrombin. *Thrombos. Diathes. haemorrh. (Stuttg.)* 2, 205 (1958).
11. Lorand, L. and J. L. G. Nilsson, Molecular approach for designing to enzymes involved in blood clotting. *Med. Chem.* 3, 415 (1972).
12. Lundblad, R. L., A rapid method for the purification of bovine thrombin and the inhibition of the purified enzyme with phenylmethylsulfonyl fluoride. *Biochem.* 10, 2501 (1971).
13. Magnusson, S., *Bovine prothrombin and thrombin.* In: *Methods in Enzymology.* S. P. Colowick and N. O. Kaplan (eds.) Vol. 19, p. 157. Academic Press, New York and London (1970).
14. Markwardt, F., Untersuchungen über Hirudin. *Naturwissenschaften* 42, 258 (1954).
15. Markwardt, F., Untersuchungen über den Mechanismus der blutgerinnungshemmenden Wirkung des Hirudins. *Naunyn-Schmiedeberg's Arch. exp. Path. Pharmak.* 229, 389 (1956).

16. Markwardt, F., Die Isolierung und chemische Charakterisierung des Hirudins. *Hoppe-Seylers Z. physiol. Chem.* 308, 147 (1957).

17. Markwardt, F., Die quantitative Bestimmung des Prothrombins durch Titration mit Hirudin. *Naunyn-Schmiedeberg's Arch. exp. Path. Pharmak.* 232, 487 (1958).

18. Markwardt, F., Versuche zur pharmakologischen Charakterisierung des Hirudins. *Naunyn-Schmiedeberg's Arch. exp. Path. Pharmak.* 234, 516 (1958).

19. Markwardt, F., Der Hirudintoleranztest. *Klin. Wschr.* 37, 1142 (1959).

20. Markwardt, F., *Blutgerinnungshemmende Wirkstoffe aus blutsaugenden Tieren.* Fischer, Jena (1963).

21. Markwardt, F., *Hirudin as an inhibitor of thrombin.* In: *Methods in Enzymology.* S. P. Colowick and N. O. Kaplan (eds.) Vol. 19, p. 924. Academic Press, New York and London (1970).

22. Markwardt, F., Synthetische Proteaseninhibitoren als Antikoagulantien. *Nova Acta Leopoldina N. F.* 202, 36 (1971).

23. Markwardt, F., Gerinnungsphysiologische Analyse der Wirkung synthetischer Thrombininhibitoren. *Thrombos. Diathes. haemorrh. (Stuttg.)* 27, 99 (1972).

24. Markwardt, F., J. Hoffmann and E. Körbs, The influence of synthetic thrombin inhibitors on the thrombin-antithrombin reaction. *Thrombos. Res.* 4, 343 (1973).

25. Markwardt, F. and H.-P. Klöcking, The antithrombotic effect of synthetic thrombin inhibitors. *Thrombos. Res.* 1, 243 (1972).

26. Markwardt, F. and H. Landmann, *Blutgerinnungshemmende Proteine, Peptide und Aminosäurederivate.* In: *Handbuch der experimentellen Pharmakologie.* F. Markwardt (Ed.) Vol. 27, p. 76. Springer, Berlin, Heidelberg, New York (1971).

27. Markwardt, F., H. Landmann and P. Walsmann, Comparative studies on the inhibition of trypsin, plasmin and thrombin by derivatives of benzylamine and benzamidine. *Eur. J. Biochem.* 6, 502 (1968).

28. Markwardt, F. and E. Leberecht, Untersuchungen über den blutgerinnungshemmenden Wirkstoff der Tabaniden. *Naturwissenschaften* 46, 17 (1959).

29. Markwardt, F., M. Richter, P. Walsmann and H. Landmann, The inhibition of trypsin, plasmin and thrombin by benzyl 4-guanidinobenzoate and 4'-nitrobenzyl 4-guanidinobenzoate. *FEBS Letters* 8, 170 (1970).

30. Markwardt, F., G. Schäfer, H. Töpfer and P. Walsmann, Die Isolierung des Hirudins aus medizinischen Blutegeln. *Pharmazie* 22, 239 (1967).

31. Markwardt, F. and E. Schulz, Über einen Hemmstoff des Gerinnungsfermentes Thrombin aus blutsaugenden Raubwanzen (Reduviiden). *Naturwissenschaften* 47, 43 (1960).

32. Markwardt, F., G. Wagner, P. Walsmann, H. Horn and J. Stürzebecher, Inhibition of serine proteinases by amidinophenyl esters of aromatic carbonic acids. *Acta biol. med. germ.* 28, K 19 (1972).

33. Markwardt, F. and P. Walsmann, Die Reaktion zwischen Hirudin und Thrombin. *Hoppe-Seylers Z. physiol. Chem.* 312, 85 (1958).

34. Markwardt, F. and P. Walsmann, Untersuchungen über den Mechanismus der Antithrombinwirkung des Heparins. *Hoppe-Seylers Z. physiol. Chem.* 317, 64 (1959).

35. Markwardt, F. and P. Walsmann, Reindarstellung und Analyse des Thrombininhibitors Hirudin. *Hoppe-Seylers Z. physiol. Chem.* 348, 1381 (1967).

36. Markwardt, F. and P. Walsmann, Über die Hemmung des Gerinnungsfermentes Thrombin durch Benzamidinderivate. *Experientia (Basel)* 24, 25 (1968).

37. Markwardt, F., P. Walsmann and H.-G. Kazmirowski, Untersuchungen über den Einfluß von Ring-Substitutionen auf die thrombinhemmende Wirkung von Benzylamin- und Benzamidinderivaten. *Pharmazie* 24, 400 (1969).

38. Markwardt, F., P. Walsmann and H. Landmann, Hemmung der Thrombin-, Plasmin- und Trypsinwirkung durch Alkyl- und Alkoxybenzamidine. *Pharmazie* 25, 551 (1970).

39. Markwardt, F., P. Walsmann, M. Richter, H.-P. Klöcking, J. Drawert and H. Land-mann, Aminoalkylbenzolsylfofluoride als Fermentinhibitoren. *Pharmazie* 26, 401 (1971).

40. Markwardt, F., P. Walsmann, J. Stürzebecher, H. Landmann and G. Wagner, Synthetische Inhibitoren von Serinproteinasen. 1. Mitteilung: Über die Hemmung von Trypsin, Plasmin und Thrombin durch Ester der Amidino- und Guanidinobenzoe-säuren. *Pharmazie* 28, 327 (1973).

41. Schwick, H.-G. and N. Heimburger: Biochemie der Antithrombine. *Thrombos. Diathes. haemorrh.* (Stuttg.) Suppl. 44,5 (1971).

42. Seegers, W. H., D. Heene, E. Marciniak, N. Ivanovic and M. J. Caldwell, Sensitivity of thrombin and autoprothrombin C to selected enzyme inhibitors. *Life Sci.* 4, 425 (1965).

43. Seegers, W. H., M. Yoshinari and R. H. Landaburu, Antithrombin as substrate for the enzyme thrombin. *Thrombos. Diathes. haemorrh. (Stuttg.)* 4, 293 (1960).

44. Walsmann, P. and F. Markwardt, Über die Biochemie des Thrombins. *Pharmazie* 23, 597 (1968).

45. Walsmann, P., M. Richter and F. Markwardt, Inaktivierung von Trypsin und Thrombin durch 4-Amidinobenzolsulfofluorid und 4-(2-Aminoäthyl)-benzol-sulfofluorid. *Acta biol. med. germ.* 28 577, (1972).

PART TWO

# PIVKA-11

# POSTRIBOSOMAL SYNTHESIS OF PROTHROMBIN
# UNDER THE INFLUENCE OF VITAMIN K[1]

J. W. SUTTIE

The only known function of vitamin K in mammals is to promote the synthesis of certain blood clotting factors. In the absence of the vitamin, or in the presence of its antagonists, prothrombin and the other 'K dependent' clotting factors (Factors VII, IX, and X) are not synthesized. The molecular mechanism by which vitamin K functions to support the production of these plasma proteins has not been elucidated, but a substantial amount of current data strongly suggests that the metabolic step involved is postribosomal. Some earlier reports did suggest (Olson, 1964) that the rate of prothrombin production is regulated by an effect of vitamin K on DNA transcription. These observations appear to have been adequately refuted (Suttie, 1967; Lowenthal and Simmons, 1967; Hill et al., 1968) and subsequent investigations have centered around two alternate hypotheses: 1) That the vitamin acts at a ribosomal site to regulate the *de novo* rate of prothrombin synthesis; or 2) that it functions postribosomally in a metabolic step which converts a precursor protein, which can be produced in the absence of the vitamin, to active prothrombin.

The possibility that a precursor protein was involved in the formation of prothrombin was first suggested by the nature of the plasma prothrombin response observed (fig. 1) when vitamin K is administered to vitamin K deficient, hypoprothrombinemic rats. There is a lag period where no increase in plasma prothrombin is seen, followed by a rapid burst of plasma prothrombin occurring 30-60 min after vitamin administration (Pyörälä, 1965; Bell and Matschiner, 1969; Hill et al., 1968; Suttie, 1970). About half of the normal levels of prothrombin are restored in the first hour, and this is followed by a slow return to normal concentrations. The appearance of plasma prothrombin is preceded (Shah and Suttie, 1972) by the transient

1. Previously unpublished research reported here was supported by the College of Agricultural and Life Sciences, University of Wisconsin, Madison, and in part by a grant AM-14881 from the National Institutes of Health.

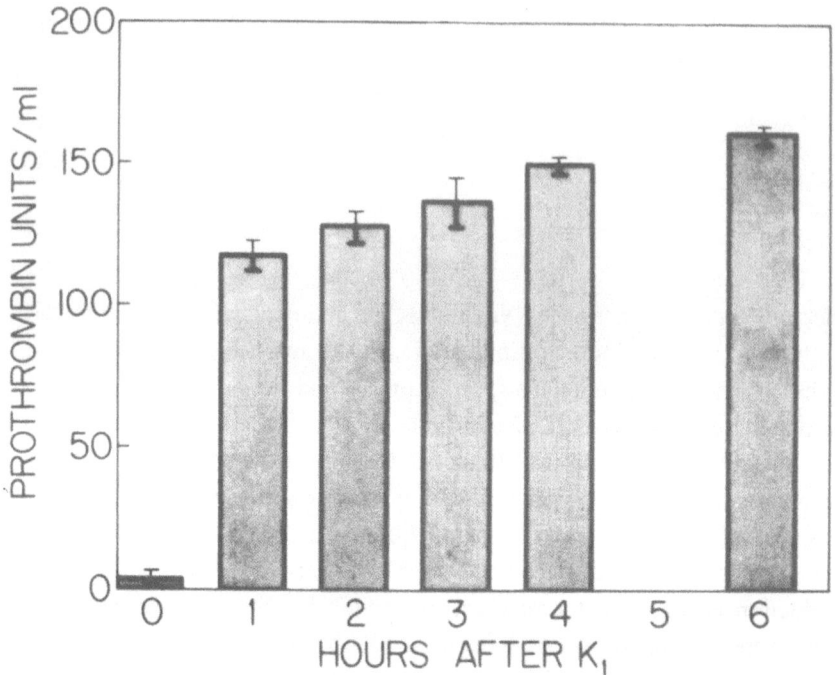

*Fig.* 1. Response of vitamin K deficient hypoprothrombinemic rats to vitamin K. Rats were given vitamin K at O time and blood sampled at hourly intervals. Plasma prothrombin concentrations in normal vitamin K sufficient rats are from 200-220 units/ml. Redrawn from Suttie (1970).

appearance of prothrombin in the crude microsomal fraction of the liver. Microsomal prothrombin concentrations peak at about 10 min after administration of vitamin K to hypoprothrombinemic rats (fig. 2) and then fall during the period that prothrombin begins to appear in the plasma. The nature of this response strongly suggests that there is a pool of some precursor in the hypoprothrombinemic rat which can be converted to prothrombin in a vitamin K dependent step, and when this pool is depleted, the rate of synthesis will decrease and become equal to the rate of precursor production.

Further evidence that there was a precursor protein involved was obtained when a number of investigators (Bell and Matschiner, 1969; Hill et al., 1968; Suttie, 1970) demonstrated that the initial period of rapid prothrombin synthesis observed in the hypoprothrombinemic rat following vitamin K stimulation was decreased only slightly if the protein synthesis inhibitor cycloheximide was administered prior to the vitamin. The small increase

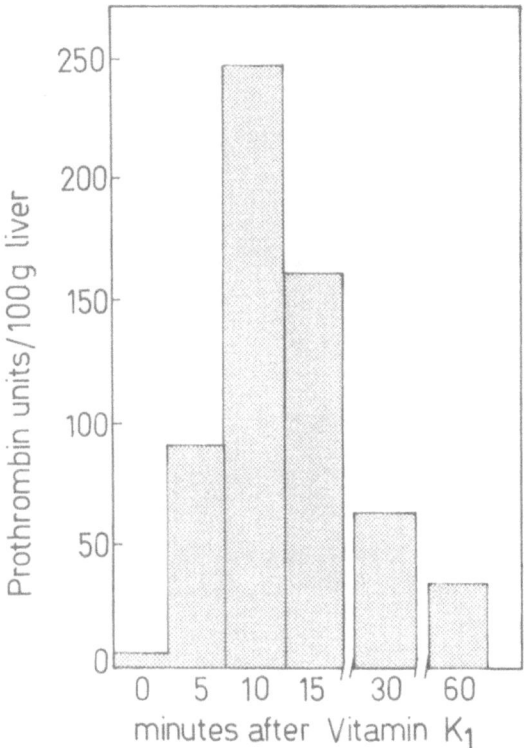

*Fig.* 2. Effect of vitamin K administration on liver prothrombin concentrations. Vitamin K deficient rats were given vitamin K at O time, killed at the times indicated and prothrombin concentrations in liver microsomal preparations assayed. Increases in plasma prothrombin concentrations in these rats are first detectable at about 30 min while the microsomal prothrombin concentration has peaked, but is falling at this time. Redrawn from Shah and Suttie (1972).

in plasma prothrombin which is usually seen between the first and second hour after vitamin administration is, however, blocked by the same dose of cycloheximide. These results (fig. 3) strongly suggest that protein synthesis is not required for the vitamin dependent step in prothrombin synthesis, and that the conversion of precursor to prothrombin proceeds at a rate which rapidly depletes the precursor pool. Subsequent synthesis is then dependent on continual ribosomal production of the precursor. Studies of prothrombin production in perfused livers, and factor VII production in liver slices, liver microsomal preparations, or isolated liver cells have also been carried out. In most, but not all cases, the use of inhibitors of protein biosynthesis in

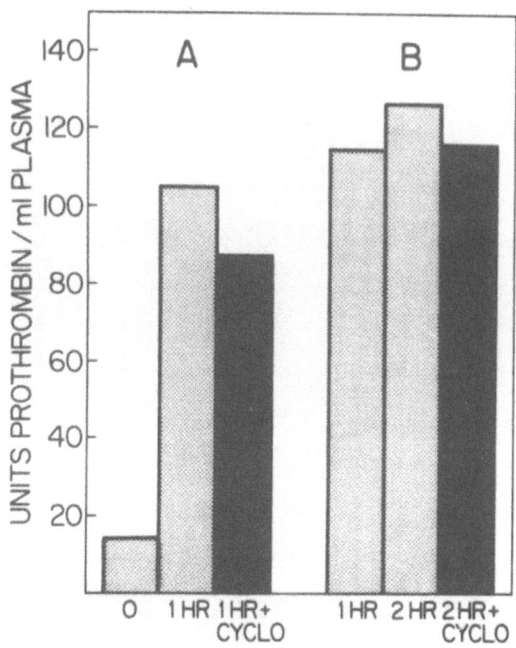

Fig. 3. Effect of cycloheximide on vitamin K stimulated prothrombin production. Vitamin K deficient rats were given vitamin K and the plasma prothrombin concentrations were measured at O time and 1 hour (Expt. A) or at 1 hour and 2 hours (Expt. B) after vitamin administration. When administered, cycloheximide was given 30 min prior to the 1 hour response period being studied. The shaded bars represent animals given only the vitamin, and the dark bars vitamin plus cycloheximide. Redrawn from Suttie (1970).

these systems supported the concept of a liver precursor of prothrombin, and a postribosomal vitamin dependent site.

These studies have been recently reviewed in more detail elsewhere (Suttie, 1974). Although these studies which utilized inhibitors of protein biosynthesis in both intact animals and various *in vitro* systems strongly suggested that protein synthesis was not involved in the vitamin K dependent step of prothrombin synthesis, they were not definitive. More conclusive and direct evidence for the presence of a precursor was obtained by Shah and Suttie (1971) when they demonstrated that the plasma prothrombin produced when hypoprothrombinemic rats are given vitamin K did not contain radioactive amino acids if these were administered at the same time as the vitamin. These data, which are summarized in table 1, provided direct evidence that the prothrombin formed in the presence of cycloheximide did not contain newly synthesized protein, and strongly suggested that it must have been derived from an existing precursor pool.

*Table* 1. Amino acid incorporation into prothrombin.

| Treatment of vitamin K deficient rat | Plasma prothrombin (units/ml) | [$^{14}$C] Dpm in Prothrombin | $\dfrac{\text{Dpm in prothrombin}}{\text{units of Prothrombin}}$ |
|---|---|---|---|
| Vitamin K | 134 | 124 | 1.7 |
| Cycloheximide + vitamin K | 87 | 4 | 0.1 |

Vitamin K-deficient rats were administered a [$^{14}$C] amino acid mix at 0 time and at 30 min. They were given vitamin K 10 min after the first amino acid dose. Cycloheximide (5 mg/kg) was administered 20 min prior to the first dose of amino acid mix. Blood was drawn 60 min after vitamin K was given. A crude prothrombin preparation was obtained by BaSO$_4$ absorption of the plasma and elution with citrate. This eluate was subjected to acrylamide gel electrophoresis, and the prothrombin band was cut from the gel and the radioactivity in it determined. For details of the procedure see Shah and Suttie (1971).

If the vitamin had initiated *de novo* synthesis of prothrombin, and for some reason cycloheximide administration was not effectively blocking prothrombin synthesis, the newly formed prothrombin should have contained a high level of radioactivity. Additional experiments indicated when radioactive amino acids were administered to hypoprothrombinemic rats prior to cycloheximide and vitamin K administration, the prothrombin subsequently formed did contain radioactive amino acids. This observation suggested that the precursor protein pool was rapidly being synthesized, and could then be converted to prothrombin in a step which did not require protein synthesis.

The hypothesis that vitamin K acts at a postribosomal site in prothrombin synthesis has been strengthened by observations that the plasma of man or animals treated with coumarin anticoagulants contains a protein which is in many ways similar to prothrombin. The existence of such a protein was first demonstrated by indirect means in the plasma of human patients receiving anticoagulant therapy by Hemker et al. (1963), and later a protein which was antigenetically similar to prothrombin, but lacked biological activity was found in such plasma by a number of workers. The discovery of these abnormal prothrombins, which are called PIVKAs (Protein Induced by Vitamin K Absence) by some workers, and a description of their properties has been treated in detail by others in this symposium (Lavergne, 1975;

Stenflo, 1975; Menaché, 1975) and will not be reviewed here. The bovine preparation has been most extensively studied, both by Stenflo's group (Stenflo, 1972; Stenflo and Ganrot, 1972, 1973; Bjork and Stenflo, 1973) and in our laboratory (Nelsestuen and Suttie, 1972a, b). The results of these studies have indicated that this protein is chemically indistinguishable from prothrombin except in its inability to adsorb to insoluble barium salts and to bind calcium ions in solution. As calcium is required to hold prothrombin to a phospholipid surface during normal activation by factor Xa (Gitel et al., 1973) the lack of this binding prevents its activation at a reasonable rate by the normal activation mechanism. Prothrombin can also be activated by a number of snake venoms including that from *Echis carinatus* (Schieck et al. 1972). The abnormal bovine prothrombin can be activated by *Echis carinatus* venom which clearly demonstrates that it contains the thrombin portion of prothrombin, and that its lack of biological activity is the result of a defect in the activation step.

These observations suggest that the vitamin K-sensitive step in prothrombin synthesis involves either the attachment of some unrecognized calcium binding prosthetic group to a liver precursor, or the modification of some amino acid residues to form the calcium binding site on the precursor. Support for this view has come from the recent isolation (Nelsestuen and Suttie, 1973) of a tryptic peptide from normal bovine prothrombin which will adsorb to insoluble barium salts and which will bind to calcium ions in solution. This peptide cannot be isolated from preparations of the bovine abnormal prothrombin. It is located in the non-thrombin portion of prothrombin, and contains a high proportion of acidic amino acid residues. The peptide has a calculated molecular weight of 3100 daltons based upon its amino acid composition, but a molecular weight of 4400 daltons based on a dry weight determination, and an anomalously high apparent molecular weight on molecular sieve columns. Its ability to bind to calcium ions or barium salts appears to be a function of a very acidic non-peptide prosthetic group covalently attached to the peptide. This observation would be consistent with Stenflo's (1973) report that he has obtained different peptide maps following thermolysin digestion of the amino terminal portion of normal compared to abnormal prothrombin, and Magnusson's (1973) report of the isolation of some extremely acidic peptides from tryptic digests of prothrombin. On the basis of these observations we have postulated that vitamin K functions in a metabolic step which is either required in the synthesis of this prosthetic group from some metabolite pool, or more likely we think, in the step where this group is attached to the precursor peptide to produce biologically active prothrombin.

The hypothesized liver precursor of prothrombin should have many of the same properties as the abnormal plasma prothrombin (PIVKA II) and such a protein has now been identified (Suttie, 1973b). Microsomes were isolated from warfarin-treated rats, solubilized with detergent, and this microsomal extract treated with Echis carinatus venom. The results, summarized in table 2, show that the amount of microsomal prothrombin decreased when

Table 2. Prothrombin and prothrombin precursor activities in rat liver microsomal extracts.

| Treatment | Plasma prothrombin (units/ml) | Activity in microsomal extract (units/ml) | |
| --- | --- | --- | --- |
| | | Prothrombin | Precursor |
| Control | 218 ± 12 | 2.1 ± 0.1 | 1.9 ± 0.3 |
| Warfarin | 32 ± 6 | <1 | 8.7 ± 0.6 |
| Warfarin + vitamin K | 136 ± 3 | 1.9 ± 0.1 | 0.6 ± 0.1 |
| Warfarin + vitamin K + cycloheximide | 104 ± 3 | 2.0 ± 0.1 | 1.1 ± 0.2 |

Prothrombin activity was measured by standard methods, and precursor activity was measured by incubating the microsomal extracts with Echis carinatus venom and then adding this activated mixture to a buffered fibrinogen acacia mixture. These clotting times were converted to thrombin units by comparison to a standard curve prepared by dilution of NIH standard thrombin. Measurements were made one hr after vitamin K was administered. All values are means ± S.E. for 6 rats per group. For details of the assay and treatment of the animals, see Suttie (1973b).

warfarin was administered, and the amount of thrombin-like activity liberated by Echis carinatus treatment ('precursor activity') increased. Similar results were seen when the animals were made vitamin K deficient or treated with a second anticoagulant, 2-chloro-3-phytyl-1,4-napthhoquinone. The microsomal precursor activity increased rapidly and leveled off after about 4 hours when warfarin was administered, and increased over a period of days when rats were placed on a vitamin K deficient diet. The amount of microsomal precursor decreases rapidly (fig. 4) when vitamin K is injected, and as its level falls, the amount of microsomal prothrombin increases and then falls as it moves out of the liver into the plasma. The precursor protein will react with an antibody prepared against rat prothrombin, but differs from prothrombin in that it will not adsorb onto barium salts, and can easily be

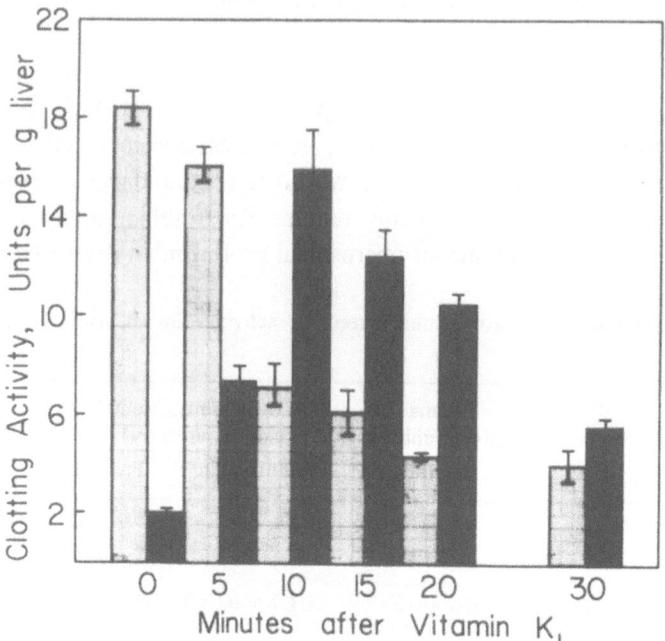

*Fig.* 4. Response of liver microsomal precursor and prothrombin concentrations to vitamin K administration. Rats which had been treated with warfarin 18 hours previously were given an intravenous injection of vitamin K and killed at the times indicated. Precursor activity (shaded bars) and prothrombin activity (dark bars) were assayed as microsomal extracts. The extract was treated with $BaSO_4$ to remove prothrombin before assaying for precursor activity. From Shah et al. (1973).

separated from prothrombin electrophoretically or by chromatography on DEAE-cellulose (Shah et al., 1973).

We have found (table 3) that a similar activity can be demonstrated in liver microsomes prepared from warfarin treated chicks, rabbits, guinea pigs, mice, hamsters, and dogs, but not in the liver microsomes obtained from calves treated with dicumarol. This raises the possibility that in a species like the bovine, and possibly the human, the precursor, or some further modification of it, does not build up in the liver but is excreted into the plasma as an abnormal prothrombin (PIVKA II). The corollary to this would be that those species which show an increase in liver precursor would not excrete an abnormal plasma prothrombin. We have, however, found some abnormal prothrombin in the plasma of most species, but not to the extent that it is found in bovine plasma.

Initial attempts to purify the rat liver precursor in our laboratory took

*Table* 3. Abnormal plasma prothrombin and liver prothrombin precursor in various species.

| | Abnormal prothrombin (% control prothrombin) | Liver precursor (U/g liver) |
|---|---|---|
| Rat | 5 | 15 |
| Cow | 84 | < 2 |
| Mouse | 17 | 11 |
| Hamster | < 5 | 12 |
| Guinea pig | < 5 | 5 |
| Rabbit | < 5 | 21 |
| Dog | < 5 | 10 |
| Chick | 32 | 19 |

All species were treated with anticoagulant to achieve a plasma prothrombin concentration of less than 20%. Abnormal prothrombin was measured as the amount of thrombin activity that could be generated in $BaSO_4$ adsorbed plasma by *E. carinatus* treatment, compared to the amount in normal plasma of that species. Liver precursor was measured as previously described (Suttie, 1973b) in liver microsomes prepared from each species (Carlisle *et al.* 1975).

advantage of the observation that this protein would react with rat prothrombin antibody. Microsomes from warfarin treated rats were salt washed, solubilized in Triton X-100, and fractionated with ammonium sulfate. The proteins were then passed through a column prepared by covalently attaching rat prothrombin antibody to an agarose matrix. After the column was washed to remove non-specifically bound proteins, the antigenically active material was eluted with a high concentration of $MgCl_2$. When this material was subjected to preparative scale isoelectrofocusing it was clear that our preparation contains at least two distinctly different proteins with precursor activity. One of these had a pI of 7.2, while the other had a pI of 5.8. The more acidic protein behaved on gel filtration columns as if it had a molecular weight much larger than rat prothrombin, which has been reported to be 85,000 daltons (Li and Olsen, 1967). Insufficient amounts of these proteins to adequately characterize them were obtained by this procedure, and in an effort to obtain larger quantities of pure precursor, it is now being purified by more conventional techniques.

By a combination of molecular sieve and modified Sephadex column chromatography, it has been possible (fig. 5) to obtain a preparation where the major protein with precursor activity has a pI of 5.8 and an apparent molecular weight of about 80,000. There is also a second component of the precursor activity with a pI of about 6.2. Both of these components have a tendency to aggregate to higher molecular weight forms, and they

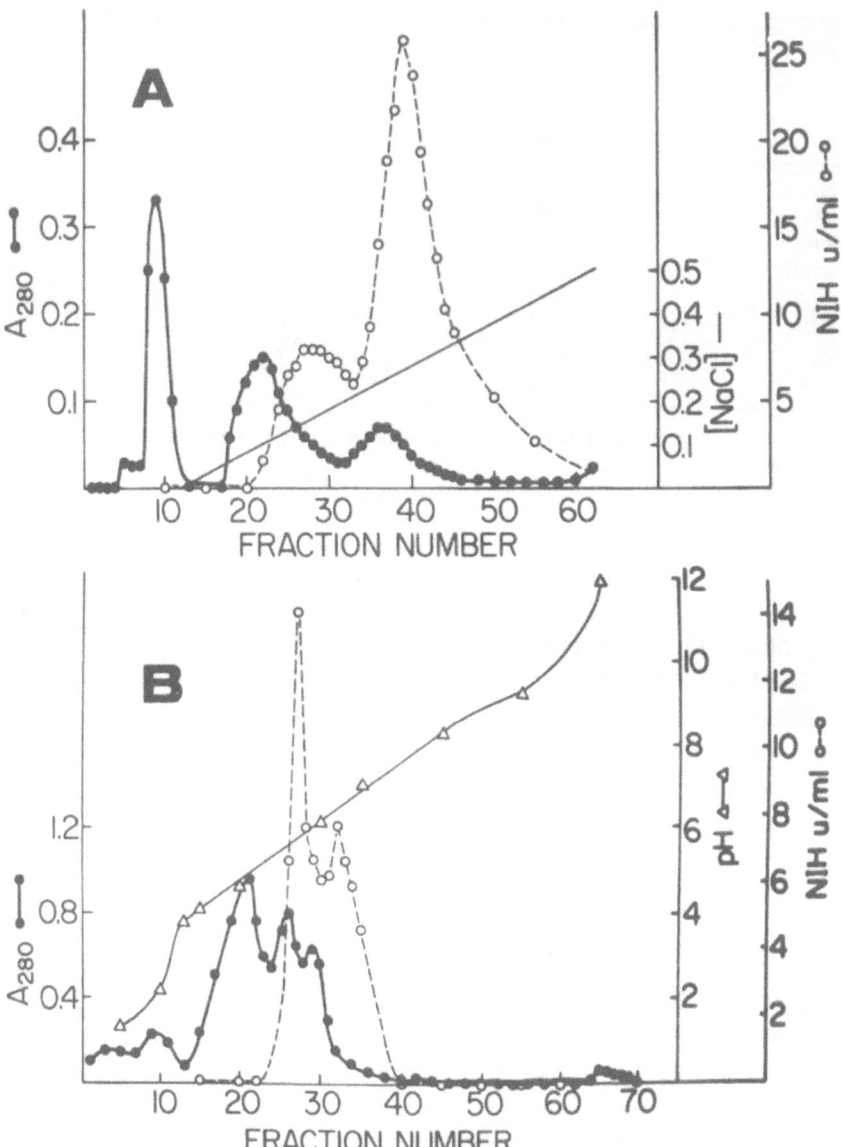

*Fig.* 5. Purification of rat liver precursor activity. Microsomes obtained from warfarin treated rats were washed with 1 M NaCl and solubilized in Trition X-100. A 0-70% $(NH_4)_2SO_4$ cut of this preparation was subjected to sequential gel filtration on agarose A 5 M and A 0.5 M columns. The precursor peak from the second column was subjected to (A) chromatography on QAE Sephadex in 0.05 M, pH 7.8. imidazole with a NaCl gradient, or (B) isoelectrofocusing over a pH 3.5-10 range in a sucrose gradient. In a separate experiment, material from the trailing edge of the second (major) peak in column A was isoelectrofocused and found to contain only the pI 5.8 (major) species of precursor (Grant et al., 1974).

may in fact be the same proteins that were obtained in the form of a 200,000 molecular weight oligomer from the antibody column. The major component (pI of 5.8) can be cleaved with thrombin to yield a 55,000 molecular weight fragment which would correspond to intermediate I of prothrombin activation. It can also be degraded (Esmon *et al.*, 1975) with *E. carinatus* venom or taipan venom to yield what appears to be rat thrombin. Morrissey et al. (1973) have purified a protein from liver microsomes of warfarin treated rats which has properties similar to our precursor preparations, and which they call isoprothrombin. This protein, which had a molecular weight of 85,000 daltons, could be autodigested to a 73,000 molecular weight species and could be digested with *E. carinatus* venom to a 55,000 molecular weight species. Olson et al. (1974) have suggested that this material is not a precursor of prothrombin, but rather an alternate gene product that is expressed in the absence of vitamin K or in the presence of warfarin. Our more recent preparations have been carried out with the extensive use of inhibitors of proteolysis and much less of the pI 7.2 protein with precursor activity has been seen. This makes it even more more likely that this protein is a degradation product, and that it is not on the main pathway to prothrombin formation. The significance of the high molecular weight precursors which were observed in the early studies is not yet clear. These proteins may have simply represented some type of stable aggregation of lower molecular weight precursors. This aggregation may have been to other proteins, lipids, or detergent, but was probably not a self aggregation. There is some indication that the amount of this higher molecular weight material is a function of the ionic strength of the buffers used, which would support the aggregation theory. It is also possible that the primary gene product is a higher molecular weight species and that it is subjected to limited proteolysis to form the true precursor. Final determinations of the molecular weight of a precursor protein will, of course, depend on its purification in sufficient amounts to characterize it more completely. The presence of a higher molecular weight precursor would be consistent with the demonstration that there are cellular precursors to the peptide hormone insulin (Steiner and Oyer, 1967) and parathyroid hormone (Cohn et al., 1972, Kemper et al., 1972) and claims of some type of liver precursor to serum albumin (Judah et al., 1973; Russell and Geller, 1973).

An alternate explanation of the data which strongly support a postribosomal action of vitamin K has been put forth by Olson, (Olson et al., 1974, Morrissey et al., 1973). He suggested that thrombin containing protein in warfarin treated rat liver (isoprothrombin) is not on the pathway to prothrom-

bin production, but rather, is a gene product which is induced or repressed
at the translational level in a reciprocal manner to prothrombin by warfarin
and vitamin K. There are a number of observations which raise serious
questions regarding this hypothesis. The level of precursor in the liver falls
within minutes after vitamin K is administered. If this does not represent
conversion of precursor to prothrombin it must be postulated that the
vitamin also increases the rate of turnover of this protein. The alternate gene
product theory questions the entire concept of a precursor and assumes that
the regulation of prothrombin production is based on its rate of *de novo*
synthesis. Such a hypothesis is not consistent with the cycloheximide effects
which have been discussed, nor with the available data on amino acid incorporation into prothrombin. The general *de novo* synthesis hypothesis is
supported by observations of the effects of vitamin K in an isolated perfused
rat liver system (Kipfer and Olson, 1970; Li et al., 1970), and by the observations that the *in vitro* rate of microsomal prothrombin synthesis is increased when the microsomes are isolated from previously hypoprothrombinemic rats which were administered vitamin K before they were killed
(Johnston and Olson, 1972a, b). Alternate explanations of this observation
are however available (Suttie, 1973a).

The weight of evidence at the present time would appear to support the
more straightforward explanation of the data, that is, that the thrombin containing protein seen in rat liver is a precursor to prothrombin. Final proof of
this hypothesis will, of course, depend upon the isolation of this protein in a
pure form, and the demonstration that it can be converted to prothrombin
in an *in vitro* system. This has not been accomplished, but some progress has
been made. We have recently shown that postmitochondrial supernates prepared from vitamin K deficient rats will produce prothrombin in an *in vitro*
incubation system (fig. 6). For maximum activity it is necessary to administer
vitamin K to the hypoprothrombinemic rats a few minutes before they are
killed. Once prothrombin synthesis is initiated, however, it will continue in
an *in vitro* incubation. The system requires an energy source and $O_2$ and is
not inhibited by cycloheximide (table 4). The amount of prothrombin which
is produced is equivalent to about 30% of the precursor which was present at
the time the incubation was started. The response is maximum in those preparations containing microsomes from rats which had converted about 30%
of the total precursor to prothrombin before they were killed. We have had
only partial success in initiating prothrombin synthesis by the *in vitro* addition of vitamin K to microsomal preparations from vitamin K deficient
rats, nor have we observed an appreciable increase in prothrombin when

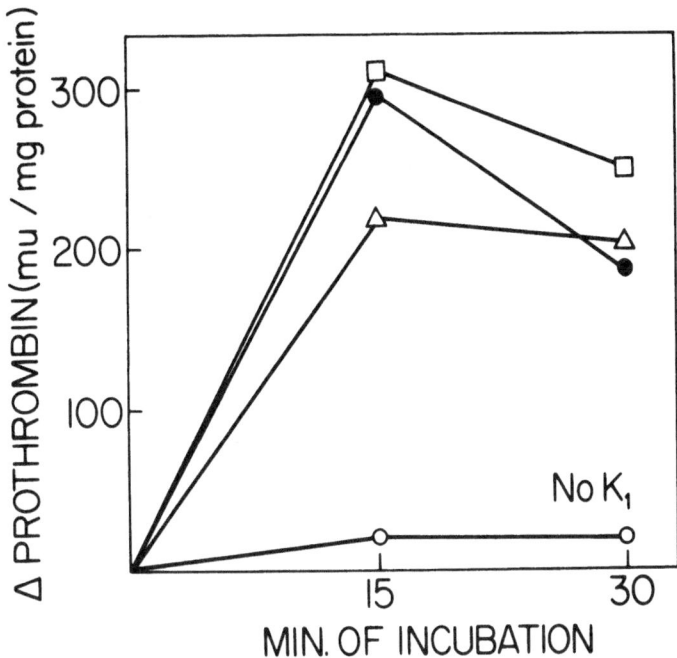

*Fig. 6. In vitro* synthesis of prothrombin. Microsomes were isolated from vitamin K deficient rats given vitamin K just prior to being killed, and incubated under the conditions described in the legend to Table 4. The curves shown are for three individual vitamin K treated rats, and for one deficient rat not given the vitamin (Shah and Suttie, 1974).

*Table* 4. Requirements for microsomal prothrombin synthesis.

| Incubation Conditions | Prothrombin Produced (% of complete system) |
|---|---|
| Postmitochondrial supernate | 5 |
| Complete system | 100 |
| −ATP, PC, CPK | 31 |
| −GTP | 108 |
| −KCl | 51 |
| −Mg(Ac)₂ | 35 |
| + Cycloheximide (100 µg/ml) | 94 |

Microsomal preparations were obtained from vitamin K deficient rats given vitamin K just prior to being killed. Prothrombin activity (2 stage) was measured at the start and finish of a 15 min incubation at 37°. The initial prothrombin concentration was 270 mU/mg protein, and increase during incubation in the complete system was 144 mU/mg. The complete system contained: 1 mM ATP, 10 mM PC, 50 µg CPK, 0.4 mM GTP, 50 mM KCl, 2.5 mM Mg(Ac)₂, 20 mM imidazole pH 7.2, and 200 mM sucrose (Shah and Suttie, 1974).

microsomes from normal rats are incubated. Although this system is far
from defined, its characteristics do strongly support the precursor theory of
prothrombin production. Little prothrombin is formed unless the microsomes have high levels of precursor before incubation. The conditions of
incubation are not suitable for active amino acid incorporation, the production is not inhibited by cycloheximide, and yet, prothrombin is being produced in an energy dependent manner. This seems possible only if the vitamin
K sensitive site was associated with some postribosomal event.

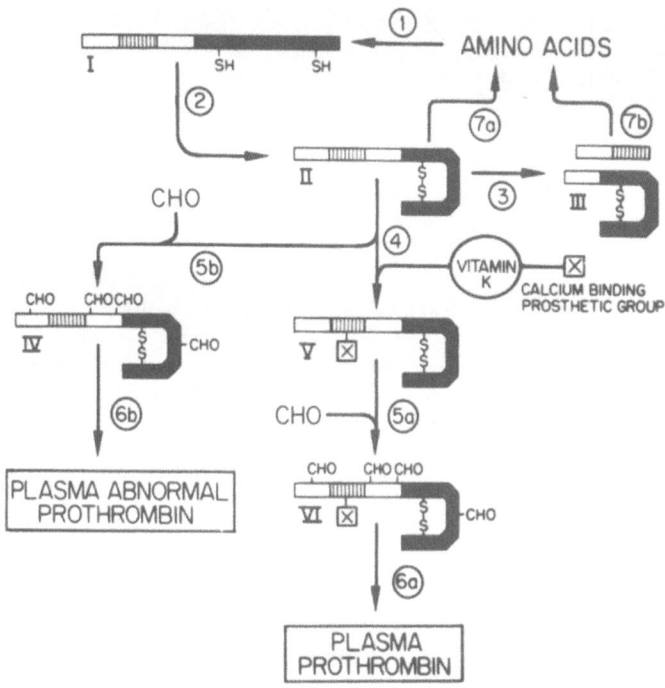

Fig. 7. The precursor theory of prothrombin production. It is assumed that steps 1 and 2
peptide bond formation and disulfide bond formation, are independent of vitamin K, and
that II (the major precursor) is continually being degraded to amino acids (step 7a) as is
any other cellular protein. Molecule III is included because of our data which indicate
that there is a molecule less acidic than prothrombin with precursor activity. This molecule
may, however, arise during purification and not exist in appreciable quantities in the liver.
The vitamin K dependent step (4) is shown here as the attachment of the prosthetic group
(X) to the precursor (II), but it could be a step in the synthesis of the group. The available
data would suggest that vitamin K dependent step is prior to prothrombin glycosylation
(step 5a) but steps 4 and 5 could be interchanged. In the figure the solid bar represents the
thrombin portion of the molecule, and the portion with vertical lines represents the calcium
binding peptide which has been isolated. The number and position of the carbohydrate
chains, disulfide bonds and prosthetic group are meant to be diagrammatic only.

The data which have been reviewed above are consistent with the preliminary model of prothrombin production which is presented in figure 7. The model is not meant to imply anything about the chemical nature of the calcium binding group which is attached to convert the precursor to prothrombin. The diagram indicates that modification of the precursor to form prothrombin occurs prior to glycosylation. The available data would tend to support this order, but do not definitively settle the question. This model also assumes that the pI 7.2 protein we have seen is not on the pathway to prothrombin, but rather, is on a degradative pathway. Although it is possible that this protein represents one of the first breakdown products of intracellular turnover of the precursor, there are data which indicate that much of this protein is formed during the initial stages of our isolation procedure. The model illustrated in this diagram does not account for the proteins we have observed with molecular weights which appear to be in excess of that of prothrombin. It is not clear at this time if these proteins are merely aggregates of lower molecular weight proteins, or if they are in fact larger molecular weight precursors which must be cleaved before they become the true prothrombin precursor. In any event, this model proposes a hypothesis which appears to be open to direct experimental attack.

### REFERENCES

1. Bell, R. G. and J. T. Matschiner, Synthesis and destruction of prothrombin in the rat. *Arch. Biochem.* 135, 152-159 (1969).
2. Bjork, I. and J. Stenflo, A conformational study of normal and dicoumarol-induced prothrombin. *FEBS Lett.* 32, 343-346 (1973).
3. Carlisle, T. L., D. V. Shah, R. Schlegel and J. W. Suttie, Plasma abnormal prothrombin and microsomal prothrombin precursor in various species. *Proc. Soc. Exp. Biol. Med.* 148, 140-144 (1975).
4. Cohn, D. V., R. R. MacGregor, L. L. H. Chu, J. R. Kimmel and J. W. Hamilton, Calcemic fraction A: biosynthetic peptide precursor of parathyroid hormone. *Proc. nat. Acad. Sci.* 69, 1521-5525 (1972).
5. Gitel, S. N., W. G. Owen, C. T. Esmon and C. M. Jackson, A polypeptide region of bovine prothrombin specific for binding to phospholipids. *Proc. nat. Acad. Sci.* 70, 1344-1348 (1973).
6. Grant, G. A., C. T. Esmon and J. W. Suttie, *Unpublished data* (1974).
7. Hemker, H. C., J. J. Veltkamp, A. Hensen and E. A. Loeliger, Nature of prothrombin biosynthesis: preprothrombinaemia in vitamin K deficiency. *Nature* 200, 589-590 (1963).
8. Hill, R. B., S. Gaetani, A. M. Paolucci, P. B. RamaRao, R. Alden, G. S. Ranhotra, D. V. Shah, V. K. Shah and B. C. Johnson, Vitamin K and biosynthesis of protein and prothrombin. *J. biol. Chem.* 243, 3930-3939 (1968).
9. Johnston, M. F. M. and R. E. Olson, Studies of prothrombin biosynthesis in cell-free

systems. II. Incorporation of L-[$^{14}$C] leucine into prothrombin by rat liver microsomes. *J. biol. Chem.* 247, 3994-4000 (1972a).

10. Johnston, M. F. M. and R. E. Olson, Studies of prothrombin biosynthesis in cell-free systems. III. Regulation by vitamin K and warfarin of prothrombin biosynthesis in rat liver microsomes. *J. biol. Chem.* 247, 4001-4007 (1972b).

11. Judah, J. D., M. Gamble and J. H. Steadman, Biosynthesis of serum albumin in rat liver: evidence for the existence of 'proalbumin'. *Biochem. J.* 134, 1083-1091 (1973).

12. Kemper, B., J. F. Habener, J. T. Potts and A. Rich, Proparathyroid hormone: identification of a biosynthetic precursor to parathyroid hormone. *Proc. nat. Acad. Sci.* 69, 643-647 (1972).

13. Kipfer, R. K. and R. E. Olson, Reversal by vitamin K of cycloheximide inhibited biosynthesis of prothrombin in the isolated perfused rat liver. *Biochem. biophys. Res. Commun.* 38, 1041-1048 (1970).

14. Lavergne, J. M., Metabolism of PIVKA-II in man. *This volume* p. 183 (1975).

15. Li, L. F., R. K. Kipfer and R. E. Olson, Immunochemical measurement of vitamin K-induced biosynthesis of prothrombin in the isolated perfused rat liver. *Arch. Biochem.* 137, 494-499 (1970).

16. Li, L. F. and R. E. Olson, Purification and properties of rat prothrombin. *J. biol. Chem.* 242, 5611-5616 (1967).

17. Lowenthal, J. and E. L. Simons, Failure of actinomycin D to inhibit appearance of clotting activity by vitamin K in vitro. *Experientia* 23, 421 (1967).

18. Magnusson, S., Primary structure studies on thrombin and prothrombin. *Thrombos. Diathes. haemorrh.* Suppl. 54, 31-35 (1973).

19. Menaché, D., Human coumarin prothrombin. *This volume* p. 159 (1975).

20. Morrissey, J. J., J. P. Jones and R. E. Olson, Isolation and characterization of isoprothrombin in the rat. *Biochem. biophys. Res. Commun.* 54, 1075-1082 (1973).

21. Nelsestuen, G. L. and J. W. Suttie, The purification and properties of an abnormal prothrombin protein produced by dicumarol-treated cows. A comparison to normal prothrombin. *J. biol. Chem.* 247, 8176-8182 (1972a).

22. Nelsestuen, G. L. and J. W. Suttie, Mode of action of vitamin K. Calcium binding properties of bovine prothrombin. *Biochemistry* 11, 4961-4964 (1972b).

23. Nelsestuen, G. L. and J. W. Suttie, The mode of action of vitamin K. Isolation of a peptide containing the vitamin K dependent portion of prothrombin. *Proc. nat. Acad. Sci.* 70, 3366-3370 (1973).

24. Olson, R. E., Vitamin K induced prothrombin formation: antagonism by actinomycin D. *Science* 145, 926-928 (1964).

25. Olson, R. E., R. K. Kipfer, J. J. Morrissey and S. R. Goodman, Function of vitamin K in prothrombin synthesis. *Thrombos. Diathes. haemorrh.* Suppl. In press (1974).

26. Pyörälä, K., Determinants of the clotting factor response to warfarin in the rat. *Ann. Med. Expt. Biol. Fenniae* 43, (Suppl. 3) (1965).

27. Russell, J. H. and D. M. Geller, Rat serum albumin biosynthesis: evidence for a precursor. *Biochem. biophys. Res. Commun.* 55, 239-245 (1973).

28. Schieck, A., F. Kornalik and E. Habermann, The prothrombin-activating principle from Echis carinatus Venom 1. Preparation and biochemical properties. *Naunyn-Schmiedeberg's Arch.* 272, 402-416 (1972).

29. Shah, D. V. and J. W. Suttie, Mechanism of action of vitamin K: evidence for the conversion of a precursor protein to prothrombin in the rat. *Proc. nat. Acad. Sci.* 68, 1653-1657 (1971).

30. Shah, D. V. and J. W. Suttie, The effect of vitamin K and warfarin on rat liver prothrombin concentrations. *Arch biochem.* 150, 91-95 (1972).

31. Shah, D. V. and J. W. Suttie, *Unpublished data* (1974).

32. Shah, D. V., J. W. Suttie and G. A. Grant, A rat liver protein with potential trombin

activity: properties and partial purification *Arch. Biochem.* 159, 483-491 (1973).

33. Steiner, D. F. and P. E. Oyer, The biosynthesis of insulin and a probable precursor of insulin by a human islet cell adenoma. *Proc. nat. Acad. Sci.* 57, 473-480 (1967).

34. Stenflo, J. Vitamin K and the biosynthesis of prothrombin. II. Structural comparison of normal and dicoumarol-induced bovine prothrombin. *J. biol. Chem.* 147, 8167-8175 (1972).

35. Stenflo, J., Vitamin K and the biosynthesis of prothrombin. III. Structural comparison of an NH$_2$ terminal fragement from normal and from dicoumarol-induced bovine prothrombin. *J. biol. Chem.* 248, 6325-6332 (1973).

36. Stenflo, J., Chemical properties of PIVKA-II. *This volume* p. 152 (1975).

37. Stenflo, J. and P. O. Ganrot., Vitamin K and the biosynthesis of prothrombin. I. Identification and purification of a dicoumarol-induced abnormal prothrombin from bovine plasma. *J. biol. Chem.* 247, 8160-8166 (1972).

38. Stenflo, J. and P. O. Ganrot., Binding of Ca$^{2+}$ to normal and dicoumarol-induced prothrombin. *Biochem. biophys. Res. Commun.* 50, 98-104 (1973).

39. Suttie, J. W., Control of prothrombin and factor VII biosynthesis by vitamin K. *Arch. Biochem*, 118, 166-171 (1967).

40. Suttie, J. W., The effect of cycloheximide administration on vitamin K-stimulated prothrombin formation. *Arch. Biochem.* 141, 571-578 (1970).

41. Suttie, J. W., Vitamin K and prothrombin synthesis. *Nutr. Rev.* 31, 105-109 (1973a).

42. Suttie, J. W., Mechanism of action of vitamin K: demonstration of a liver precursor of prothrombin. *Science* 179, 192-193 (1973b).

43. Suttie, J. W., Metabolism and properties of a liver precursor to prothrombin. *Vitamins and Hormones* 32. In press (1974).

*Note added in proof:* The vitamin K dependent *in vitro* production of prothrombin in microsocial preparations from vitamin K deficient rats has now been demonstrated. (*Biochem. Biophys. Res. Commun.* 60, 1397-1402 (1974) cf. p. 146).

# STRUCTURAL COMPARISON OF NORMAL
## AND DICOUMAROL-INDUCED PROTHROMBIN

JOHAN STENFLO

Normal biosynthesis of prothrombin and of Factor VII, IX and X requires vitamin K. The vitamin exerts its effect in a posttranscriptional step, i.e. after completion of the polypeptide chain there are vitamin K dependent metabolic steps in which some prosthetic group is attached to the polypeptide chain or some amino acid is modified (1-3). Vitamin K deficiency or administration of the vitamin K antagonist dicoumarol results in the biosynthesis of abnormal prothrombin, Factor VII, IX and X[1], all of which appear to lack biological activity (4-10). These abnormal coagulation factors are probably precursors of the biologically active ones (11, 12). In the human and bovine species they appear in the blood, whereas in the rat at least the abnormal prothrombin does not appear in the blood but is instead retained within the liver cells (12). In contrast with the normal vitamin K dependent coagulation factors, the abnormal ones do not bind $Ca^{2+}$ (5, 13, 14). They nevertheless have the same main antigenic determinants as their biologically, active counterparts (7-10). Figure 1 shows the appearance of abnormal prothrombin obtained from a cow receiving dicoumarol treatment.

The identification of the biologically inactive dicoumarol-induced prothrombin made it urgent to define the structural difference between normal and abnormal prothrombin. Knowledge of this difference would facilitate the work aiming at a better understanding of the mode of action of vitamin K. It would probably also shed light on the structures responsible for the binding of $Ca^{2+}$ and thereby help to reveal the mechanism of activation of prothrombin. In order to obtain the amounts of material necessary for a structural comparison most work has hitherto been done on bovine material (1-3, 7-9).

Rapid activation of prothrombin requires adsorption of it to the surface of phospholipids to secure a high local concentration of the reactants capable

1. PIVKA ll, Vll, IX and X (PIVKA, abbrevation for proteins induced by vitamin K absence) according to the nomenclature of Hemker (10).

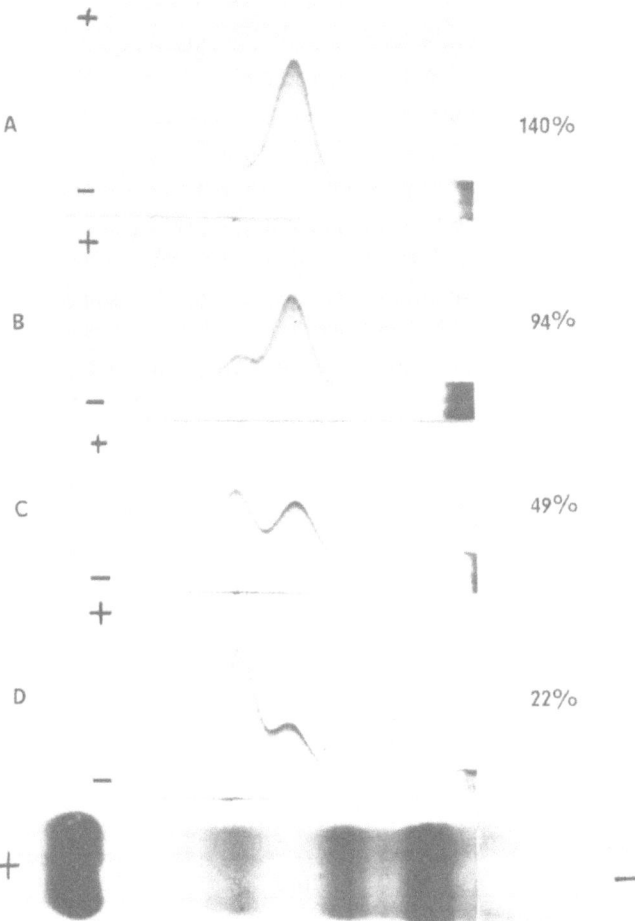

*Fig.* 1. Crossed immunoelectrophoretic patterns of bovine plasmas obtained during treatment with dicoumarol. Prothrombin activities in per cent of a standard is given to the right. Electrophoresis was run in 0.075 M barbital buffer, 2 mM in calcium lactate, pH 8.6. A. Sample obtained before administration of dicoumarol: B, C and D samples obtained 2, 4 and 7 days after the beginning of dicoumarol treatment. The electrophoretic pattern of a bovine plasma is included as a reference.

of counterbalancing the action of the plasma protease inhibitors, and the presence of Factor X and V. The adsorption of the prothrombin molecules to the phospholipid requires $Ca^{2+}$ ions, which appear to form bridges between negatively charged groups in prothrombin and in the phospholipid (15, 16). The non-activation of abnormal prothrombin appears to be due to the fact that it does not bind $Ca^{2+}$. This is corroborated by the observation that activation of abnormal prothrombin by non-physiological activators, such as trypsin, results in the formation of a normal amount of thrombin (9).

Normal prothrombin binds approximately 10 $Ca^{2+}$, whereas abnormal prothrombin binds at most one $Ca^{2+}$ (13, 14, 17). It has been demonstrated by isolation of fragments produced by thrombin digestion of prothrombin (2, 17) that the $Ca^{2+}$ binding groups in normal prothrombin reside in the $NH_2$-terminal part of the protein. Thrombin cleaved prothrombin into two fragments, of which the $NH_2$-terminal, smaller one (MW approximately 25,000) bound $Ca^{2+}$, while the larger one did not. The small fragment contained only one methionine residue. Hence, cyanogen bromide cleavage gave two fragments. The smaller of these fragments, which was isolated by gel chromatography, contained approximately the 75 $NH_2$-terminal amino acid residues of intact prothrombin. The fragment bound $Ca^{2+}$, while the corresponding fragment from abnormal, dicoumarol-induced prothrombin did not (fig. 2). Judging from electrophoretic, immunochemical and peptide mapping experiments (2, 18) the large fragment produced by thrombin digestion and the large cyanogen bromide fragment from normal prothrombin did not differ from the corresponding fragments from dicoumarol-induced prothrombin.

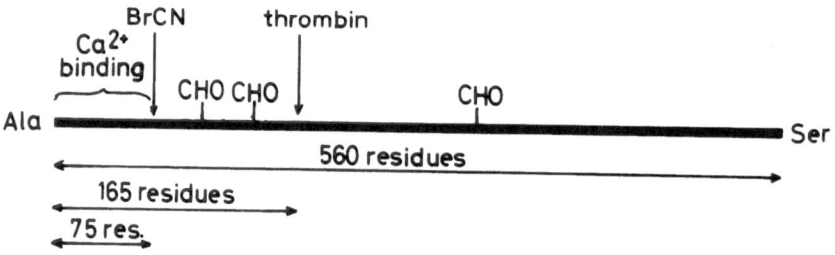

*Fig.* 2. Structure of prothrombin. The points of cleavage by thrombin and cyanogen bromide are indicated by arrows. The vitamin K-dependent $Ca^{2+}$-binding structures are in the $NH_2$-terminal part of the polypeptide chain.

The $NH_2$-terminal cyanogen bromide fragment from normal and that from abnormal prothrombin, which differed from each other in $Ca^{2+}$ ion binding, had identical amino acid compositions and both lacked carbohydrate (18). But distinct differences were observed between peptide maps prepared from tryptic digests of the completely reduced and carboxymethylated fragments (fig. 3). The peptide map of the fragment from abnormal prothrombin contained three peptides, which appeared to have no counterparts in the peptide map of the fragment from normal prothrombin (A4 to

A6)[2]. Furthermore, one anodal peptide in normal prothrombin which stained faintly yellow (N2) had a higher anodal electrophoretic mobility at pH 6.5 than a peptide with identical staining characteristics from abnormal prothrombin (A2; fig. 3).

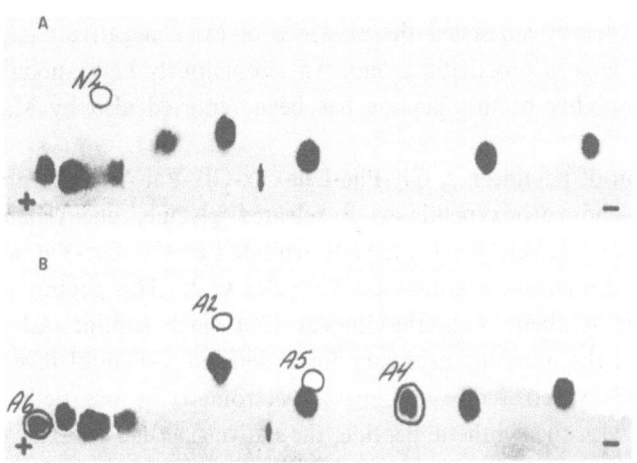

*Fig.* 3. Peptide maps of $NH_2$-terminal cyanogen bromide fragments of normal prothrombin (A) and dicoumarol-induced prothrombin (B). The electrophoresis was run at pH 6.5.

```
1          5              10              15             20
Ala-Asn-Lys-Gly-Phe-Leu-Glu-Glu-Val-Arg-Lys-Gly-Asn-Leu-Glu-Arg-Glu——Leu-Glu-Glu-Pro—— —— ——
       N1                  N2             N3                    N4
       A1                  A2             A3      A5               A6
                                              A4
```

*Fig.* 4. $NH_2$-terminal sequence of prothrombin according to Heldebrant et al. (19). Peptides from normal prothrombin are denoted N and those from abnormal prothrombin A.

The peptides, which differed between normal and abnormal prothrombin, were isolated on a preparative scale by high voltage electrophoresis and gel chromatography on Sephadex G 25. The partial or entire amino acid sequences of the peptides were determined by dansyl-Edman degradations in order to ascertain the position of the peptides in the prothrombin sequence (fig. 4) published by Heldebrant et al. (19). In this way it was established that peptides N2 and A2, despite their different electrophoretic mobilities, constituted residues 4-10 in normal and in abnormal prothrombin respectively

2. Peptides from normal prothrombin are designated N .......... and those from abnormal prothrombin A .........

(18). Furthermore, it was found that, judging from the diagram given by Offord (20), peptide A2 had an electrophoretic mobility consistant with its amino acid composition if residues 7 and 8 were glutamic acid. On the other hand, the electrophoretic mobility of peptide N2, whose amino acid composition was identical with that of A2, was too high for its amino acid composition, and thereby suggested the existence of extra negative charges, presumably due to a prosthetic group. An anomalously high anodal electrophoretic mobility of this peptide has been reported also by Magnusson et al. (1).

Digestion of peptide N2, Gly-Phe-Leu-Glx-Glx-Val-Arg with aminopeptidase M and carboxypeptidase B released glycine, phenylalanine and arginine quantitatively, leaving the tetrapeptide Leu-Glx-Glx-Val, which was isolated by gel chromatography on Sephadex G 25. This peptide was compared with synthetic Leu-Glu-Glu-Val (21) since peptide A2 was not available in the amounts necessary for a detailed structural investigation. From NMR spectroscopy and mass spectrometry it was deduced that, compared with the synthetic peptide, the native one had an extra carboxyl group on the γ-carbon on each of the two glutamic acid residues, i.e. the native peptide contained two residues of the hitherto unidentified amino acid, γ-carboxy-glutamic acid (3, amino, 1, 1, 3-propanetricarboxylic acid: figure 5; see ref. 21) instead of two glutamic acid residues.

$$\begin{array}{c} \text{HOOC} \quad \text{COOH} \\ \diagdown \diagup \\ \text{CH} \\ | \\ \text{CH}_2 \\ | \\ \text{H}_2\text{N}-\text{CH}-\text{COOH} \end{array}$$

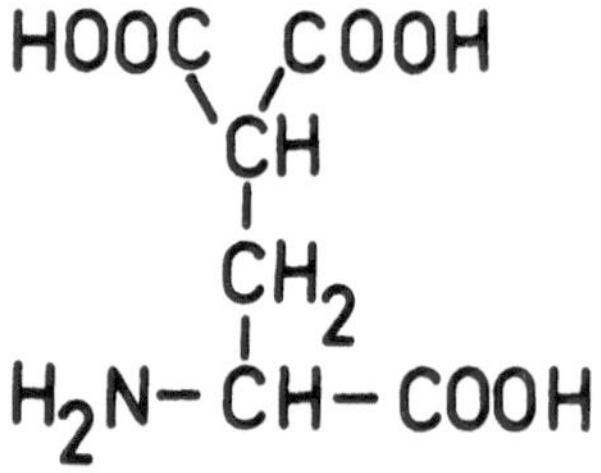

*Fig.* 5. Structure of γ-carboxyglutamic acid.

Peptide N4 (residues 12 to approximately 34) was isolated from a thermolysin digest of a tryptic peptide (not visible in fig. 3). Judging from the amino acid composition of the peptide, it derives from the same part of the prothrombin sequence as the peptide Nelsestuen and Suttie recently isolated from a tryptic digest of intact prothrombin by adsorption to barium citrate (3). In the dicoumarol-induced prothrombin peptide N4 is corresponded by at least three peptides (A4 to A6). Peptide N4 contains two arginine residues inaccessible to trypsin and is very resistant to digestion with neutral protease. Comparison of the electrophoretic mobility, at pH 6.5, of peptide N4 in buffers with and without $Ca^{2+}$ indicated that the peptide bound $Ca^{2+}$, as suggested from the barium citrate adsorption experiments by Nelsestuen and Suttie (3). The high $Ca^{2+}$ affinity of this peptide and its resistance to digestion with proteolytic enzymes suggests that it contains several γ-carboxyglutamic acid residues.

Trypsin cleaved normally at the arginine and lysine residues in abnormal prothrombin (fig. 4) and the resulting peptides had electrophoretic mobilities consistant with their amino acid compositions. Therefore, no evidence is available for the presence of γ-carboxyglutamic acid residues in the abnormal prothrombin, i.e. abnormal prothrombin has glutamic acid in the positions where normal prothrombin has γ-carboxyglutamic acid. The structural studies thus show that the differences between the two prothrombins are confined to the $NH_2$-terminal parts of the polypeptide chains. This is further substantiated by the finding that when activated with non-physiological activators, such as trypsin, abnormal prothrombin gives rise to a normal amount of thrombin (9), which is derived from the COOH-terminal part of prothrombin.

The two adjacent carboxyl groups in γ-carboxyglutamic acid give these residues a far higher affinity for $Ca^{2+}$ than the corresponding glutamic acid residues in dicoumarol-induced prothrombin. Owing to its low $Ca^{2+}$ affinity abnormal prothrombin is not adsorbed to the phospholipids on which the activation of prothrombin is known to occur in physiological systems.

So far, all available evidence indicates that the γ-carboxyglutamic acid residues are the only vitamin K dependent structures in prothrombin. It therefore appears that vitamin K is involved in the carboxylation of some glutamic acid residues in the $NH_2$-terminal part of prothrombin. The mechanism of this reaction is not known.

Recently two of the other vitamin K dependent coagulation factors, IX and X, have been characterized chemically (22-25). Like prothrombin they bind $Ca^{2+}$, but the abnormal forms synthetized under the influence of dicoumarol do not (10). The amino acid sequence of the $NH_2$-terminal part of Factor IX and that of the light chain of Factor X have been determined. Both sequences show considerable homologies with the $NH_2$-terminal sequence of prothrombin (26). This suggests that Factor IX and X also contain γ-carboxyglutamic acid residues.

## REFERENCES

1. Magnusson, S., Third Congress, International Society of Thrombosis and Haemostasis, Washington. D.C. (1972). *Thrombos. Diather. haemorr.* Suppl. 54, p. 31 (1973).
2. Stenflo, J., *J. biol. Chem.* 248, 6325-6332 (1973).
3. Nelsestuen, G. L. and J. W. Suttie, *Proc. nat. Acad. Sci.* 70, 3366-3370 (1973).
4. Niléhn, J. E. and P. O. Ganrot, *Scand. J. clin. Lab. Invest.* 22, 17-22 (1968).
5. Ganrot, P. O. and J. E. Niléhn, *Scand. J. clin. Lab. Invest.* 22, 23-28 (1968).
6. Josso, F., J. M. Lavergne, M. Goualt, D. Prou-Wartelle and J. P. Soulier, *Thrombos. Diathes. haemorrh.* 20, 88-98 (1968).
7. Stenflo, J., *Acta chem. scand.* 24, 3762-3763 (1970).
8. Stenflo, J. and P. O. Ganrot, *J. biol. Chem.* 247, 8160-8166 (1972).
9. Nelsestuen, G. L. and J. W. Suttie, *J. biol. Chem.* 247, 8176-8182 (1972).
10. Reekers, P. P. M., M. J. Lindhout, B. H. M. Kop-Klaassen and H. C. Hemker, *Biochim. biophys. Acta* 317, 559-562 (1973).
11. Shah, D. V. and J. W. Suttie, *Proc. nat. Acad. Sci.* 68, 1653-1657 (1971).
12. Suttie, J. W., *Science* 179, 192-194 (1972).
13. Nelsestuen, G. L. and J. W. Suttie, *Biochemistry* 11, 4961-4964 (1972).
14. Stenflo, J. and P. O. Ganrot, *Biochem. biophys. Res. Commun.* 50, 98-104 (1973).
15. Bull, R. K., S. Jeyous and P. G. Barton, *J. biol. Chem.* 247, 2747 (1972).
16. Gitel, S. N., W. G. Owen, C. T. Esnouf and C. M. Jackson, *Proc. nat. Acad. Sci.* 70, 1344-1348 (1973).
17. Benson, B. J., W. Kisiel and D. J. Hanahan, *Biochim. biophys. Acta* 329, 81-87 (1973).
18. Stenflo, J., *J. biol. Chem.* 249, 5527-5535 (1974).
19. Heldebrant, C. M., C. Noyes, H. S. Kingdon and K. G. Mann, *Biochem. biophys. Res. Commun.* 54, 155-160 (1973).
20. Offord, R. E., *Nature* 211, 591-593 (1966).
21. Stenflo, J., P. Fernlund, W. Egan and P. Roepstorff, *Proc. nat. Acad. Sci.* 71, 2730-2733 (1974).
22. Jackson, C. M., *Biochemistry* 11, 4873-4881 (1972).
23. Fujikawa, K., M. E. Legay and E. W. Davie, *Biochemistry* 11, 4882-4891 (1972).
24. Fujikawa, K., M. E. Legay and E. W. Davie, *Biochemistry* 11, 4892-4898 (1972).
25. Titani, K., M. A. Hermodson, K. Fujikawa, L. H. Ericsson, K. A. Walsh, H. Neurath and E. W. Davie, *Biochemistry* 11, 4899-4903 (1972).
26. Fujikawa, K., M. H. Coan, D. L. Eufield, K. Titani, L. H. Ericsson and W. E. Davie, *Proc. nat. Acad. Sci.* 71, 427-430 (1974).

# PRELIMINARY STUDIES ON
# HUMAN COUMARIN PROTHROMBIN

DORIS MENACHE, MARIE-CLAUDE GUILLIN,
CATHERINE BOYER AND NICOLE CESBRON

The coagulation and immunological characteristics of chromatographed human coumarin prothrombin were determined and compared to normal chromatographed human prothrombin.

Coumarin prothrombin was isolated using plasma derived from patients under either dicoumalone or ethylbiscoumacetate treatment. Patients were selected on the basis of a prothrombin level of less than 30 per cent of normal when measured by a one stage assay. In accordance with what has already been widely reported (2, 6, 13) barium citrate and barium sulfate were found unable to remove coumarin prothrombin from citrated plasma. However, coumarin prothrombin proved to be adsorbable on to barium sulfate when oxalated plasma was used instead of citrated plasma. The blood derived from the treated patients was thus collected on a mixture of ammonium and potassium oxalate.

In order to identify the prothrombin induced in coumarin treated patients and to follow its isolation and purification, advantage was taken of four characteristics that have been ascribed to this protein: 1) its precipitation in agarose gel with anti-human normal prothrombin antiserum (7); 2) its distinctive electrophoretic mobility which is not calcium ions dependent (2, 4, 6, 13); 3) its inability to be converted to thrombin by physiological activators (6, 8, 13); 4) its conversion to thrombin-coagulase by staphylocoagulase (11).

MATERIALS AND METHODS

The various steps of the preparation were followed by prothrombin determination using four different techniques: a) one stage prothrombin assay (10); b) two stage prothrombin assay (14); c) staphylocoagulase assay (12);

d) crossed immunoelectrophoresis in agarose using a rabbit antihuman normal prothrombin antiserum (5, 13).

In a first step normal prothrombin was removed by adsorption on to small amounts of barium sulfate, the amount of barium sulfate used varied according to the prothrombin level found and corresponded in mg per ml to the percentage of prothrombin activity. In the supernatant plasma, prothrombin activity when measured by a one stage assay and Factor VII, X and IX activities were in the range of zero to 1 per cent of normal. After removal of fibrinogen in the supernatant plasma by bentonite adsorption (4 mg/ml), prothrombin activity when measured by a one stage assay was completely removed. However, prothrombin activity could still be measured using staphylocoagulase and immunological techniques. This activity which corresponds to coumarin prothrombin proved to be adsorbable on to large amounts of barium sulfate (100 mg/ml). After elution into 0.18 M Na Citrate (pH adjusted to 8.5) coumarin prothrombin was precipitated with ethanol to a final concentration of 25 per cent. The precipitate was dissolved in 0.022 M Tris Cl-0.15 M NaCl buffer pH 7.4 and chromatographed on DEAE cellulose using a linear gradient (0.022 M Tris Cl-0.15 M NaCl pH 7.4-0.066 M Tris Cl-0.50 M NaCl pH 7.4). Those fractions containing coumarin prothrombin were concentrated in a Diaflo ultrafiltration cell (PM 10).

## RESULTS

The degree of purification of coumarin prothrombin was followed using Laurell's quantitative technique and the results expressed as antigen units per mg protein (arbitrarily 1 ml of undiluted normal plasma was defined as containing 100 units of prothrombin antigen). A mean of 250 fold purification was obtained when chromatographed coumarin prothrombin was compared to the starting material after removal of normal prothrombin by barium sulfate and bentonite adsorptions.

Using a similar linear gradient on DEAE cellulose the elution profile obtained when coumarin prothrombin was subjected to column chromatography was compared to that obtained with normal prothrombin. Both preparations were separated in two absorbance peaks (fig. 1). The fractions eluted were screened for prothrombin antigen like material according to Nelsestuen and Suttie (6). Coumarin prothrombin was eluted in a peak ahead of the one found for normal prothrombin (0.23-0.30 M versus 0.30-0.36 M).

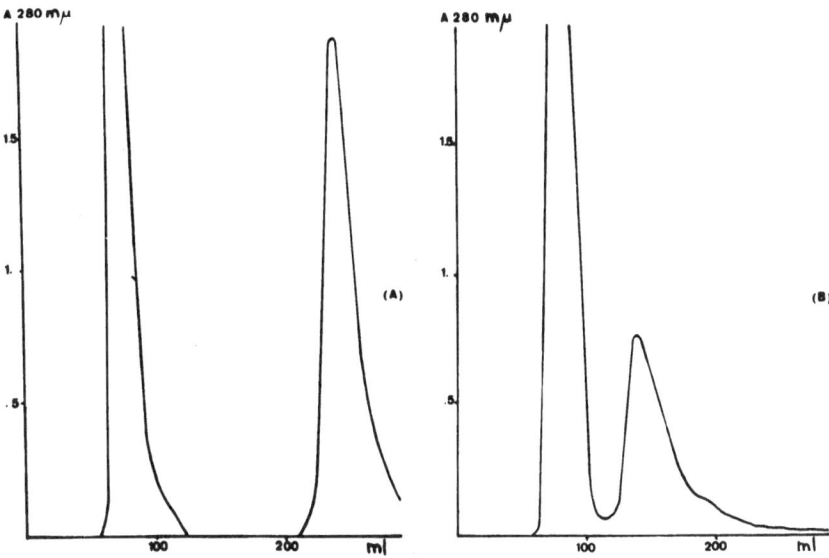

*Fig.* 1. DEAE cellulose chromatography of human normal (A) and coumarin (B) prothrombin: 100 mg of protein in 10 ml were applied to the column (2 × 30 cm). Linear gradient (0.022 M Tris Cl-0.15 M NaCl pH 7.4 — 0.066 M Tris Cl-0.50 M NaCl pH 7.4). Flow rate 25 ml per hour.

Immunological and coagulation studies were performed on the chromatographed material and compared with normal prothrombin. On double diffusion, no difference could be visualized between normal and coumarin prothrombin. Antihuman normal prothrombin antiserum gave a precipitin line with coumarin prothrombin which was in complete identity with normal plasma and plasma from coumarin treated patients. Partial identity with spur formation was obtained between coumarin prothrombin and normal serum, whereas complete identity was obtained with serum derived from coumarin treated patients indicating that this latter serum contains intact coumarin prothrombin. Partial identity with spur formation was also obtained between coumarin prothrombin and normal human thrombin in the same way as for normal prothrombin. On crossed immunoelectrophoresis when tested against antihuman normal prothrombin antiserum, the electrophoretic mobility of coumarin prothrombin unlike prothrombin was not modified by the addition of calcium ions. Coumarin prothrombin had a slightly faster electrophoretic mobility than normal prothrombin indicating that the protein was not able to bind calcium. This inability of binding to calcium is not related to an alteration of the prothrombin molecule due to barium sulfate adsorption and citrate elution since it has been shown (1) that adsorption on to barium sulfate of normal prothrombin does not modify its ability to bind calcium.

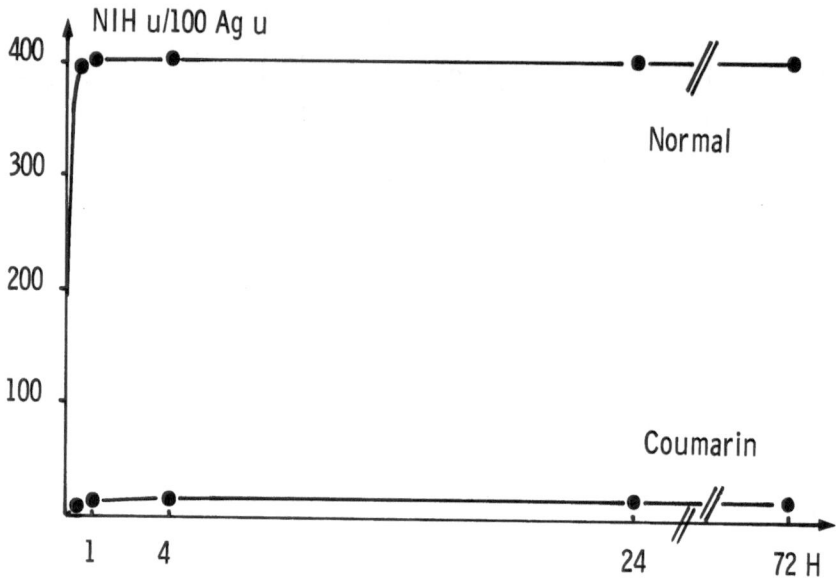

*Fig.* 2. Prothrombin: Physiological activation. Each sample contains 100 prothrombin antigen units per ml. Two stage assays were performed according to Ware and Seegers (14) with the following modifications: the prothrombin activation mixture consisted of human brain thromboplastin, human serum devoid of prothrombin, and bovine factor V preparation; the generated thrombin was measured on human fibrinogen derived from previously adsorbed plasma. A reference curve was derived using NIH thrombin (lot B3). Maximum thrombin units generated: Normal = 380 NIH u/100 Ag u; Coumarin = 10 NIH u/100 Ag u.

Coagulation studies revealed that coumarin prothrombin could not be activated by physiological activators (fig. 2) using a two stage assay, and following thrombin generation up to 72 hours. Conversion to thrombin was possible by non-physiological activators such as staphylocoagulase and

Echis carinatus venom. The rate of conversion with staphylocoagulase was similar for both types of prothrombin (fig. 3). Using the venom, the rate of thrombin generation was slower for coumarin prothrombin than for normal prothrombin (fig. 4). The amounts of thrombin generated (per 100 antigen units) measured until a maximum was reached, were almost similar for cou-

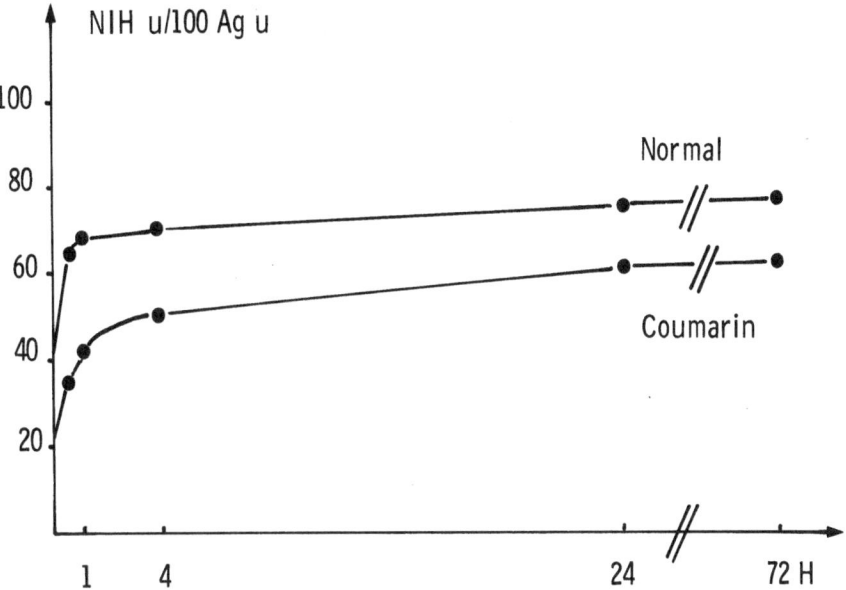

*Fig.* 3. Prothrombin: Staphylocoagulase activation. Each sample contains 100 prothrombin antigen units per ml. To 2 ml of staphylocoagulase were added 2 ml of the sample to be assayed diluted 1 in 20 in 0.022 M Tris Cl-0.15 M NaCl buffer pH 7.4. Incubation of the mixture was performed at room temperature. At different time intervals 0.4 ml of the mixture was added to 0.1 ml of bovine fibrinogen at a concentration of 0.4 per cent clottable fibrinogen (w/v). The clotting times were recorded. Thrombin activity was expressed as NIH equivalent units using NIH thrombin as reference on the same bovine fibrinogen solution. Maximum thrombin units generated: Normal = 75 eq NIH u/100 Ag u; Coumarin = 61 eq NIH u/100 Ag u.

marin and normal prothrombin under staphylocoagulase activation whereas the amounts of thrombin generated for coumarin prothrombin under the action of the venom were less than for normal prothrombin.

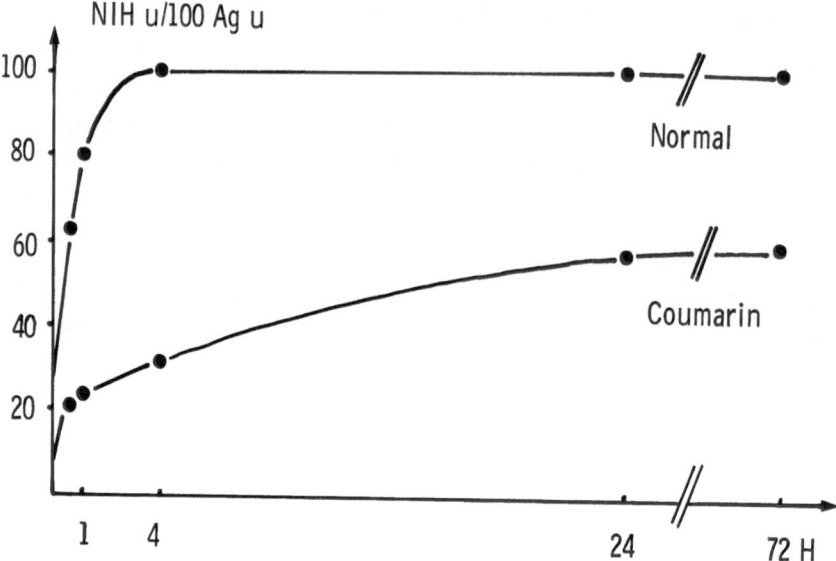

*Fig.* 4. Prothrombin: Echis carinatus activation. Each sample contains 100 prothrombin antigen units per ml. 0.1 ml of venom (1 mg/ml) was added to 0.9 ml of the diluted sample to be assayed. At various time intervals 0.1 ml of the mixture was added to 0.4 ml of human fibrinogen at 0.25 per cent concentration (w/v). Thrombin activity was expressed as NIH units using NIH thrombin as reference on the same human fibrinogen.

CONCLUSION

Separation of human coumarin- from normal prothrombin was achieved owing to the differential affinity of these two proteins to barium sulfate.

The electrophoretic mobility in the presence of calcium ions and the immunological studies performed on chromatographed human coumarin prothrombin showed that it had the same characteristics as those previously reported by Josso et al. (3) for the abnormal prothrombin detected in the native plasma of patients under vitamin K antagonist therapy and by Stenflo and Ganrot (13) for the purified preparation derived from dicoumarol treated cows.

Coagulation studies showed that human coumarin prothrombin was not able to be converted to thrombin by physiological activators. These results are in accordance with those previously reported for purified prothrombin derived from dicoumarol treated cows by Nelsestuen and Suttie (6); Stenflo and Ganrot (13) and also on the preparation derived from dicoumarol treated rats by Shah and Suttie (8). Studies on the activation of coumarin prothrombin indicated that the protein could generate thrombin in the presence of non physiological activators such as staphylocoagulase and echis carinatus venom. The property of generating thrombin with prothrombin specific venoms has previously been reported by Nelsestuen and Suttie (6) for the abnormal prothrombin derived from dicoumarol treated cows. However the specific thrombin activity obtained in this case was much higher than for human coumarin prothrombin. This discrepancy could be due to species specificity or to the fact that our preparation is less purified and/or partially altered during the isolation procedure.

The distinctive features of human coumarin prothrombin when compared to the purified preparation derived from dicoumarol treated cows is that human coumarin prothrombin was found to have less binding capacity to DEAE cellulose than normal prothrombin. This behavior is similar to the observation reported by Shah, Suttie and Grant (9) concerning the rat liver precursor protein.

The results obtained on dicoumarol prothrombin derived from treated patients, cow and rat show some difference which might probably be related to species specificity. This problem remains to be elucidated.

ACKNOWLEDGEMENTS

Supported by grant C.R.A.T. n° 71.2.415.1 from Institut National de la Santé et de la Recherche Médicale, Paris.

We are indebted to Miss Dominique Bertrand for skilful technical assistance.

REFERENCES

1. Cesbron, N., C. Boyer, M. C. Guillin and D. Menache, Human coumarin prothrombin. Chromatographic, coagulation and immunologic studies. *Thrombos. Diathes. haemorrh.* 30, 437 (1973).
2. Ganrot, P. O. and J. E. Nilehn, Plasma prothrombin during treatment with dicoumarol. II. Demonstration of an abnormal prothrombin fraction. *Scand. J. clin. Lab. Invest.* 22, 23 (1968).
3. Josso, F., J. M. Lavergne, M. Gouault, O. Prou-Wartelle and J. P. Soulier, Différents états moléculaires du Facteur II (Prothrombine). Leur étude à l'aide de la staphylocoagulase et d'anticorps anti-facteur II. I. Le facteur II chez les sujets traités par les antagonistes de la vitamine K. *Thrombos. Diathes. haemorrh.* 20, 88 (1968).
4. Josso, F., J. M. Lavergne and J. P. Soulier, Les dysprothrombinémies constitutionnelles et acquises. *Nouv. Rev. franc. Hémat.* 10, 633 (1970).

5. Laurell, C. B., Antigen-antibody crossed electrophoresis. *Analyt. Biochem.* 10, 358 (1965).

6. Nelsestuen, G. L. and J. W. Suttie, The purification and properties of an abnormal prothrombin protein produced by dicoumarol-treated cows. *J. biol. Chem.* 247, 8176 (1972).

7. Nilehn, J. E. and P. O. Ganrot, Plasma prothrombin during treatment with dicoumarol. I. Immunochemical determination of its concentration in plasma. *Scand. J. clin. Lab. Invest.* 22, 17 (1968).

8. Shah, D. V. and J. W. Suttie, Mechanism of action of vitamin K: evidence for the conversion of a precursor protein to prothrombin in the rat. *Proc. nat. Acad. Sci.* 68, 1653 (1971).

9. Shah, D. V., J. W. Suttie and G. A. Grant, A rat liver protein with potential thrombin activity: properties and partial purification. *Arch. Biochem.* 159, 483 (1973).

10. Soulier, J. P. and M. J. Larrieu, Nouvelle méthode de diagnostic de l'hémophilie. Dosage des facteurs anti-hémophiliques A et B. *Sang* 24, 3 (1953).

11. Soulier, J. P. and O. Prou-Wartelle, Etude comparative des taux de cofacteur de la staphylocoagulase (C.R.F.) et des taux de facteur II (Prothrombine) dans diverses conditions. *Nouv. Rev. franc. Hémat.* 10, 41 (1970).

12. Soulier, J. P. and O. Prou-Wartelle, Dosage de l'activité 'prothrombine coagulase'. *Nouv. Rev. franc. Hémat. 10*, 41 (1970).

13. Stenflo, J. and P. O. Ganrot, Vitamin K and the biosynthesis of prothrombin. I. Identification and purification of a dicoumarol-induced abnormal prothrombin from bovine plasma. *J. biol. Chem.* 247, 8160 (1972).

14. Ware, A. G. and W. H. Seegers, Two-stage procedure for the quantitative determination of prothrombin concentration. *Amer. J. clin. Path.* 19, 741 (1949).

# PROTHROMBIN METABOLISM IN HEALTHY SUBJECTS AND IN TWO PATIENTS WITH CONGENITAL HYPOPROTHROMBINEMIA

J. ROUVIER[1], D. COLLEN[2], A. C. W. SWART[3] AND M. VERSTRAETE

ABSTRACT

The metabolism of human prothrombin labeled with radioactive iodine was studied in 16 healthy subjects and in two patients with congenital hypoprothrombinemia. The purified prothrombin was of high specific activity (2,000-2,450 Iowa units per mg), devoid of factors VII, IX and X activity and homogeneous on immunoelectrophoresis, polyacrylamide gel electrophoresis and sodium dodecylsulfate polyacrylamide gel electrophoresis. The labeled prothrombin had the same specific activity and was indistinguishable from the prothrombin in plasma by immunoelectrophoresis and Sephadex gel filtration.

The purified prothrombin behaved as a homogeneous protein in the turnover experiments. The radioactivity data were fitted by a sum of two exponential terms and the metabolism of prothrombin was represented by a two compartment mathematical model.

The results in the 16 normal subjects were: plasma prothrombin concentration 13.2 $\pm$ 1.6 mg/100 ml plasma; plasma radioactivity half-life 3.04 $\pm$ 0.28 days; intravascular fraction 0.58 $\pm$ 0.05; fractional catabolic rate 0.40 $\pm$ 0.04 of the plasma pool per day, absolute catabolic (synthetic) rate 2.27 $\pm$ 0.34 mg/kg per day, fractional transcapillary efflux rate 0.44 $\pm$ 0.18 of the plasma pool per day. Circulating large-molecular weight degradation products of labeled prothrombin could not be detected by Sephadex gel filtration.

The plasma disappearance rate of prothrombin activity after transfusion

1. Research fellow at the laboratory of Blood Coagulation, Leuven, supported in part by a fellowship of the Union Clinique Belge (U.C.B.); present address: U.A.M.I. Rivadavia Peralta Ramos, Las Heras 2670, Buenos Aires, Argentina.
2. Aangesteld navorser N.F.W.O.
3. Lab. of blood coagulation biochemistry, U.M.C., Leiden, the Netherlands.

of 500 ml fresh plasma in two patients with congenital hypoprothrombinemia was very similar to the plasma disappearance rate of radioactivity in the controls. The identical behavior of labeled prothrombin and the unfractionated prothrombin in fresh plasma was further evidenced by a similar disappearance rate of both radioactivity and enzymatic activity after simultaneous infusion of plasma and labeled prothrombin in one of the hypoprothrombinemic patients.

INTRODUCTION

The metabolism of prothrombin has recently been investigated in normal (1-3), hypocoagulable (2) and hypercoagulable (4) conditions in humans. However, it remains to be demonstrated that the purified labeled prothrombins used, were handled by the organism in the same way as untreated native prothrombin in fresh plasma. Furthermore, the prothrombin preparations used were highly contaminated with factor VII, IX and X activity.

In the present study, we report data on the kinetics of prothrombin synthesis and catabolism in normal subjects, using a highly purified labeled prothrombin preparation devoid of factors VII, IX and X activity.

The biological integrity of the labeled prothrombin was investigated by comparing its turnover rate with the disappearance rate of prothrombin activity after transfusion of fresh plasma in two patients with congenital hypoprothrombinemia.

METHODS

*Laboratory procedures*
The following laboratory determinations were performed: prothrombin one stage (5) and two stage (6) method, factor VII (7), factor IX (8), factor X (9), fibrinogen (10, 11), activated partial thromboplastin time (12). Prothrombin was also assayed by the immunologic method of Laurell (13), using a monospecific rabbit antiserum raised against purified prothrombin. Gel filtrations on Sephadex G-200 were performed on 2.5 × 45 cm columns using a 0.15 M NaCl-0.01 M citrate buffer pH 7.5. Immuno electrophoresis was performed according to Scheidegger (14), crossed immunoelectrophoresis by the method of Laurell (15), polyacrylamide gel electrophoresis at pH 8.3 according to Davis (16) with the use of a single 5% polyacrylamide

gel and continuous 0.05 M Tris-0.3 M glycine buffer and SDS-polyacrylami-
de gel electrophoresis with 7% gels as described by Weber and Osborn (17).

*Preparation and characterization of prothrombin*
Human prothrombin was purified from fresh or fresh frozen ACD plasma
according to the method of Shapiro and Waugh (18), involving successive
adsorptions on DEAE cellulose and barium citrate, followed by precipitation with ammonium sulfate. The resulting material, 'Step 3 prothrombin'
contained 300-500% (mean 375%) of the prothrombin activity of pooled
normal plasma per absorbancy unit at 280 nm (A.U.) or 950-1,600 (mean
1,180) Iowa units of prothrombin per A.U. and 300-500% (mean 370%) of
the factor IX activity of pooled normal plasma per A.U., indicating about
375-fold purification of both components. The mean contaminating factor
VII and X activity was 60% of pooled normal plasma per A.U. Sephadex
G-100 gel filtration ('step 4'), performed as described by Shapiro and Waugh
(18) resulted in a further purification but did not separate factors II and IX
activity. After labeling of this material and injection in man, the plasma
radioactivity disappearance curve gradually levelled off from the sixth day
after injection of the tracer, which is indicative of contamination with protein with a longer half-life.[3]

Therefore, prothrombin was further purified by gel filtration on Sephadex G-100 in 0.1 M $K_2HPO_4$-0.1 M $KH_2PO_4$ buffer, pH 6.8, and by hydroxylapatite chromatography according to Swart (19). The prothrombin rich
fractions after Sephadex G-100 gel filtration, 'Step 4 prothrombin', were adsorbed on a 1 × 20 cm hydroxylapatite column, equilibrated with 0.1 M
$K_2HPO_4$-0.1 M $KH_2PO_4$ and eluted by a linearly increasing ionic strength
gradient obtained with 150 ml 0.1 M $K_2HPO_4$-0.1 M $KH_2PO_4$ as starting
buffer and 150 ml 0.25 M $KH_2PO_4$-0.25 M $K_2HPO_4$ as limiting buffer. The
buffers used in the last two steps were prepared with sterile pyrogen-free
water. This purified material 'Step 5 prothrombin' contained 1,450-1,800
(mean 1680) Iowa units prothrombin per A.U. or 2,000-2,450 (mean 2280)
Iowa units per mg protein (extinction coefficient $A_{280nm}^{1\%} = 13.6$ (18)) and
was devoid of factor VII, IX or X activity. No thrombin activity could be
measured. The recovery from plasma, based on prothrombin activity determinations, was approximately 15%.

SDS polyacrylamide gel electrophoresis of this material, in the presence
of dithiothreitol showed a single component with an estimated molecular

3. According to Dr. Shapiro this preparation yields straight semilogarithmic disappearance curves up to over 10 days after injection (personal communication).

weight of 72,500 (fig. 1). Polyacrylamide gel electrophoresis at pH 8.3 revealed one band and also in some cases a trace component with a slower mobility. Immunoelectrophoresis against a rabbit antiserum raised against this material revealed a single precipitin line.

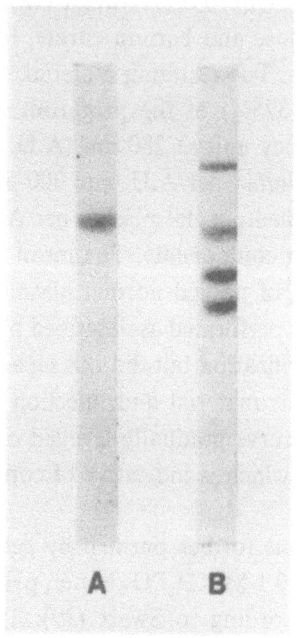

*Fig.* 1. Sodium dodecylsulfate (SDS) – polyacrylamide gel electrophoresis.
A. Step 5 prothrombin
B. Reference mixture containing phosphorylase A (MW 94,000) and reduced fibrinogen (alpha chain, MW 70,900; beta chain, MW 60,400 and gamma chain, MW 50,700).

Step 5 prothrombin was labeled with $Na^{131}I$ or $Na^{125}I$ by a slightly modified method of McFarlane (20), in which radioactive iodine was generated by adding radioactive NaI to an acid mixture of KI and $KIO_3$. The reagents were mixed in a small plastic beaker. Unbound iodide was removed by passage through a $1.5 \times 3$ cm column of Amberlite IRA 401 (Rohm and Haas Co., Philadelphia, Pa.). The solution was then mixed with human serum albumin to a concentration of 4 g/100 ml, sterilized by filtration, placed in sterile siliconized vials, frozen at $-20°C$ and kept at this temperature until used. The preparations were shown to be sterile and free of pyrogens. The average substitution level was 0.25 atoms of iodine per molecule of prothrombin. No changes in the biological activity of prothrombin could be

detected after iodination, nor in the turnover characteristics by storage at
$-20°C$ for up to 3 months.

## Metabolic studies

These studies were carried out in 16 normal subjects and in 2 patients with
congenital hypoprothrombinemia. Results of routine hematologic tests and
complete coagulation analysis were normal in all control subjects. The patients with congenital hypoprothrombinemia were studied at the University
of Nijmegen. Their coagulation defect has been described previously (21).
Both subjects had a prothrombin level of 4 to 6 per cent of normal by two
stage prothrombin assay and by quantitative immunoelectrophoresis according to Laurell. All subjects received 500 mg of potassium iodide or 20
drops of Lugol solution before the injection of labeled prothrombin and
once daily during the study. Approximately 20 μCi (less than 1 mg) of the
labeled homologous prothrombin solution was injected intravenously in the
control subjects and in one patient with hypoprothrombinemia. In the two
hypoprothrombinemic patients the metabolism of untreated prothrombin
was studied after transfusion of 500 ml fresh plasma by enzymatic and
immunologic prothrombin assay. No side effects were noted in any of the
subjects after the infusion of plasma or labeled prothrombin. Blood samples
(20 ml) were drawn on trisodium citrate (final concentration 0.315 per cent)
10 min after the end of the injection or 30 min after the end of the transfusion in the patients and at different time intervals thereafter for up to at least
7 days, with a minimum of 9 blood samples from each subject. Pooled urine
samples were collected each 24 hr throughout the observation period in
some of the subjects.

Two ml of each of the following were pipetted in duplicate into counting
tubes: radioactive plasma, plasma supernatant after protein precipitation
with an equal volume of 10% trichloroacetic acid, and urine. After completion of the experiment, the radioactive aliquots were measured in a well type
scintillation counter (Gamma Guard Autowell Counting System[4]) with a
sensitivity of approximately 625,000 cpm/μ Ci against a background of 30
cpm.

## Analysis of tracer data

The tracer data were analyzed using a two compartment mammillary model
(22, 23) for the metabolism of prothrombin. The plasma radioactivity data

4. Tracerlab, Mechelen, Belgium.

versus time were fitted with a sum of 2 exponential terms $x(t) = C_1e^{-at_1} + C_2e^{-at_2}$ by graphical curve peeling on semilogarithmic paper (see legend fig. 4). From the coefficients and exponents of this function estimations of the radioactivity distribution ratio $(\frac{EV}{IV})$ between the extravascular (EV) and intravascular pool (IV), the fractional transcapillary transfer rate constant $(k_{12})$ and the fractional catabolic rate constant $(k_{10,p})$ can be obtained using the formulae given elsewhere (26).

In the subjects in whom quantitative urine collections were obtained the fractional catabolic rate constant $(k_{10,u})$ was also determined from the ratio of the daily urinary radioactivity to the corresponding mean plasma radioactivity (24), corrected for delay in urinary excretion of iodide (25).

The plasma volume was obtained from the total radioactivity injected, divided by the concentration of plasma radioactivity in the first sample, corrected for the dilution caused by added anticoagulant.

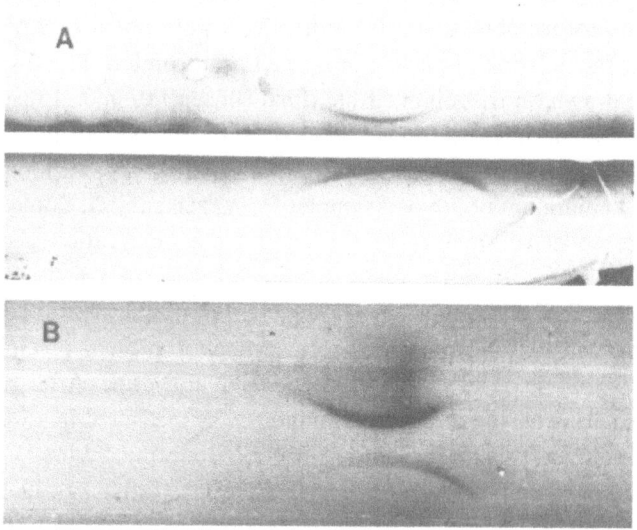

*Fig.* 2. Immunoelectrophoresis and autoradiography.
A. Immunoelectrophoresis using a specific antiprothrombin. Upper well: 4 µl of a mixture of plasma and a trace amount of labeled prothrombin.
Lower well: 4 µl of a mixture of purified prothrombin (1.15 mg/ml) and a trace amount of labeled prothrombin.
Slit: 50 µl rabbit antiserum against purified prothrombin.
B. Autoradiography of A.

RESULTS

*Physicochemical properties of labeled prothrombin*
Immunoelectrophoresis of a mixture of labeled and unlabeled step 5 prothrombin showed a single precipitin line in the same relative position as the precipitin line obtained with plasma (fig. 2). Autoradiography showed a concentration of isotope in the precipitin line.

Polyacrylamide gel electrophoresis at pH 8.3 of a mixture of labeled and unlabeled prothrombin showed one main protein band. The main protein band contained 97% of the total radioactivity of the gel.

Sephadex G-200 gel filtration of a mixture of labeled prothrombin and normal plasma showed a single radioactivity peak at the same elution volume as the enzymatic prothrombin activity in plasma (fig. 3).

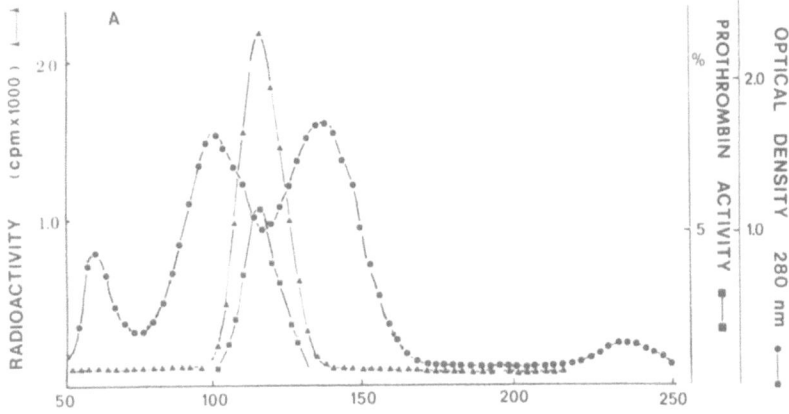

*Fig.* 3. Sephadex G-200 gel filtration of a mixture of 3 ml human plasma with a trace amount of labeled prothrombin.

*Prothrombin metabolism in control subjects*
Table 1 summarizes the clinical and laboratory data in the normal subjects. The mean plasma prothrombin concentration as measured by the two stage prothrombin time was 301 ± 37 Iowa units per ml or 13.2 ± 1.3 mg per 100 ml. A conversion factor of 2280 Iowa units per mg of prothrombin as obtained from our purified preparations was used to convert enzymatic prothrombin activity to protein concentration. The plasma prothrombin concentration measured by the immunoelectrophoretic technique of Laurell (13), using a monospecific rabbit serum raised with step 5 prothrombin was 13.3 ± 1.3 mg/100 ml. Daily fluctuations of the prothrombin levels in

*Table* 1. Clinical and laboratory data on the control subjects.

| | Age (y) | Weight (kg) | Plasma prothrombin Enzymatic assay | | Immuno assay mg/100 ml | Plasma volume ml/kg |
|---|---|---|---|---|---|---|
| | | | Iowa U/ml | mg/100 ml | | |
| JV | 32 | 68 | 335 | 14.7 | – | 43 |
| JR | 32 | 86 | 315 | 13.8 | – | 36 |
| NB | 26 | 74 | 310 | 13.6 | 15.1 | 38 |
| DH | 25 | 71 | 310 | 13.6 | 15.3 | 37 |
| MV | 45 | 92 | 315 | 13.9 | 12.9 | 41 |
| RV | 28 | 67 | 305 | 13.3 | 12.9 | 35 |
| JL | 48 | 70 | 300 | 13.1 | 11.6 | 35 |
| AV | 59 | 74 | 310 | 13.6 | 11.6 | 45 |
| JC | 57 | 49 | 315 | 13.9 | 12.9 | 38 |
| GM | 23 | 81 | 310 | 13.6 | 13.3 | 47 |
| PS | 35 | 51 | 385 | 16.9 | 13.9 | 51 |
| DC | 30 | 85 | 271 | 11.9 | – | 31 |
| GB | 26 | 88 | 236 | 10.4 | – | 39 |
| SJ | 29 | 65 | 261 | 11.5 | – | 40 |
| NS | 25 | 66 | 230 | 10.0 | – | 39 |
| RV | 30 | 75 | 303 | 13.3 | – | 33 |
| Mean | 34 | 73 | 301 | 13.2 | 13.3 | 39 |
| SD | 11 | 12 | 37 | 1.6 | 1.3 | 5 |

*Table* 2. Prothrombin tracer data on the control subjects.

| | $x(t) = C_1 e^{-a t_1} + C_2 e^{-a t_2}$ | | | | |
|---|---|---|---|---|---|
| | $C_1$ | $a_1$ | $C_2$ | $a_2$ | t 1/2 for $a_1$ (days) |
| JV | 0.50 | 0.23 | 0.50 | 1.40 | 3.00 |
| JR | 0.54 | 0.26 | 0.46 | 1.40 | 2.65 |
| NB | 0.45 | 0.21 | 0.55 | 1.25 | 3.25 |
| DH | 0.41 | 0.21 | 0.59 | 1.40 | 3.30 |
| MV | 0.52 | 0.20 | 0.48 | 1.15 | 3.50 |
| RV | 0.45 | 0.21 | 0.55 | 1.15 | 3.35 |
| JL | 0.43 | 0.24 | 0.57 | 0.92 | 2.85 |
| AV | 0.50 | 0.24 | 0.50 | 1.73 | 2.85 |
| JC | 0.52 | 0.23 | 0.48 | 1.15 | 3.00 |
| GM | 0.49 | 0.23 | 0.51 | 1.38 | 3.00 |
| PS | 0.50 | 0.19 | 0.50 | 1.26 | 3.60 |
| DC | 0.56 | 0.26 | 0.44 | 1.31 | 2.71 |
| GB | 0.55 | 0.25 | 0.45 | 0.97 | 2.79 |
| SJ | 0.49 | 0.23 | 0.51 | 2.24 | 3.00 |
| NS | 0.47 | 0.24 | 0.53 | 2.04 | 2.88 |
| RV | 0.47 | 0.24 | 0.53 | 1.98 | 2.95 |
| Mean | 0.49 | 0.23 | 0.51 | 1.42 | 3.04 |
| SD | 0.04 | 0.02 | 0.04 | 0.38 | 0.28 |

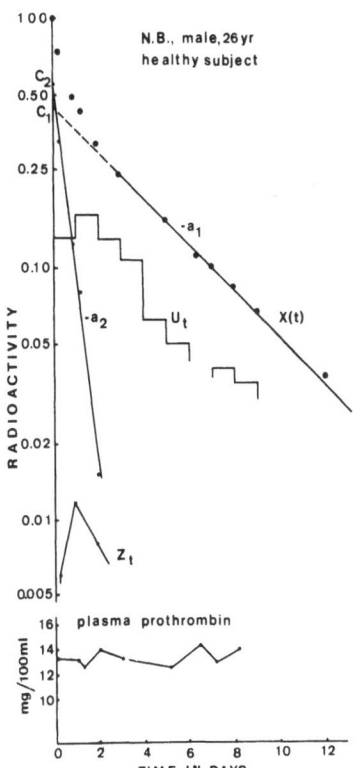

*Fig*. 4. Prothrombin metabolism in a control subject.

x(t) : plasma radioactivity

u(t) : fractional daily urinary excretion of label

z(t) : non-TCA precipitable radioactivity in plasma.

Graphical curve peeling in a sum of two exponential terms. The linear terminal portion of the plasma radioactivity curve x(t) is extrapolated to the ordinate to obtain the intercept $C_1$. The slope of this line is $-a_1$. By subtracting the extrapolated line from the original curve $x(t)-C_1e^{-a_1t}$, a new line is obtained $C_2e^{-a_2t}$ for which the slope $-a_2$ and the intercept value $C_2$ are determined.

plasma were negligible. It is therefore reasonable to assume that the subjects were in steady state with respect to prothrombin metabolism, inferring that the amount of prothrombin synthesized daily equaled the amount catabolized.

Results of a representative study are visualized in figure 4. Similar results were obtained in all subjects. The plasma radioactivity x(t) versus time could readily be approximated by a sum of two exponential terms, using data up to approximately 10 days after injection of the tracer. The tracer data are summarized in table 2. The mean value of the equation, describing the evolution of plasma radioactivity was $x(t) = 0.49e^{-0.23t} + 0.51e^{-1.42t}$. The plasma radioactivity half-life after equilibration was $3.04 \pm 0.28$ days.

The amount of non-TCA precipitable radioactivity in plasma never exceeded 2% of the total plasma radioactivity which it paralleled after the first day. Except for the first day, the daily urinary excretion of label was approximately a constant fraction of the corresponding mean plasma radioactivity. During the first day, a smaller radioactivity fraction was excreted probably due to equilibration of released isotope with the body iodide pool. The absence of a high excretion of label during the first day indicated that the initial fall in plasma radioactivity was mainly due to transfer of labeled prothrombin to the extravascular compartment and not to rapid clearing of denatured protein.

The distribution of radioactivity in serial plasma samples was investigated by gel filtration on Sephadex G-100. Throughout the study the radioactivity was eluted in one main peak corresponding to the enzymatically measured prothrombin. A small peak, (less than 5% of total) probably re-

*Table* 3. Calculated metabolic parameters on the control subjects.

| | Fractional catabolic rate constant | | Absolute catabolic (synthetic) rate | Fractional transcapillary transfer rate constant | Intravascular fraction |
|---|---|---|---|---|---|
| | $k_{10,p}$ | $k_{10,u}$ | (mg/kg/day) | $k_{12}$ | IV |
| JV | 0.40 | − | 2.50 | 0.42 | 0.58 |
| JR | 0.42 | − | 2.06 | 0.37 | 0.63 |
| NB | 0.39 | 0.38 | 2.02 | 0.40 | 0.54 |
| DH | 0.42 | 0.37 | 2.12 | 0.49 | 0.50 |
| MV | 0.33 | 0.30 | 1.87 | 0.33 | 0.60 |
| RV | 0.38 | − | 1.75 | 0.35 | 0.55 |
| JL | 0.42 | − | 1.92 | 0.21 | 0.58 |
| AV | 0.42 | − | 2.61 | 0.56 | 0.57 |
| JC | 0.37 | − | 1.98 | 0.30 | 0.62 |
| GM | 0.40 | − | 2.56 | 0.42 | 0.58 |
| PS | 0.33 | − | 2.90 | 0.40 | 0.58 |
| DC | 0.40 | − | 2.40 | 0.32 | 0.65 |
| GB | 0.38 | − | 2.72 | 0.20 | 0.67 |
| SJ | 0.42 | − | 2.48 | 0.83 | 0.54 |
| NS | 0.45 | − | 2.07 | 0.74 | 0.53 |
| RV | 0.45 | − | 2.33 | 0.71 | 0.53 |
| Mean | 0.40 | | 2.27 | 0.44 | 0.58 |
| SD | 0.04 | | 0.34 | 0.18 | 0.05 |

presenting circulating small breakdown products and free iodide was eluted at the total volume of the column.

The metabolic parameters, calculated from the plasma and urine tracer data are summarized in table 3.

The results were as follows: fractional catabolic rate constant, as determined from the plasma disappearance rate of radioactivity ($k_{10,p}$) 0.40 $\pm$ 0.04 of the plasma pool per day and as determined from the urinary excretion of radioactivity ($k_{10,u}$) 0.35 of the plasma pool per day. The absolute catabolic (synthetic) rate, obtained by multiplying the intravascular prothrombin pool with the fractional catabolic rate constant ($k_{10,p}$) was 2.27 $\pm$ 0.34 mg/kg per day. The intravascular fraction (IV) was 0.58 $\pm$ 0.05 and the fractional transcapillary efflux rate constant ($k_{12}$) 0.44 $\pm$ 0.18 of the plasma pool per day.

*Prothrombin metabolism in the patients with hypoprothrombinemia*
The metabolism of prothrombin in the two patients with hypoprothrombinemia was studied after transfusion of 500 ml fresh plasma by serial prothrombin determinations and in one patient (L.R.) in addition by radioactivity measurements after simultaneous injection of labeled prothrombin. The transfusion resulted in an increase of the prothrombin levels from 5.7 to 15.5% in patient L.R. and from 5.8 to 18.5% in patient J.T.R. as measured by the two stage prothrombin assay, and from 6.7 to 9.9% in patient L.R. and from 4.3 to 12.7% in patient J.T.R. as measured by the height of the rockets in the immunologic assay of Laurell. However the precipitin rockets

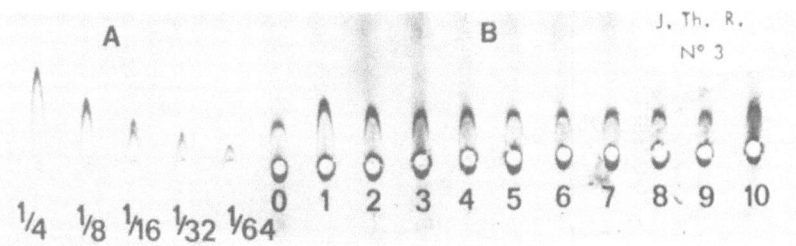

*Fig.* 5. Quantitative immunoelectrophoretic assay of prothrombin in the plasma of a patient with congenital hypoprothrombinemia before and after transfusion of 500 ml fresh plasma.
A. dilutions of pooled normal plasma
B. undiluted plasma of the patient
    0: before transfusion
    1: 30 min after the end of the transfusion
    2-10: at daily intervals after the transfusion

in the patients were broader than in normal plasma, resulting in a less precise quantitation of the immunoreactive protein from the height of the rockets (fig. 5).

The disappearance rate of the transfused prothrombin was studied by measuring the decay of the difference between the prothrombin baseline value and the prothrombin levels after transfusion of fresh plasma. Differences more than 20% above the baseline value were only obtained during the first 4 days after the transfusion. The mean values of these differences obtained in the two patients, expressed as a fraction of the difference in the first sample, are visualized in figure 6. These data show that the mean dis-

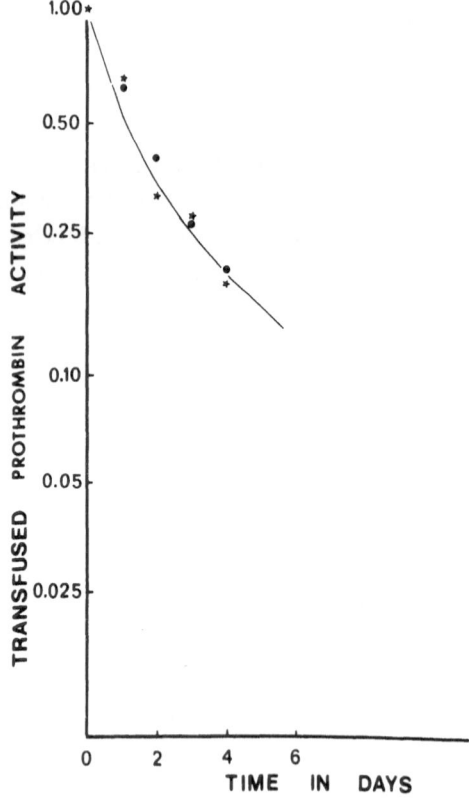

*Fig.* 6. Disappearance rate of infused prothrombin from the plasma in two patients with congenital hypoprothrombinemia.
✦ enzymatic assay, mean of the two patients.
● immunologic assay, mean of the two patients.
Solid line: mean disappearance rate of radioactivity in the control group.

appearance rate of infused unlabeled prothrombin in the patients is indistinguishable from the mean disappearance rate of labeled prothrombin in
the 16 control subjects.

The disappearance rate of infused prothrombin activity and radioactivity
from the plasma in patient L.R. is visualized in figure 7. Within the errors
of the biologic assay, no difference in the plasma disappearance rate of
unlabeled and labeled prothrombin was observed. Moreover, after equilibration, the plasma half-life of labeled prothrombin was 3.1 days, which is
the mean value obtained in the control group.

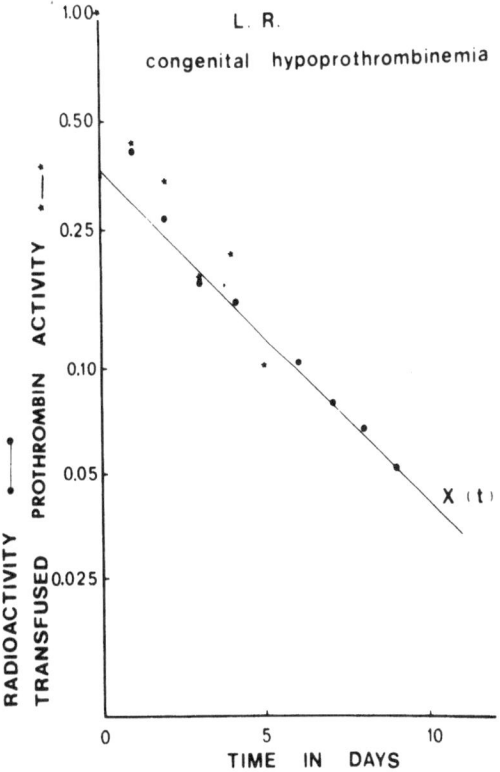

*Fig.* 7. Prothrombin metabolism in a patient with congenital hypoprothrombinemia, after
transfusion of 500 ml fresh plasma and injection of labeled prothrombin.
● plasma radioactivity.
★ enzymatic prothrombin activity: difference between measured level and baseline value.

DISCUSSION

The purity of the prothrombin preparation used in this study has been demonstrated, both before and after iodination, by its high specific activity and its homogeneous behavior on Sephadex gel filtration, immunoelectrophoresis and polyacrylamide gel electrophoresis. Biologic integrity was in vivo evidenced by absence of an initially high urinary excretion of radioactivity, and by the presence of a relatively high intravascular fraction after equilibration with the extravascular fluids. The separation of prothrombin from the other factors of the prothrombin complex by hydroxylapatite chromatography did not deteriorate the in vitro nor the in vivo characteristics of prothrombin, but instead resulted in a further purification.

The mean plasma radioactivity half-life of 3.04 ± 0.28 days in our control series is in line with the data of Shapiro and Martinez (2) obtained with step 4 prothrombin, larger than the value reported by Takeda (3) but shorter than the results obtained by Benamon-Djiane et al. (1). Direct proof that the turnover of labeled proteins reflects the metabolism of their endogenous native counterparts is difficult to obtain. However, the disappearance rate of enzymatic and immunoreactive prothrombin activity after transfusion of 500 ml fresh plasma in our two hypoprothrombinemic patients was indistinguishable from the disappearance rate of radioactivity from the plasma of the normal subjects. This finding strongly suggests identical biological behavior of the purified labeled substrate and the untreated prothrombin in plasma and is further substantiated by a similar disappearance rate of prothrombin activity and radioactivity after simultaneous transfusion of fresh plasma and injection of labeled prothrombin in one hypoprothrombinemic patient.

The normal disappearance rate of plasma radioactivity in a patient with hypoprothrombinemia clearly demonstrates that prothrombin metabolism in man follows first order kinetics over a large range of plasma prothrombin concentrations and is in line with our previous observations on the metabolism of labeled fibrinogen (26). Subsequent studies (27) have indicated that labeled prothrombin can be used as a sensitive metabolic tracer for the detection and quantitation of disturbances in the synthesis or catabolism of prothrombin.

ACKNOWLEDGEMENTS

The turnover studies in the hypoprothrombinemic patients were performed by Prof. Dr. C. Haanen and his staff at the University of Nijmegen, The Netherlands. The technical assistance of Mr. F. De Cock is gratefully acknowledged.

REFERENCES

1. Benamon-Djiane, D., J. Drouet, A. Cosson, Ch. Blatrix, D. Ménaché and F. Josso, Durée de vie chez l'homme de la prothrombine marquée par l'iode radioactif (I-131). *Rev. franç. Transfusion* 11, 129 (1968).
2. Shapiro, S. S. and J. Martinez, Human prothrombin metabolism in normal man and in hypocoagulable subjects. *J. clin. Invest.* 48, 1292 (1969).
3. Takeda, Y., Metabolism and distribution of [125]I-prothrombin in healthy men. *J. Lab. clin. Med.* 76, 1023 (1969).
4. Shapiro, S. S. and J. Martinez, The use of [125]I-prothrombin in the study of states of altered coagulability. II Congress Int. Soc. Thrombosis Haemostasis, Abstract volume, p. 164 Oslo (1971).
   p. 164 Oslo (1971).
5. Soulier, J. P. and M. J. Larrieu, Etude analytique des temps de Quick allongés. Dosage de prothrombine, de proconvertine et de proaccélerine. *Sang* 23, 549 (1952).
6. Ware, A. G. and W. H. Seegers, Two-stage procedure for quantitative determination of prothrombin concentration. *Amer. J. clin. Path.* 19, 471 (1949).
7. Vermylen, J., M. Verstraete and I. Brosens, Effect of dydrogesterone (Duphaston) on haemostasis and liver function. *J. Obstet. Gynaec.* 79. In press. (1975).
8. Soulier, J. P. and M. J. Larrieu, Nouvelle méthode de diagnostic de l'hémophilie Dosage des facteurs antihémophiliques A et B. *Sang* 24, 205 (1953).
9. Bachmann, F., F. Duckert and E. Koller. The Stuart-Power assay and its clinical significance. *Thrombos. Diathes. haemorrh.* 2, 24 (1958).
10. Vermylen, C., R. de Vreker and M. Verstraete, A rapid enzymatic method for assay of fibrinogen: the fibrin polymerization time (F.P.T. Test). *Clin. chim. Acta* 8, 418 (1963).
11. Blombäck, B. and M. Blombäck, Purification of human and bovine fibrinogen. *Arkiv Kemi* 10, 415 (1956).
12. Proctor, R. R. and S. I. Rapaport, The partial thromboplastin time with Kaolin. A simple screening test for first stage plasma clotting factor deficiencies. *Amer. J. clin. Med.* 36, 212 (1961).
13. Laurell, C. B., Quantitative estimation of proteins by electrophoresis in agarose gel containing antibodies. *Analyt. Biochem.* 15, 45 (1966).
14. Scheidegger, J. J., Une micro-méthode de l'immuno-électrophorèse. *Int. Arch. Allergy* 7, 103 (1955).
15. Laurell, C. B., Quantitative estimation of proteins by electrophoresis in agarose gel containing antibodies. *Analyt. Biochem.* 15, 45 (1966).
16. Davis, B. J. Disc electrophoresis. II. Method and application to human serum proteins, *Ann. N.Y. Acad. Sci.* 121, 404 (1964).
17. Weber, K. and M. Osborn, The reliability of molecular weight determinations by dodecyl sulfate-polyacrylamide gel electrophoresis. *J. biol. Chem.* 244, 4406 (1969).
18. Shapiro, S. S. and F. Waugh, The purification of human prothrombin. *Thrombos. Diathes. haemorrh.* 16, 469 (1966).

19. Swart, A. C. W., *Studies on the purification and separation of blood coagulation factors II, VII, IX and X*. Ph. D. Thesis, University of Leiden (1971).
20. McFarlane, A. S., Efficient trace-labeling of proteins with iodine. *Nature* (Lond.) 182, 53 (1958).
21. Hart, H. Ch. and E. A. Loeliger, In: Genetics and the interaction of blood clotting factors. *Thrombos. Diathes. haemorrh.* Suppl. 17, p. 209 (1966).
22. Matthews, C. M. E., The theory of tracer experiments with $^{131}$I-labelled plasma proteins. *Phys. Med. Biol.* 2, 36 (1957).
23. Berman, S. and R. Schoenfeld, Invariants in experimental data on linear kinetics and the formulation of models. *J. appl. Physics* 27, 136 (1956).
24. Campbell, R. M., D. P. Cuthbertson, C. M. E. Matthews and A. S. McFarlane, Behaviour of C-14 and I-131 labeled protein in the rat. *Int. J. appl. Radiat.* 1, 66 (1965).
25. Reeve, E. B. and J. E. Roberts, The kinetics of the distribution and breakdown of $^{131}$I-albumin in the rabbit. *J. gen. Physiol.* 43, 415 (1959).
26. Tytgat, G., D. Collen and J. Vermylen, Metabolism and distribution of fibrinogen. II. Fibrinogen turnover in polycythaemia, thrombocytosis, haemophilia A, congenital afibrinogenaemia and during streptokinase therapy. *Brit. J. Haemat.* 22, 701 (1972).
27. Collen, D., J. Rouvier and M. Verstraete, Metabolism of iodine-labeled plasminogen and prothrombin in liver cirrhosis. *Clin. Res.* 20, 483 (1972).

# METABOLISM OF PIVKA II IN MAN

J. M. LAVERGNE AND F. JOSSO

In 1963, Hemker and coworkers postulated from kinetic data that oral anti-coagulation using Vitamin K antagonists induced the synthesis of a biolog-ically inactive prothrombin precursor (1). Since 1968 it has been demons-trated that the decrease of plasma prothrombin activity in subjects under-going oral anticoagulant therapy was accompanied by the appearance in plasma of an abnormal component, immunogically undistinguishable from prothrombin but lacking its biological activity: preprothrombin or PIVKA II (2, 3, 4). It was assumed that this precursor was converted into active prothrombin in the liver cell by a Vitamin K dependant system.

The main characteristics of PIVKA II are as follows: 1) apparent immu-nochemical identity with normal prothrombin; 2) lack of affinity for pro-thrombinase; 3) ability to form a fibrinogen-fibrin converting complex with staphylocoagulase, 4) unability to bind calcium ions.

The aim of the present study was to follow the fate of plasma PIVKA II during coumarin therapy and after Vitamin K administration. To achieve this purpose it was necessary to be able to perform a specific assay of plasma PIVKA II and therefore to separate this component from normal prothrom-bin. Oxalated plasma was used as starting material and normal prothrombin was adsorbed by small amounts of $Ca_3 (PO_4)_2$ until its level was lower than 2 per cent, as measured by a one-stage clotting assay. To achieve complete depletion of prothrombin without any loss of PIVKA II, the necessary amount of the adsorbant was a function of the prothrombin concentration in the sample. This amount was never higher than 3 mg per ml. Then it was possible to apply an immunochemical prothrombin (i.e. PIVKA II) assay to the supernatant (fig. 1).

Two kinds of experiments were carried out.

1. The respective fates of plasma prothrombin and PIVKA II were followed under sustained administration of acenocoumarol with subsequent vitamin K injection.

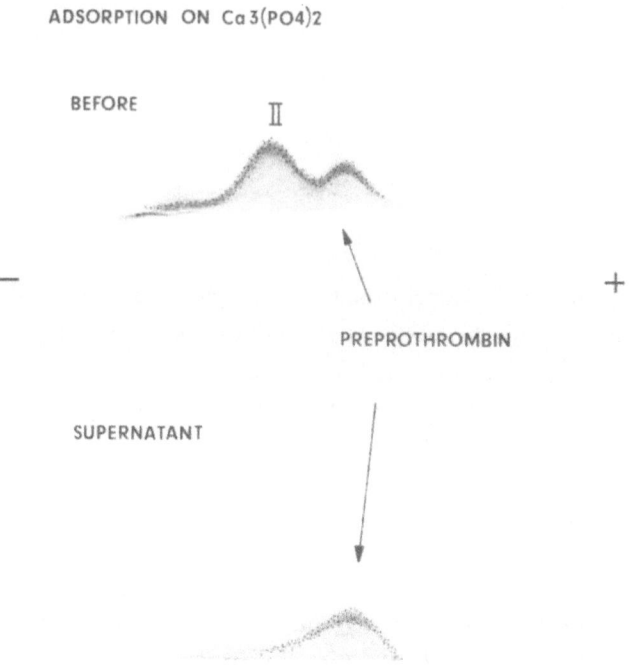

*Fig.* 1. Separation of PIVKA II (preprothrombin) from prothrombin in plasma during coumarin-therapy: antigen-antibody crossed electrophoresis against antiprothrombin antibodies, before and after tricalcium phosphate adsorption.

2. The effect of Vitamin K injection on plasma prothrombin level was measured with and without previous acenocoumarol administration.

1. VARIATIONS OF PLASMA PIVKA II LEVELS UNDER ORAL ANTICO-AGULATION

One normal adult subject was given acenocoumarol (4 mg per os daily) until the four vitamin K dependant factors reached a constant level, as tested by the one-stage clotting assay: between 12 per cent for factor VII and 24 per cent for factor X. At day 11 acenocoumarol was stopped and a single intra-venous 25 mg dose of Vitamin $K_1$ was given. The plasma prothrombin level was followed using three different methods: one stage clotting assay, staphy-locoagulase assay and immunoassay (fig. 2).

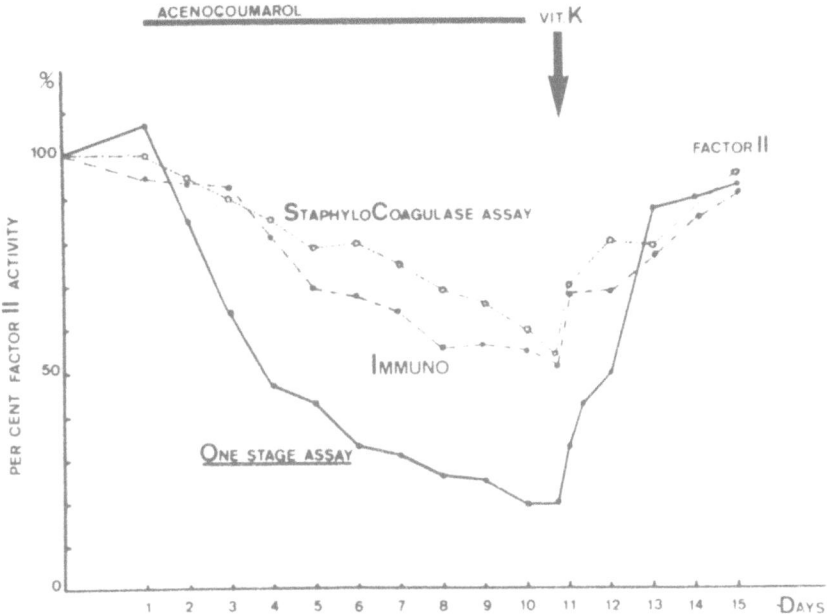

*Fig.* 2. Behaviour of plasma factor II, during oral anticoagulation. At D11 the treatment was stopped and a single intravenous 25 mg dose of vitamin $K_1$ was given.

As previously reported immuno assay and staphylocoagulase assay gave the same results which were always higher than those of the one stage assay. However, the total immunoreactive material did not remain constant but decreased slowly. This finding was confirmed without exception in every patient we tested during oral anticoagulant therapy. The half-life of plasma prothrombin biological activity, as tested by one stage clotting assay, was 72 hours (fig. 3A).

On each daily sample, the respective concentrations of prothrombin and PIVKA II were tested, using immuno assay performed before and after tricalcium phosphate adsorption (fig. 4). PIVKA II appeared in plasma as soon as the anticoagulation was started and its concentration progressively increased until a plateau was reached, persisting as long as a constant dose of anticoagulant was maintained. The half-time of the plasma PIVKA II increase was about 18 hours (fig. 3A).

Once acenocoumarol administration stopped, Vitamin $K_1$ injection was followed by two distinct phenomena (fig. 3B). A sharp increase in plasma prothrombin level was observed during the first hours, demonstrated as well by clotting assay as by immuno assay, followed by a slower increase. At

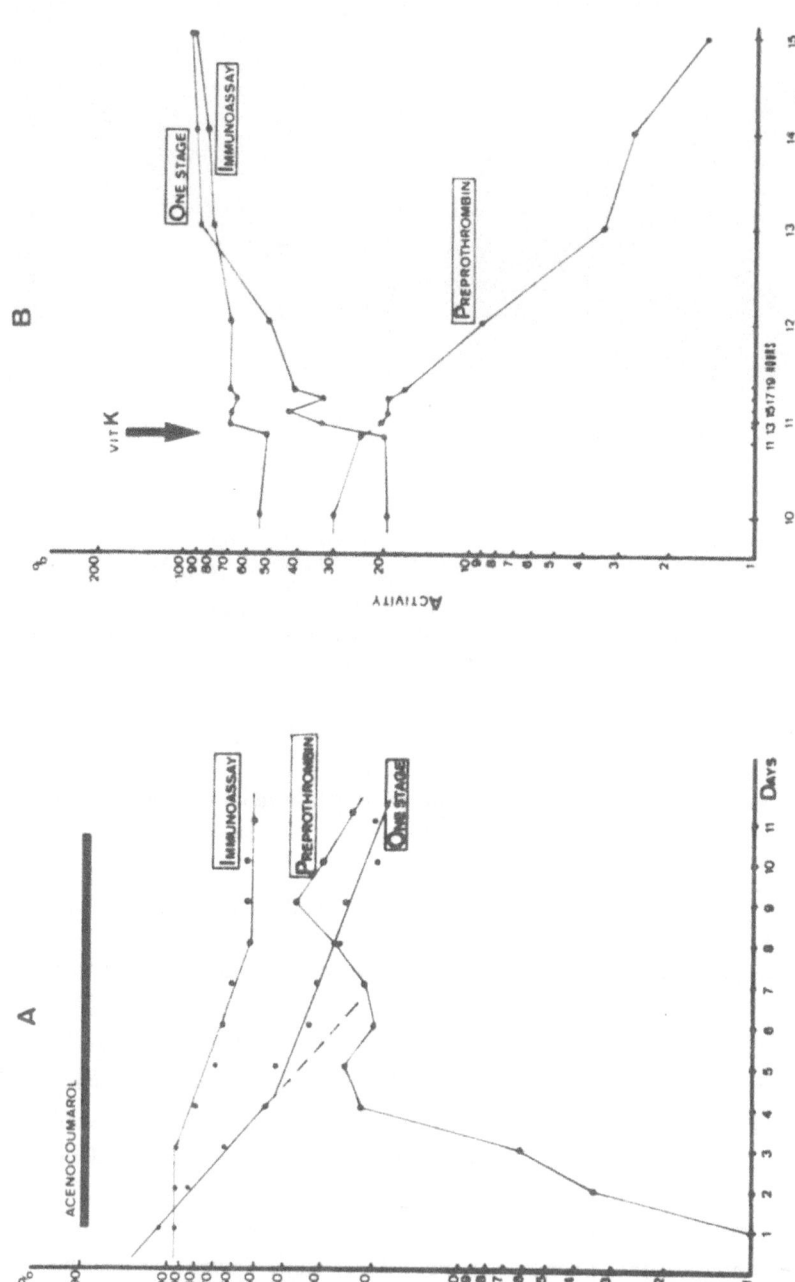

*Fig.* 3. Kinetics of active prothrombin (one stage clotting assay) and PIVKA II or preprothrombin (specific immunochemical assay) compared with total prothrombin antigen (immuno assay). Preprothrombin levels are expressed with reference to plasma prothrombin antigen in normal plasma.

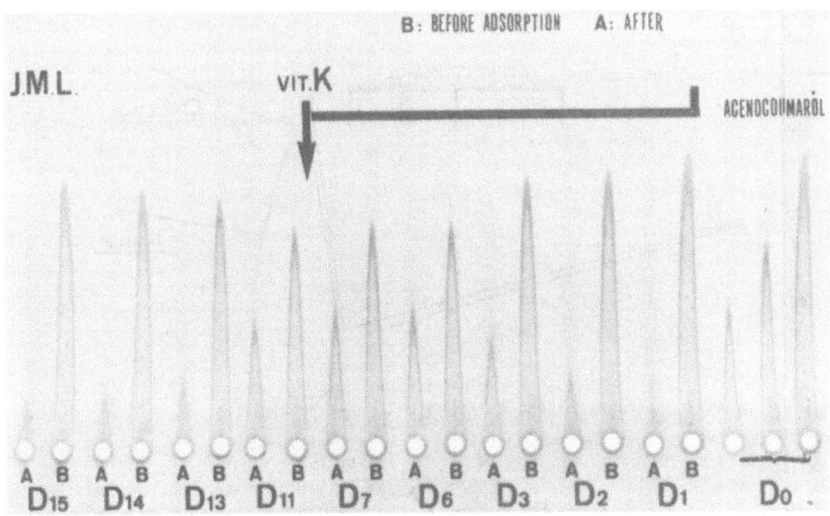

*Fig.* 4. Plasma prothrombin immuno assay.
B: Total prothrombin antigen amount before adsorption by tricalcium phosphate.
A: PIVKA II in the supernatant after adsorption.

the same time plasma PIVKA II level regularly decreased with a half-life of 18 hours. There was no fall of plasma PIVKA II level corresponding to the sharp increase of the prothrombin level.

## 2. EFFECT OF VITAMIN $K_1$ ON PROTHROMBIN LEVEL

Two groups of normal subjects received intravenously 25 mg Vitamin $K_1$, the first group without any previous treatment, the second after a 6 mg acenocoumarol administration for a one day period. In the first experiment, without anticoagulant therapy, Vitamin $K_1$ injection was not followed by any increase of plasma prothrombin level. In the second group, plasma prothrombin level slightly decreased after acenocoumarol administration and then sharply increased above the baseline value after Vitamin $K_1$ injection (fig. 5).

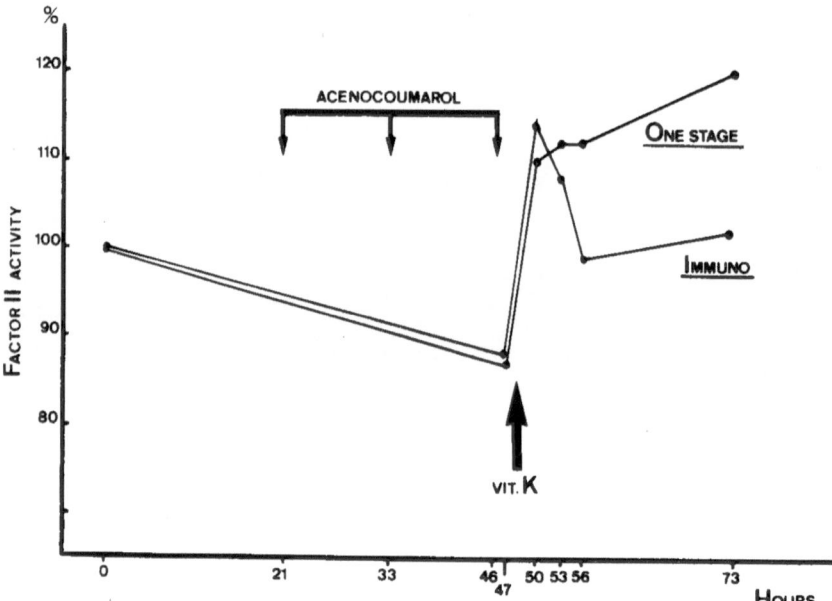

*Fig. 5.* Factor II response to vitamin K₁ injection after a short acenocoumarol intake:
mean of four experiments in normal adult subjects.

## DISCUSSION

PIVKA II appears in plasma in the first hours following the start of anticoagulant therapy, as already shown by Brozovic and Gurd (5). Then its
level increases progressively to reach a plateau. PIVKA II turn-over rate
seems to be much higher than that of prothrombin if one compares the respective half-lifes of the two components: about 18 hours for PIVKA II and
at least 72 hours for prothrombin.

In normal subjects Vitamin K administration does not affect plasma prothrombin level. But in coumarin treated subjects Vitamin K induces a very
rapid increase of plasma prothrombin level, as already demonstrated by
Van der Meer (6). This early increase is not due to the conversion of plasma
PIVKA II into prothrombin since the circulating level of this component
is not affected by the prothrombin variations. Moreover, after a short administration of coumarin drugs, Vitamin K injection raises plasma prothrombin level above its baseline value. These data are compatible with the
hypothesis of a coumarin-induced intracellular storage of a prothrombin

precursor which would be available for a rapid conversion into active pro-thrombin by vitamin K.

Most of the experimental data collected in animals are in good agreement with such an hypothesis: presence in coumarin-treated rat plasma of a pro-tein resembling inactive prothrombin, with a much higher turn-over rate than that of normal prothrombin (7); failure of blocking by actinomycine D (8) or cycloheximide (9, 10, 11) the response to Vitamin K in coumarin treated animals; presence in liver microsomes of Vitamin K deficient rats of a precursor able to generate thrombin activity with Echis carinatus venom (12). However, other authors have failed to find an appreciable amount of immunologically reactive intracellular material in coumarin treated animals: dog liver cells (13); rat liver microsomes (14). Discrepan-cies between these various results could be related to some differences in specificity and sensibility of the methods used.

Analysis of our data allows to propound a model for the regulation of prothrombin synthesis in man. In the hepatocyte, PIVKA II is converted into active prothrombin by a Vitamin K dependant system. In Vitamin K deficiency (or during oral anticoagulation) PIVKA II accumulates in the hepatocyte and then gains access to plasma. This storage suggests that PIVKA II passes through the cell membrane more slowly than prothrombin does.

In such a situation Vitamin K injection allows the rapid conversion of the intracellular precursor into active prothrombin with concomitant increase of plasma prothrombin level.

Although the sum of PIVKA II and prothrombin in plasma is always lower than the normal prothrombin level, the short half-life of PIVKA II impli-cates that the synthesis rate of this precursor is much higher under coumarin therapy than in the steady state. Such a phenomenon could be explained by the experiments reported by Karpatkin and Karpatkin (15). These investi-gations showed that injection to normal rabbits of coumarin-treated rabbit plasma was able to raise the plasma prothrombin level in the injected animals, suggesting that the synthesis of a hormone-like component enhancing pro-thrombin synthesis would be induced by a low plasma prothrombin level.

Thus prothrombin synthesis would be regulated by a feedback mechanism acting on the synthesis rate of the precursor PIVKA II. This synthesis would be accelerated by an hormonal mediator and repressed by the intracellular level of the precursor. Such an hypothesis must be confirmed by further studies.

## REFERENCES

1. Hemker, H. C., J. J. Veltkamp, A. Hensen and E. A. Loeliger, *Nature* 200, 589 (1963).
2. Ganrot, P. O. and J. E. Nilehn, Scand. *J. clin. Lab. Invest.* 22, 23 (1968).
3. Josso, F., J. M. Lavergne, M. Gouault, O. Prou-Wartelle and J. P. Soulier, *Thrombos. Diathes. haemorrh.* 20, 88 (1968).
4. Brozovic, M. and L. Gurd, *Lancet* 11, 427 (1971).
5. Brozovic, M. and L. Gurd, *Brit. J. Haemat.*, 24, 579 (1973).
6. v. d. Meer, J., H. C. Hemker and E. A. Loeliger, *Thrombos. Diathes. haemorrh.*, suppl. 29, 4 (1968).
7. Johnson, H. V., C. Boyd, J. Martinovic, G. Valkovich and B. C. Johnson, *Arch. Biochem.* 148, 431 (1972).
8. Lowenthal, J. and E. L. Simmons, *Experientia*, 23, 421 (1967).
9. Hill, R. B., S. Gaetani, A. M. Paolucci, P. B. R. Rao, R. Alden, G. S. Ranhotra, D. V. Shaw and B. C. Johnson, *J. biol. Chem.* 243, 3, 930 (1968).
10. Bell, R. G. and J. J. Matschiner, *Arch. Biochem.* 135, 152 (1969).
11. Suttie, J. W., *Fed. Proc.* 28, 963 (1969).
12. Suttie, J. W., *Science* 1979, 192 (1973).
13. Anderson, G. F. and M. I. Barnhart, *Am. J. Physiol.* 206, 929 (1964).
14. Johnston, M. F. M. and R. E. Olson, *J. biol. Chem.* 247, 4001 (1972).
15. Karpatkin, M. and S. Karpatkin, *Brit. J. Haemat.* 24, 253 (1973).

# FACTORS INFLUENCING PROTHROMBIN COMPLEX
# CLOTTING FACTOR SYNTHESIS IN THE RAT

A. T. VAN OOSTEROM

## INTRODUCTION

The aim of this study was to quantitate the disappearance and reappearance rates of the prothrombin complex factors II, VII and X under different metabolic conditions.

The disappearance rate of the clotting factors of the prothrombin complex from the plasma, has been reported to be accelerated in men in hypermetabolic states like fever and hyperthyroidism (1), this is probably also true for other coagulation factors.

Another factor influencing the turnover of clotting factors is genetic as shown by Pyörällä (2) in different strains of rats. Also by Pyörällä (3) and recently by Matschiner and Bell (4) it was demonstrated that sex is also an important factor.

## METHODOLOGY

In the experiments presented here only male rats from a highly inbred colony of Wistar rats were used being the sixty fourth generation of brother-sister matings (5). All rats were 4 month old. Rats were made hypothyroidism by radio-chemical thyroidectomy with $J^{131}$.

After 4 weeks they were clinically hypothyrotic, as indicated by stunted growth, indolent behaviour, low voice and dull dry hair; the serum $T_3$ and $T_4$ values showed a 40 percent reduction. This hypometabolic state could be corrected by administration of thyroxin subcutaneously in a daily dosage as indicated by Cullen (6).

The dose of Warfarin (Coumadin-sodium) completely blocking the synthesis of the prothrombin complex factors in these rats, indicated by Pyörällä (3) to be above 25 micrograms per hundred gram body weight in all strains he tested, was found to be higher than 50 micrograms. To ensure complete blocking 150 micrograms per hundred gram bodyweight were administrated in all rats used for the determination of the disappearance rates. The production was studied in rats pretreated with 25, 25 and 15 micrograms per 100 gram bodyweight Warfarin on three succesive days. They were given vitamin $K_1$ when their normotest time was over 150 seconds, i.e. lower than 10 procent mean coagulation factor activity (7).

The optimal dose of vitamin $K_1$ to correct the coumarin-induced hypocoagulability was not experimentally investigated; 1.5 mg, 100 times more than advised by Pyörällä (3), per 100 gram bodyweight was given.

The factor II, VII and X assays were carried out in a one-stage method, using artifical substrate plasma's (8,9) and home-made rat-brain thromboplastin according to the method described by Owren and Aas (10) for human brain thromboplastin. Blood sampling was carried out in ether anesthetized rats by cutting of one vertebra from the tail (7).

## RESULTS AND DISCUSSION

The average disappearance rate (fig. 1), expressed as the biological half life of prothrombin, in 21 normal rats was 5.8 hours. In 21 hypothyroid rats the half life of prothrombin activity was 9.1 hours.

In 21 hypothyroid rats, substituted for two weeks with thyroxin, the half life was 6.1 hours, a value nearly the same as found in normal rats.

The same phenomenon can be seen in figure 2, for the reappearance or production of prothrombin after vitamin $K_1$ administration in 20 anticoagulated normal rats, 21 anticoagulated hypothyroid rats and 21 anticoagulated thyroxin-substituted hypothyroid rats. The thyroxin-substituted rats showed an even faster reappearance of prothrombin activity than normal rats.

The data concerning the disappearance of factor II, VII and X activity in the three groups of rats are summarized in table 1. The reversal of the ab-

Table 1. Disappearance rates of factors II, VII and X in euthyroid, hypothyroid and adequately thyroxin-substituted hypothyroid rats.

| disappearance, $T\frac{1}{2}$ (in hrs) | | |
|---|---|---|
| rats: | normal | hypothyroid | T4-substituted |
| factor II | 5.8 | 9.1 | 6.1 |
| factor VII | 3.7 | 4.7 | 3.4 |
| factor X | 4.5 | 5.8 | 4.0 |

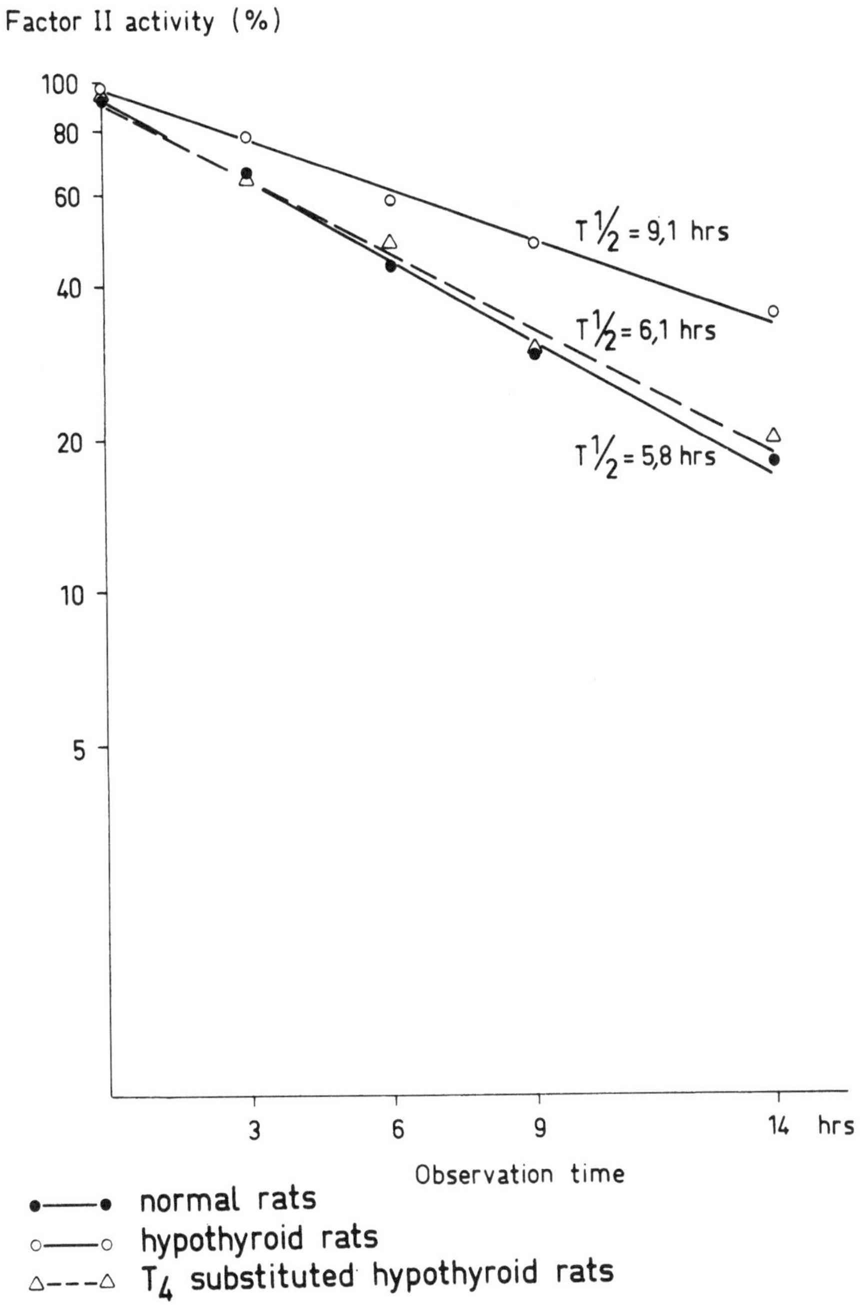

Factor II activity (%)

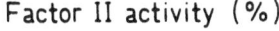

Fig. 1. Disappearance rates (T½) of factor II activity in three groups of rats, euthyroid, hypothyroid, thyroxin-substituted hypothyroid, after a complete synthesis blocking dose of coumadin-sodium (Warfarin).

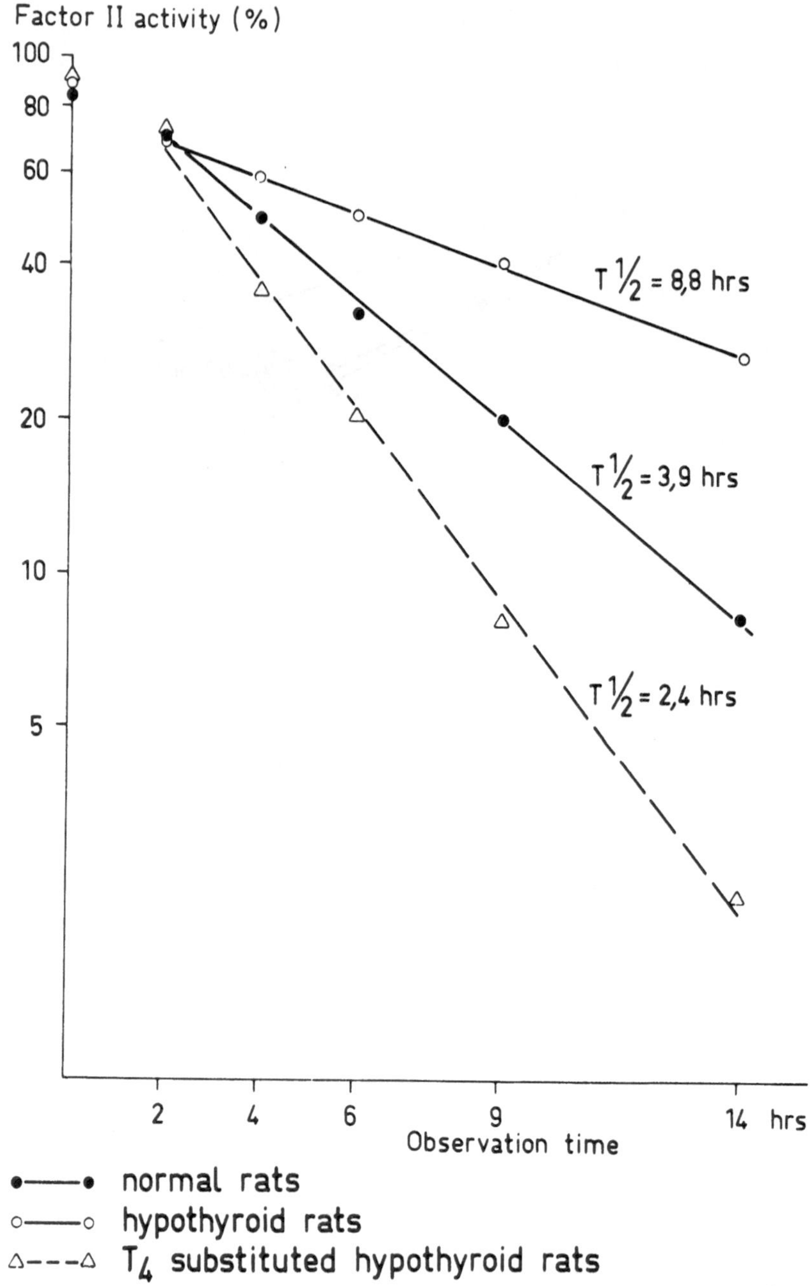

Factor II activity (%)

Fig. 2. Production of factor II activity after vitamin $K_1$ administration in the three groups of rats with coumarin-induced hypocoagulability. For the construction of the lines, each representing a reappearance $T\frac{1}{2}$, the prothrombin activity found at different times was subtracted from the pre-experimental value in each rat. The first two hours after administration of vitamin $K_1$ were omitted. The calculations used did not correct for simultaneous degradation of newly synthetized prothrombin.

normal hypothyroid state by thyroxine administration, resulting in correction of the biological half-live times, is evident.

In table 2 data are presented on reappearance rates of these coagulation factors after vitamin $K_1$ administration that show an even greater influence of hypothyroidism on production.

An interesting finding, is the consistent discrepancy between disappearance and reappearance rates (compare table 1 and 2).

This discrepancy cannot be real because it is incompatible with a stable coagulation factor activity level under normal conditions. It is not probable

*Table 2.* Production rates, expressed in reappearance $T\frac{1}{2}$, of factors II, VII and X in euthyroid, hypothyroid and adequately thyroxin-substituted hypothyroid rats.

|  | reappearance, $T\frac{1}{2}$ (in hrs) | | |
| --- | --- | --- | --- |
| rats: | normal | hypothyroid | T4-substituted |
| factor II | 3.9 | 8.8 | 2.4 |
| factor VII | 1.0 | 2.7 | 1.0 |
| factor X | 1.2 | 4.4 | 1.1 |

that the phenomenon is due to a rapid conversion of PIVKA II, VII and X retained in the liver cells because all the reappearance rates show excellent rectilinearity, nearly excluding the possibility that two mechanisms with different velocities are at work.

The different reappearance rates for the different coagulation factors also do not favour the hypothesis that PIVKA conversion by vitamin $K_1$ action is the major mechanism in restoring coagulation factor levels.

In our opinion the newly synthetized clotting factors have to be distributed over a space larger than the plasma volume, which would explain for the too high values resulting in a too short reappearance rate, due to a lag-phase in distribution. The $T\frac{1}{2}$ of disapearance on the other hand is seemingly prolonged because of supply from the extravascular space.

The hypothesis is supported by the finding of an overshoot of all three factors 6 to 14 hours after the vitamin $K_1$ administration. The factor activity levels 24 hours after the administration of vitamin $K_1$ were all completely normal, equal to the pre-experimental values and remained so.

SUMMARY

A clear cut influence of the metabolic state on both disappearance and re-appearance rates of the coagulation factors of the prothrombin complex was found in rats.

The use of genetically identical male rats made it possible to avoid longi-tudinal studies. The most intruiging finding was the discrepancy between disappearance and reappearance rates consistently observed in all groups of rats and for all three factors tested which could be caused by a constantly present but relatively slow distribution of these factors in a space larger than the plasma volume.

REFERENCES

1. Loeliger, E. A., B. van de Esch, H. C. Hemker and M. J. Mattern, *Thrombos. Diathes. haemorrh.* 10, 267 (1964).
2. Pyörällä, K. and H. R. Nevanlinna, *Ann. med. exp. Fenn.* 46, 35 (1968).
3. Pyörällä, K., *Ann. med. exp. Biol. Fenn.* 43, suppl. 3 (1965).
4. Matschiner, J. T. and R. G. Bell, *Proc. Soc. exp. Biol.* 144, 316 (1973).
5. Geertzen, H. M., F. J. G. van der Ouderaa and A. H. Kassenaar, *Acta endocrin. (Kbh.)* 72, 197 (1973).
6. Cullen, M. J., G. F. Doherey and S. H. Ingbar, *Endocrin.* 92, 1028 (1973).
7. van Oosterom, A. T. and J. J. Veltkamp, *Experientia* 30, (8), 953-955 (1974).
8. Koller, F., E. A. Loeliger and F. Duckert, *Acta haemat.* 6, 1 (1951).
9. Hemker, H. C., A. C. W. Swart and A. J. M. Alink, *Thrombos. Diathes. haemorrh.* 27, 205 (1972).
10. Owren, P. A. and K. Aas, *Scand. J. clin. Lab. Invest.* 3, 201 (1951).

# PART THREE

# CONGENITAL ABNORMALITIES

# A CONGENITALLY ABNORMAL PROTHROMBIN:
## PROTHROMBIN BARCELONA

F. JOSSO, J. M. LAVERGNE, R. BENAROUS, J. MONASTERIO DE SANCHEZ
D. LABIE AND J. TRIGINER

Plasma prothrombin is defined by several properties: conversion into thrombin by physiological prothrombinase (one-stage and two-stage assays); generation of a fibrinogen-fibrin converting activity induced by non physiological activators (trypsin, staphylocoagulase, echis carinatus venom); precipitation by monospecific antibodies allowing immunochemical assay and immunoelectrophoresis. In serum, inactive prothrombin fragments are revealed by immunochemical analysis.

In congenital prothrombin deficiency, a close relationship between the results of various clotting assays and immunochemical assay was clearly demonstrated.

In 1968, Shapiro and coll. studied a family in which eleven members had half-normal levels of prothrombin biological activity but normal quantities of immunoreactive zymogen. Presented data suggested that affected individuals were heterozygous for the synthesis of a defective prothrombin molecule (prothrombin Cardeza). The changes undergone by this molecule during activation lead to the appearance of an abnormal fragment in serum, without thrombin formation (4). In 1971, Josso and coll. reported another case of congenital dysprothrombinemia (prothrombin Barcelona) in four siblings homozygous for the defect. The main characteristics of this variant were the slowness of its conversion into trombin by prothrombinase, finally leading to a nearly complete thrombin yield, and an electrophoretic migration apparently more anodic than that of normal prothrombin (1). In 1973, two new variants were reported: prothrombins San-Juan (Shapiro and coll.) and Brussels (Kahn); recently Girolami observed a fifth case of dysprothrombinemia (prothrombin Padua). The aim of the present paper is to describe the main data collected up to now on prothrombin Barcelona.

Five years ago we had the opportunity to study a spanish family in which four siblings out of eight had a haemorrhagic syndrome resembling mild hemophilia. The affected children were two girls and two boys. The parents were unrelated.

The patients seemed to have a congenital prothrombin deficiency. One stage prothrombin assay revealed a very low activity, 5 per cent, identical in the four siblings, whereas factors VII, IX, and X were normal. However, a prothrombin assay using staphylocoagulase gave normal results and the immunochemical assay showed that the patients' plasma contained the same amount of immuno reactive material as the control plasma.

In the parents as well as in another sibling, the prothrombin level was about 60 per cent by the one-stage assay but normal by both staphylocoagulase and immunochemical assay.

Qualitative immunochemical studies showed an identity reaction between the prothrombin of normal plasma and that of the Barcelona patients. Moreover, when blood was allowed to clot in a glass tube at 37°C and serum tested 4 hours after clotting, an identity reaction was also observed between prothrombin derivatives of normal serum and that of the Barcelona patients.

Immunoelectrophoresis showed that the prothrombin migration was slightly more anodic in the patients' plasma than in normal plasma.

Regarding the biological activity, the main characteristic of this variant was the slowness of its conversion into thrombin by prothrombinase. When prothrombin was separated from the plasma antithrombins by precipitation at low ionic strength, it appeared that the patients' prothrombin could be converted into thrombin in the 'intrinsic' system with the same final yield as normal prothrombin. But, whereas normal prothrombin was converted into thrombin after 15 minutes in the experimental system used, conversion of the patient's prothrombin took six hours.

Blood from siblings and their parents was collected on ACD by plasmapheresis; plasma was frozen at −70°C immediatly after centrifugation and stored at −20°C. In order to purify the abnormal prothrombin, we used a method described in its main features by Morrison and Esnouf (2) and perfected by Shapiro (3) who kindly showed us the details of this procedure which was applied for the first time on prothrombin Barcelona in his laboratory. After barium citrate adsorption, the eluate was chromatographed on DEAE-Sephadex using a linear sodium chloride gradient in tris-citrate buffer, pH 6.5. All the experiments were carried out by processing in parallel, in two similar columns, the patient's prothrombin and the prothrombin of a normal plasma.

The abnormal prothrombin, unlike the normal one (A), was eluted in two peaks (B1 and B2). The second peak (B2), the major one, was eluted at approximately the same ionic strength as normal prothrombin (fig. 1).

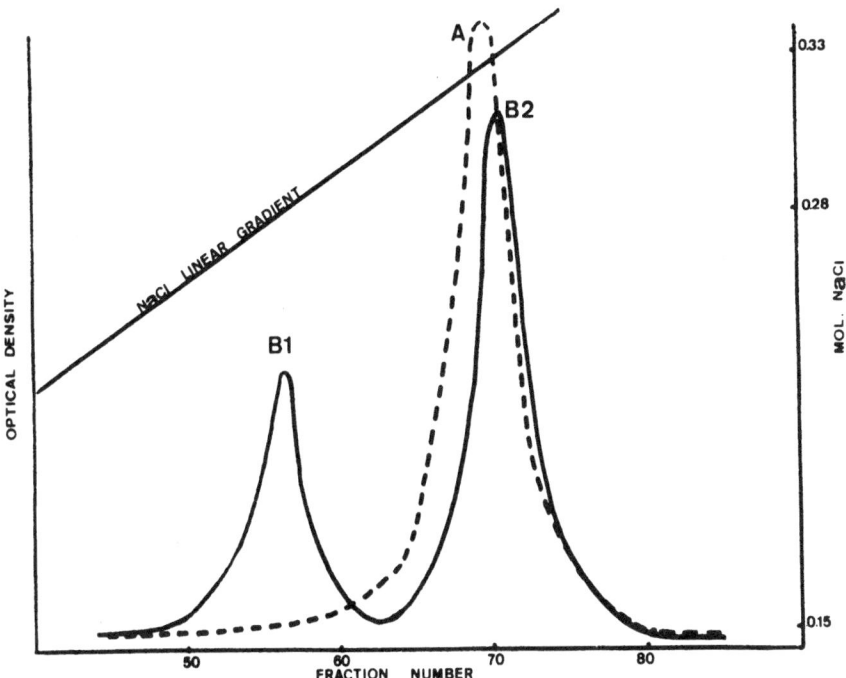

*Fig.* 1. Chromatographic pattern of the abnormal prothrombin. In dotted line, peak A obtained from normal plasma; peaks B1 and B2 are obtained from the patient's plasma.

By disc gel electrophoresis, peak B2 was essentially homogeneous, with a single band migrating slightly faster than normal prothrombin. Peak B1 showed one minor band having the same electrophoretic behaviour as the B2 band, and a major band, less anodic. These two bands reacted with anti-prothrombin antibodies (fig. 2).

SDS gel electrophoresis showed one single band in B2, with the same mobility as that of normal prothrombin, corresponding to a molecular weight of approximatively 75.000 daltons. In B1, in addition to this band, another one was observed, corresponding to a molecular weight of approximatively 32.000 daltons.

Rechromatography of B2 was carried out under the same conditions in order to determine if B1 could be due to an artefactual conversion of B2 during the chromatographic procedure. Peak B2 was recovered almost

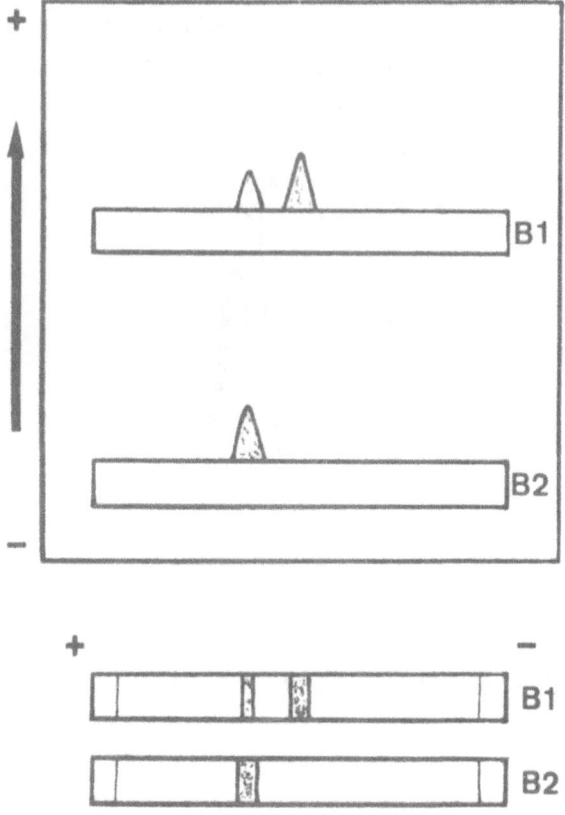

*Fig.* 2. Electrophoretic pattern of abnormal peaks B1 and B2: disc gel electrophoresis below; on the top, subsequent migration in agarose containing antiprothrombin antibodies.

quantitatively in a single peak eluted at the same ionic strength as in the previous chromatography.

Activation studies showed that the material eluted in peak B2 could be converted into thrombin much more slowly than normal prothrombin. Material eluted in peak B1 was unable to generate any thrombin activity (fig. 3).

The same procedures were applied to the plasma of each parent. In both cases two peaks were obtained at the same ionic strength as peaks B1 and B2 respectively. But the amount of material eluted in peak B1 was smaller than observed for the affected children. In the parents, B2 was heterogeneous in disc gel electrophoresis which showed two distinct bands, one migrating as normal prothrombin, the other migrating slightly faster. Activation studies performed on the mother's material showed that the thrombin

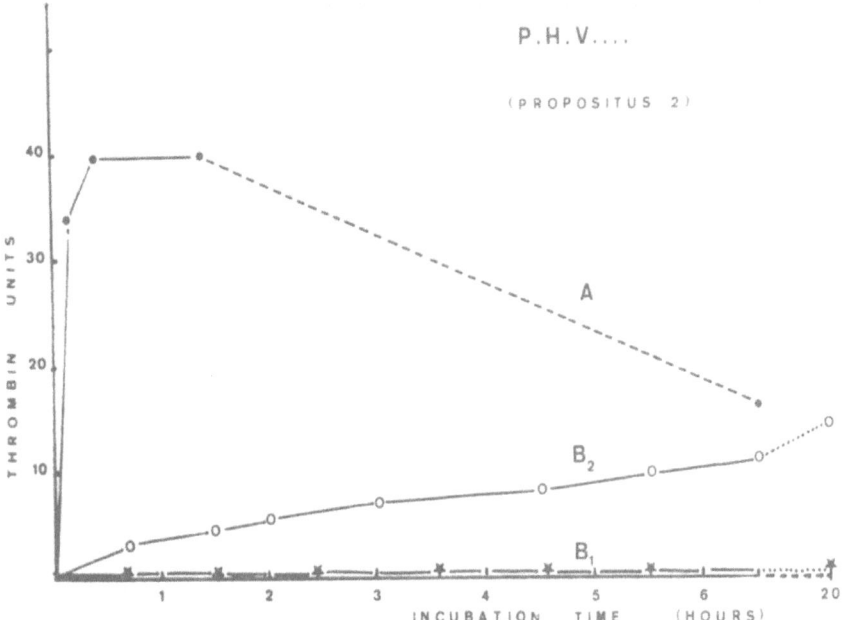

*Fig.* 3. Kinetics of the conversion of prothrombin into thrombin. Activation mixture: R.V.V., phospholipids, human factors X and V, calcium. Proteins eluted in peaks A, B1 and B2 respectively was adjusted to the same concentration in the activation mixture by reference to the immunochemical prothrombin assay.

yield was approximatively 50 per cent lower for B2 than for the normal peak A. In peak B1 no thrombin formation occurred.

In conclusion, from a genetic point of view, these data indicate clearly that the parents are identically heterozygous and the affected children homozygous for the prothrombin Barcelona trait. On the other hand the results of the chromatographic purification of the abnormal component are somewhat disturbing. The material eluted in the major peak obviously represents an abnormal prothrombin molecule. But the significance of the material eluted in the additional peak is not clear up to now. At first sight, it does not seem to be due to an artefactual formation during the purification process. This problem is now being investigated.

REFERENCES

1. Josso, F., J. Monasterio de Sanchez, J. M. Lavergne, D. Menache and J. P. Soulier, Congenital abnormality of the prothrombin molecule (factor II) in four siblings: prothrombin Barcelona. *Blood* 38, 9 (1971).

2. Morrison S. A. and M. P. Esnouf, The nature of the heterogeneity of prothrombin during Dicoumarol therapy. *Nature new biology* 242, 92 (1973).
3. Shapiro, S. S., *Personal communication.*
4. Shapiro, S. S., J. Martinez and R. R. Holburn, Congenital dysprothrombinemia: an inherited structural disorder of human prothrombin. *J. clin. Invest.* 48, 2251 (1969).

# PROTHROMBIN SAN JUAN:
# A COMPLEX NEW DYSPROTHROMBINEMIA

SANDOR S. SHAPIRO

Although genetic abnormalities of the prothrombin molecule had not been observed until five years ago, four dysfunctional variants, Prothrombins Cardeza (1), Barcelona (2), Brussels (3) and Padua (see p. 213), have been reported since that time. The first is a mutant of normal electrophoretic mobility, found so far only in the heterozygous state, the second is an anodally migrating variant, found in several siblings who appear to be homozygotes, and the third is a normal or slightly cathodally migrating protein, again found only in the heterozygous condition. In all families an autosomal mode of inheritance is present. The abnormality of biologic activation of each of these proteins is apparently distinctive.

We have observed a fourth family with genetic dysprothrombinemia present in three generations, in whom the molecular defect is apparently distinct from those previously reported. The hereditary transmission in this family is also autosomal, and we have called this abnormality Prothrombin San Juan. However, further investigation has demonstrated that the genetic defect is more complicated than in the hitherto reported cases. Some of this material has recently been reported elsewhere (4).

The 33 year old propositus of the Prothrombin San Juan defect and his 32 year old sister both have histories since childhood of severe bleeding with operations and dental extractions. Both siblings have required blood transfusions on several occasions; neither has had hemarthroses. In both siblings cessation of bleeding has occurred in response to plasma infusions. Prothrombin levels measured by a two-stage technique (5) are 47 and 39 units per ml, about 15-20% of normal. The other vitamin K dependent factors as well as general liver function studies are within the normal range. Prothrombin times range between 14 and 17 seconds, with controls of 12 seconds. Neither prothrombin level nor prothrombin time responds to vitamin K administration.

Investigation of this large family by two-stage assay revealed six indivi-

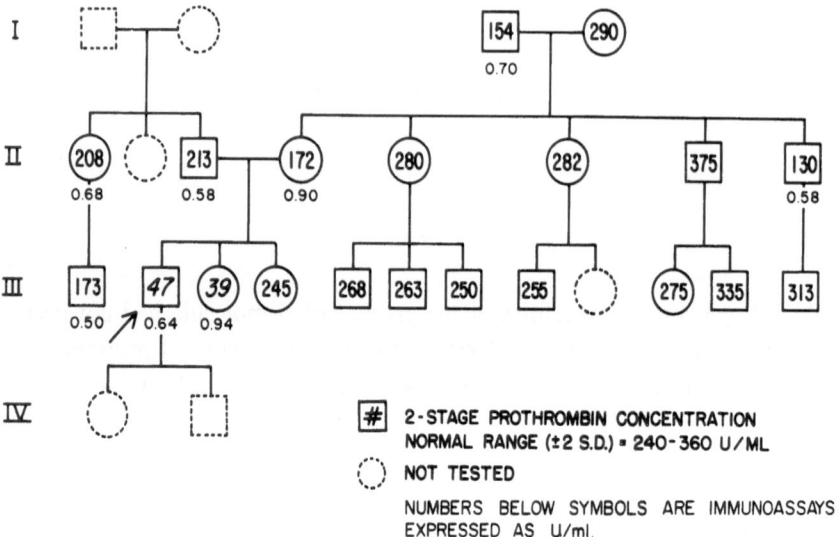

*Fig.* 1. Prothrombin San Juan family pedigree.

duals with prothrombin levels 3 standard deviations or greater below the normal mean – the patient's parents and two relatives in each of their families (fig. 1). Immunoassays were performed both by the Laurell electrophoretic (6) and by the Mancini diffusion (7) techniques so that possible assay variations dependent on molecular charge or size might be discerned. Results expressed in arbitrary units/ml with a normal mean of 1 unit/ml, were identical with both assays. The propositus and his sister have nearly normal amounts of immunoassayable prothrombin, resulting in a very high ratio of immunoassayable to bioassayable prothrombin. Their father and his two affected relatives have immunoassays more or less proportional to their bioassays, while their mother, grandfather and uncle have clearly higher levels by immunoassay than bioassay. These results strongly suggest the existence of two distinct genetic defects in the mother and father.

Crossed antigen-antibody electrophoresis performed on the plasma of the propositus, his mother and father, corroborated these suspicions (fig. 2). The propositus shows a major rapid mobility prothrombin component as well as a significant amount of a second peak of normal or nearly normal mobility. This second peak comprises perhaps 25% of the total immuno-

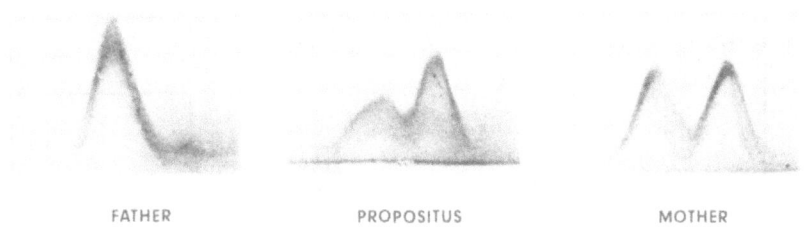

FATHER                    PROPOSITUS                    MOTHER

*Fig.* 2. Crossed immunoelectrophoresis of prothrombin San Juan.

reactive material. The propositus' mother shows two distinct prothrombin peaks of equal size, one of normal mobility and one of anodal mobility. The propositus' father, on the other hand, shows only a single prothrombin band, apparently of normal mobility.

Examination of other family members showed that the propositus' sister has a pattern similar to his, and the mother's and father's affected relatives show patterns identical respectively to their own.

In order to investigate further these anomalous patterns, another technique of prothrombin analysis was utilized. Morrison and Esnouf recently described a DEAE-Sephadex gradient chromatography technique for the purification of prothrombin from small samples of plasma (8). The gradient is a linear salt gradient from 0.15 M to 0.45 M sodium chloride, buffered with tris-citrate, pH 6.5. Almost all the material applied to this column runs through during the initial application, and prothrombin elutes as a single absorbance peak having a relatively constant specific activity of 1300-1400 two-stage units of prothrombin per unit absorbance (fig. 3a). Prothrombin Cardeza plasma cannot be resolved in this system into its normal and abnormal components (fig. 3b). Propositus plasma run in this system, however, shows a clear-cut separation into two prothrombin components (fig. 4). Each of these peaks, when concentrated and re-chromatographed, elutes as an independent entiry at its original elution position.

The major abnormal prothrombin, whose electrophoretic mobility is more anodal than normal prothrombin, is *less* tightly bound to the positively charged DEAE-Sephadex than either normal prothrombin or the second identifiable prothrombin component in the propositus. That neither of these two prothrombin peaks represents normal zymogen can be seen from the specific activity curves. The major peak has no two-stage activity, and the minor peak has greatly diminished specific activity compared to normal. The major peak does activate nearly completely with Echis carinatus venom,

ABSORBANCE
(280 nm)

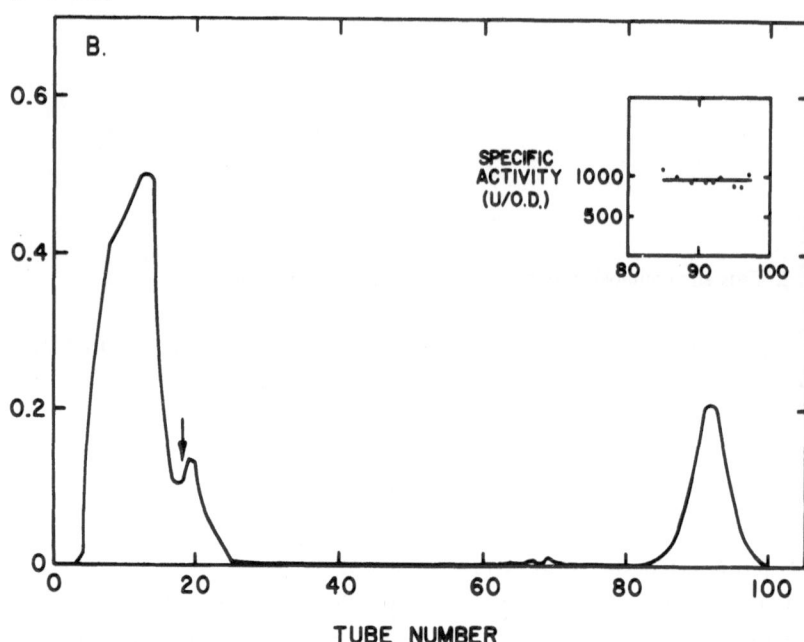

*Fig.* 3a. Column chromatography of normal prothrombin.

ABSORBANCE
( 280 nm )

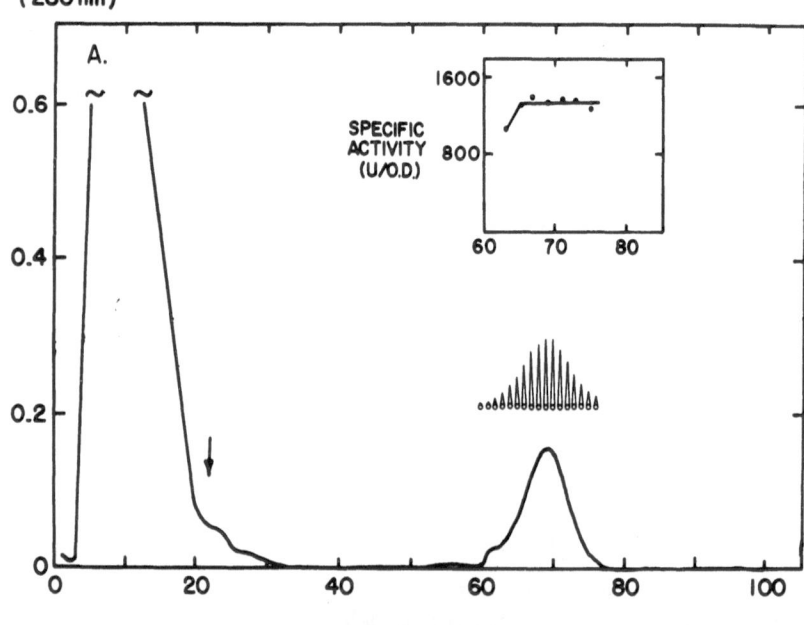

*Fig.* 3b. Column chromatography of prothrombin Cardeza.

ABSORBANCE

(280 nm)

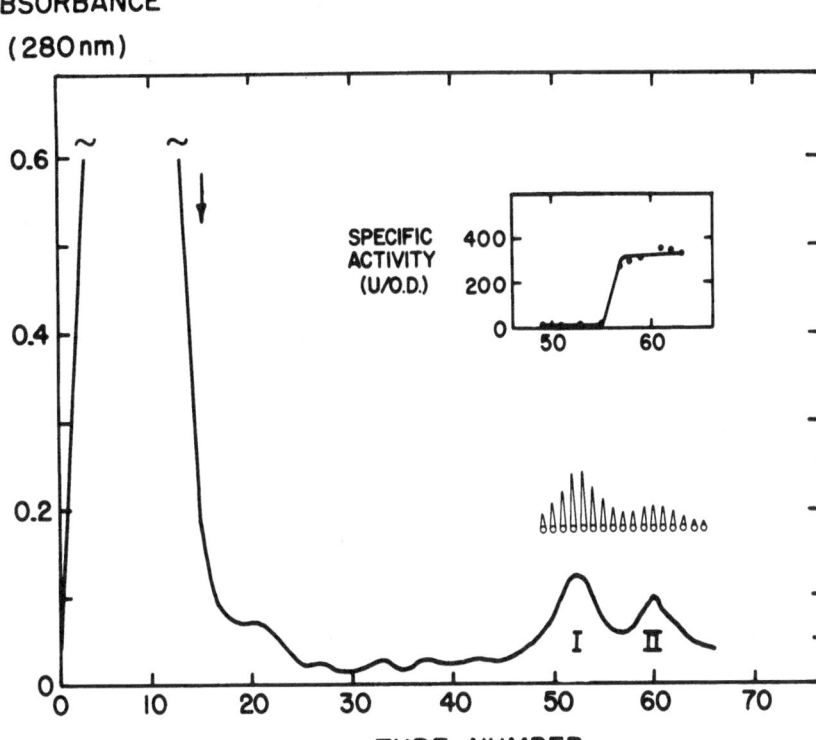

*Fig.* 4. Column chromatography of prothrombin San Juan (propositus).

a direct activator of prothrombin, whereas the minor peak activates to the same extent as with the two-stage assay. As can be seen particularly clearly from the immunochemical assays, the second peak once again represents approximately 25% of the total immunoassayable prothrombin.

Analysis of the mother's plasma is shown in figure 5. Two equal peaks of absorbance and prothrombin immunoreactivity can be identified. The first peak is identical in position and biologic reactivity to the major component seen in the propositus, while the second peak is in the position of normal prothrombin. The two-stage specific activity of this second peak is normal.

Gradient chromatography of the propositus' father's plasma is shown in figure 6. It is clear that the father also possesses two immunoreactive prothrombin components. The major component elutes in a position corresponding to normal prothrombin, but there is an only partially resolved

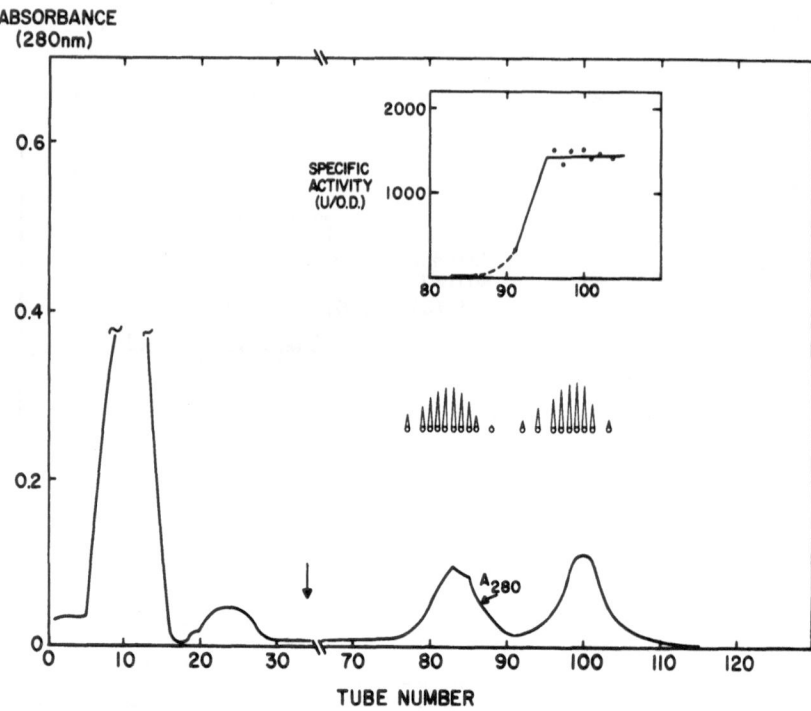

*Fig.* 5. Column chromatography of prothrombin San Juan (mother).

minor component showing as a trailing edge in this chromatogram. Specific activity measurements demonstrate clearly that the trailing edge component is of considerably lower specific activity than normal, while the leading component of the peak has essentially normal specific activity. Thus, each parent synthesizes a distinct abnormal prothrombin, in addition to the normal zymogen. The possibility exists that these two components are in some way interrelated, but experiments with separated and radiolabelled mutant prothrombins have failed to demonstrate any in vivo interconversion during prothrombin activation. These data indicate clearly that the propositus and his sister, although phenotypically homozygous, are genotypically compound heterozygotes for dysprothrombinemia. Not one but two abnormal prothrombins are present. The non-equal distribution of the two gene products in the San Juan propositus may be due to differential rates of synthesis or, as we recently demonstrated for Fibrinogen Philadelphia (9), to different rates of catabolism of the mutant proteins. Resolution of this question requires in vivo metabolic studies which are presently being planned.

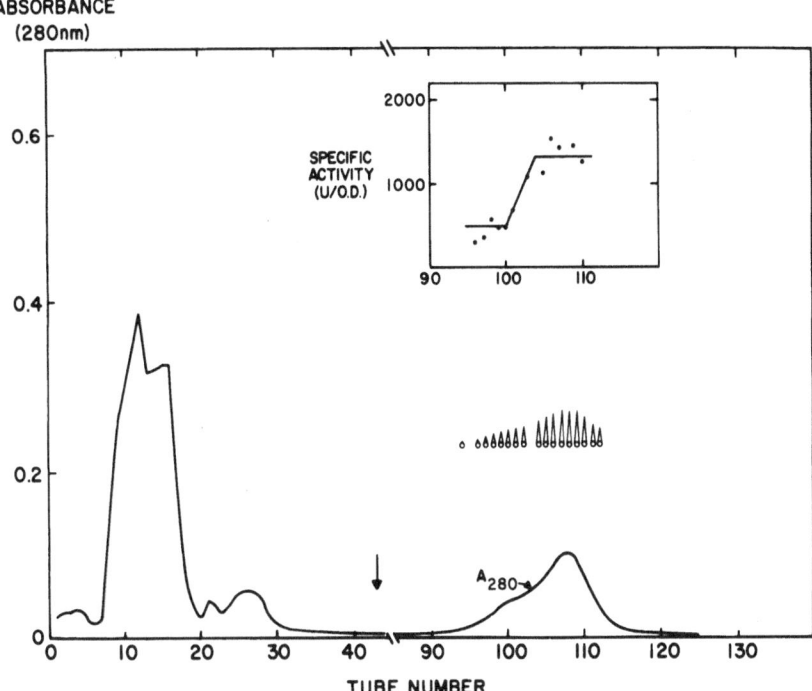

*Fig.* 6. Column chromatography of prothrombin San Juan (father).

Although perhaps not clearly demonstrated previously for a coagulation factor, compound heterozygosity for a mutant protein has been reported in several red cell enzyme deficiencies, and is, of course, well-known in the hemoglobin field.

It appears possible that, for rare mutations at least, the likelihood of two non-related individuals being carriers of the identical mutation may be considerably smaller than the likelihood of their carrying different mutations. The possibility exists, therefore, that other dysproteinemias characterized by absent biological activity may sometimes represent compound heterozygous situations. Since such natural experiments form the basis of a considerable body of our knowledge of structure-function relationships for plasma proteins in general, and blood coagulation factors in particular, the search for single amino acid substitutions in supposedly homozygous individuals must take into account the extra complexities exemplified by this study.

### REFERENCES

1. Shapiro, S. S., J. Martinez and R. R. Holburn, Congenital dysprothrombinemia: an inherited structural disorder of human prothrombin. *J. clin. Invest.* 48, 2251 (1969).
2. Josso, F., J. Monasterio de Sanchez, J. M. Lavergne, D. Menache and J. P. Soulier, Congenital abnormality of the prothrombin molecule (Factor II) in four siblings: prothrombin Barcelona. *Blood* 38, 9 (1971).
3. M. J. P. Kahn, *Abstracts of the IVth International Congress on Thrombosis and Haemostasis.* Abstract No. 228. Vienna (1973).
4. Shapiro, S. S., N. I. Maldonado, J. Fradera and S. McCord, Prothrombin San Juan: a complex new dysprothrombinemia. *J. clin. Invest.* 53, 73A (1974).
5. Shapiro, S. S. and D. F. Waugh, The purification of human prothrombin. *Thrombos. Diathes. haemorrh.* 16, 469 (1966).
6. Laurell, C. B., Quantitative estimation of proteins by electrophoresis in agarose gel containing antibodies. *Anal. Biochem.* 15, 45 (1966).
7. Mancini, G., O. Carbonara and J. F. Heremans, Immunochemical quantitation of antigens by single radial immunodiffusion. *Immunochem.* 2, 235 (1965).
8. Morrison, S. A. and M. P. Esnouf, The nature of the heterogeneity of prothrombin during dicoumarol therapy. *Nature (New Biol.)* 242, 92 (1973).
9. Martinez, J., R. R. Holburn, S. S. Shapiro and A. J. Erslev, Fibrinogen Philadelphia. A hereditary hypodysfibrinogenemia characterized by fibrinogen hypercatabolism. *J. clin. Invest.* 53, 600 (1974).

# PROTHROMBIN PADUA

ANTONIO GIROLAMI

Congenital deficiencies or abnormalities of prothrombin (factor II) are rare coagulation disorders. Only about 25 patients have been described to have congenital true hypoprothrombinemia (1, 2, 6) and only three dysprothrombinemias were so far recognized (4, 7, 8) whereas a fourth one is being investigated (5).

We have recently studied a new congenital dysprothrombinemia and wish to present here some data concerning such an abnormality which has been

☒ or ◉ = affected, symptomatic or asymptomatic, male and female ; □ or ○ = studied, normal ; ⊞ or ⊕ = not studied, asymptomatic, normal ?; ⊞ or ⊕ = deceased, asymptomatic, normal ?.

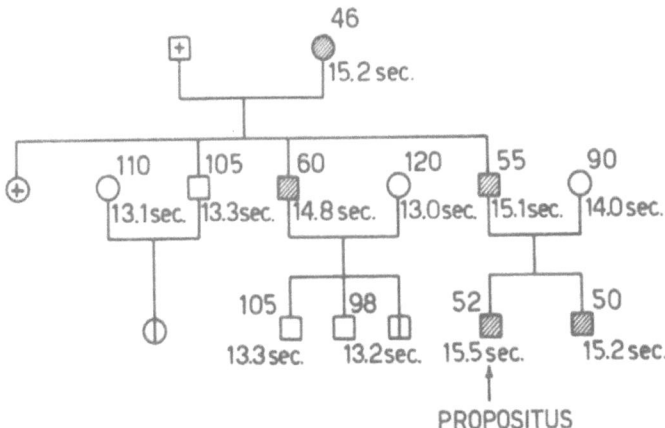

*Fig.* 1. Family pedigree. All affected members are indicated by hatching of the circles or squares. The upper numbers reported on the left or right side of each circle or square refer the one stage factor II level. The lower numbers refer to the prothrombin time in seconds. Two sisters of the paternal grandmother were also found to be affected bringing the total to 7 patients.

termed Prothrombin Padua (3). 6 members of a family are affected besides the propositus. Three of them are mildly symptomatic, whereas the other four are so far asymptomatic. The propositus is a 7 year old child who bled excessively after a tonsillectomy (fig. 1).

The parents of the propositus are not related. All patients seem to be heterozygous for the abnormality.

Prothrombin activity in the propositus and in the other affected family members, varies between 32 and 52% in several one-stage or two stage systems. The lowest level (32% of normal) is obtained using the Taipan viper venom.

The staphylocoagulase-complexed prothrombin level, on the contrary, is normal (table 1).

*Table* 1. Prothrombin assay in the propositus using different techniques. Similar values were observed in the other relatives affected.

| Method | Prothrombin level in % of normal | Thromboplastin |
|---|---|---|
| Classical one stage method | 52% | human brain |
| Iowa two-stage method | 48% | id. |
| Oxford two-stage method | 50% | id. |
| Hjort's method | 47% | id. |
| Jobin and Esnouf' method (modified) | 44% | Tiger snake venom (Notechis scutatus scutatus). Taipan viper |
| Taipan Viper venom method | 32% | venom (Oxyuranus scutellatus). |
| Staphylocoagulase method | 105% | |
| Radial Immunodiffusion method | 100% | |

Immunologically prothrombin results are also normal in several assay systems (fig. 2, 3, 4). A line of identity with normal prothrombin is seen on immunodiffusion. The immunoelectrophoretic mobility of Prothrombin Padua in plasma is identical to that of normal prothrombin both in the standard immunoelectrophoresis and in the bidimensional immunoelectrophoresis (fig. 5 and 6). The same is true after addition of calcium to the buffer.

The main feature of Prothrombin Padua seems to lie in an abnormal fragmentation of the prothrombin molecule during clotting.

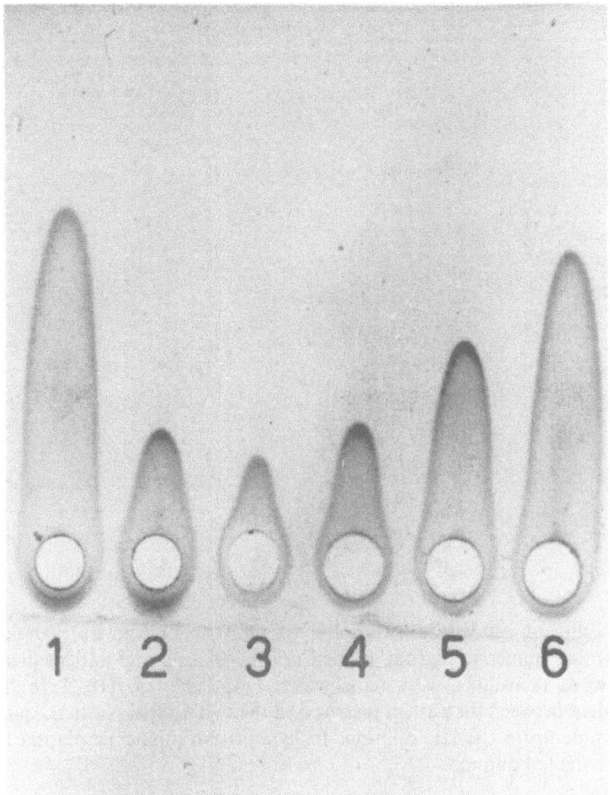

*Fig.* 2. Electroimmunoassay according to the Laurell's technique. Well n° 1 contains 1:2 diluted patient plasma; well n° 2 contains undiluted hypoprothrombinemic plasma, wells 3, 4, 5 and 6 contain Dade normal plasma diluted 1:16, 1:8, 1:4, and 1:2, respectively.

Serum immunoelectrophoresis reveals the presence of three separate precipitates as compared to a single, irregular band seen in normal serum. One of the three peaks seen in the patient serum appears equivalent to the normal ,,pro-piece'': of the other two precipitates, one is more anodal and one is more cathodal in position, as compared to the ,,pro-piece'' (fig. 7).

In the Clarke-Freeman bidimensional immunoelectrophoresis five distinct bands are evident as compared with 3 bands normally seen in normal serum.

The three peaks normally seen in normal serum are termed A, B and C. Two of the peaks (A and C) seen in propositus serum are similar to their normal counterparts. The second normal peak or precipitate (B) is absent and is substituted, in the patient serum, by three abnormal precipitates

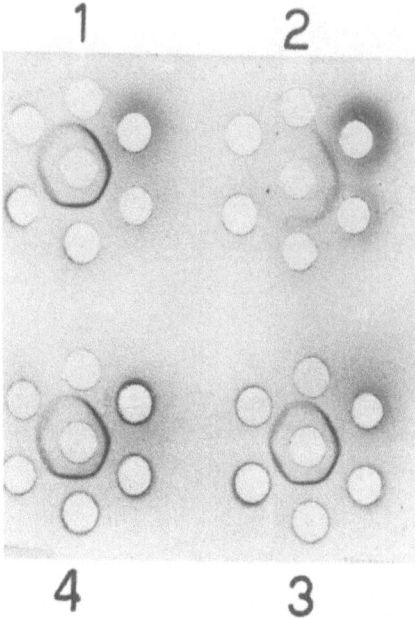

*Fig.* 3. Immunodiffusion studies in (from left to right and clockwise): Dade normal plasma, hypoprothrombinemic plasma, pooled normal plasma and patient plasma. The dilutions used in each instance were (clockwise): 1:1, 1:2, 1:4, 1:8, 1:16, 1:32. No difference is evident between the patient plasma and the two normal plasmas. In all cases a precipitate is visible up to the last dilution. In hypoprothrombinemic plasma a band is visible only up to the 1:4 dilution.

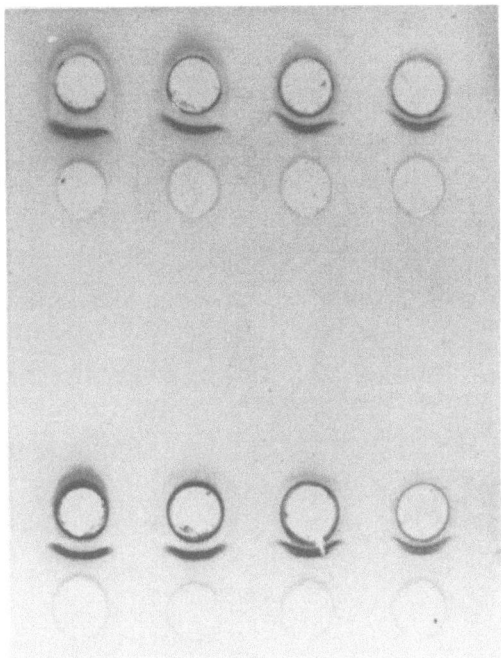

*Fig.* 4. Cross-over electrophoresis (electrosyneresis) of patient plasma (top) and Dade normal plasma (bottom). No difference between the two plasmas was noted in any of the dilutions used (1:1, 1:2, 1:4 and 1:8).

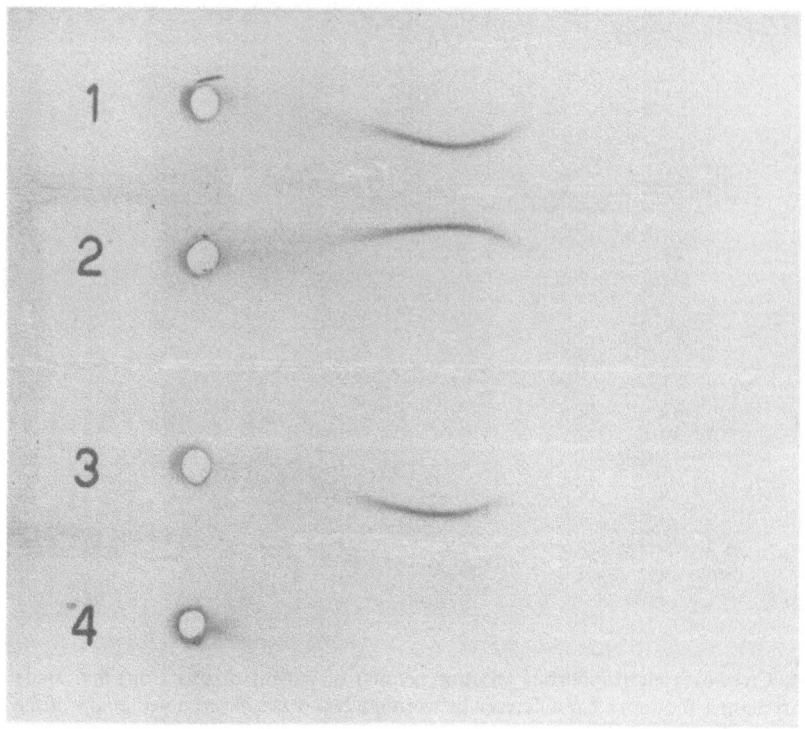

*Fig.* 5. Immunoelectrophoresis of: 1) pooled normal plasma; 2) patient plasma; 3) Dade normal plasma and 4) hypoprothrombinemic plasma. In 4 the band is absent or barely visible. The addition of calcium to the buffer had no effect on the shape or mobility of the propositus prothrombin band as compared to the normal counterparts.

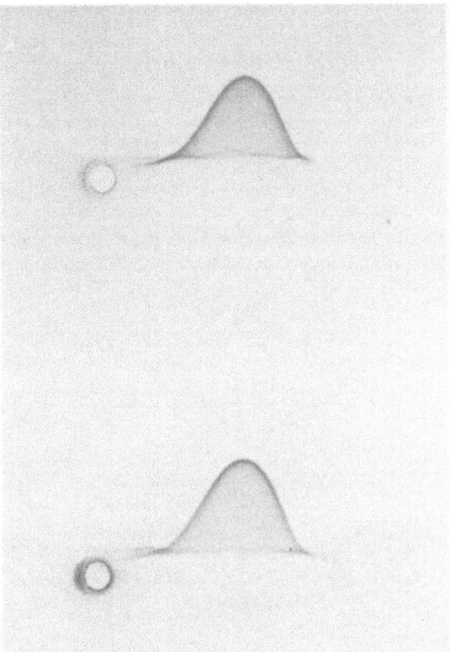

*Fig.* 6. Bidimensional immunoelectrophoresis of patient plasma (top) and of pooled normal plasma (bottom). No difference in mobility is noted.

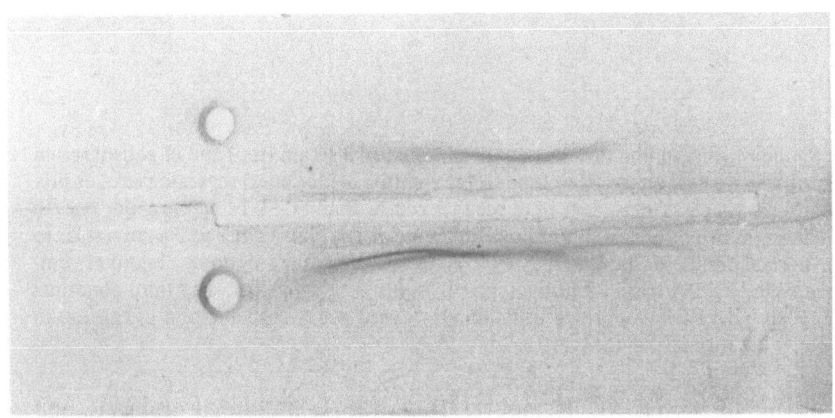

*Fig.* 7. Immunoelectrophoresis of normal serum and patient serum. Only one band, even though somewhat irregular, is seen in normal serum (upper run). In patient serum; on the contrary, three distinct bands are visible (lower run). One of these bands is approximately equivalent to the normal 'pro-piece'; of the other two, one is more cathodal and one more anodal in position.

The addition of calcium to the buffer did not alter the pattern obtained as compared to the normal counterparts.

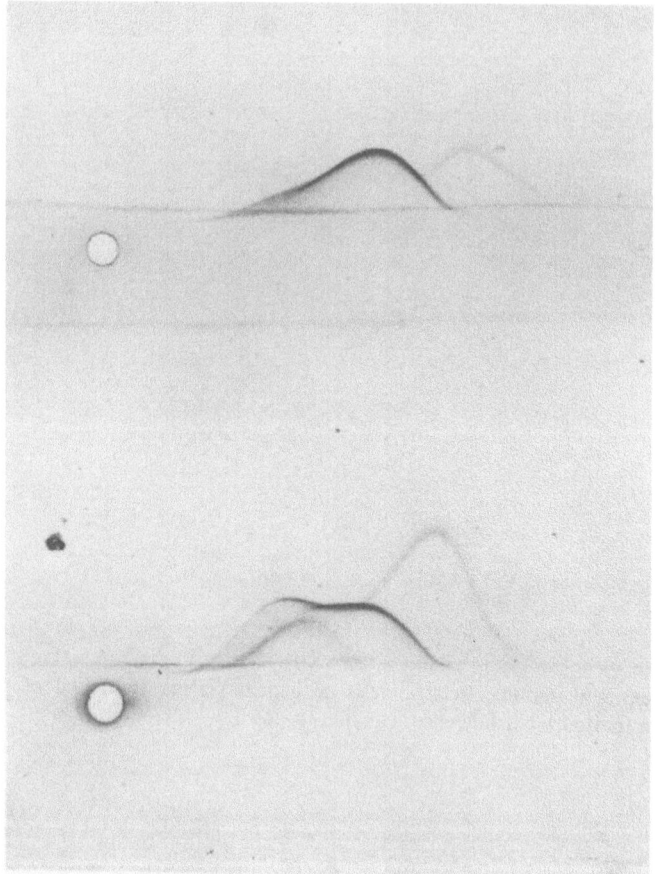

*Fig.* 8. Bidimensional immunoelectrophoresis of normal serum (top) and of patient serum
(bottom). In normal serum three (one major and two lighter ones) separate peaks or precipitates are visible. These peaks have been termed A, B and C; B being the major one. In
patient serum five distinct peaks or precipitates are visible. The lighter peaks are similar to
their normal counterparts. The major precipitate is substituted by three abnormal components ($B_1$, $B_2$, $B_3$) two of which ($B_1$ and $B_3$) seem fused together. The third abnormal
component ($B_2$) is circumscribed below the two fused peaks. The addition of calcium to
the buffer has no effect on the pattern.

which may be termed $B_1$, $B_2$ and $B_3$. Two of these abnormal peaks ($B_1$ and
$B_3$) appear to be partially fused together, whereas the second one ($B_2$) is
circumscribed below the two fused peaks (fig. 8).

Prothrombin Padua seems to be different from the other dysprothrombinemias. The main distinctive features of the five dysprothrombinemias so
far described are shown in table 2.

*Table 2.* Main features of the dysprothrombinemias so far studied.

| Anomaly | Patients described | Factor II biological activity | Factor II immunological assay | Staphylocoagulase factor II assay | Immunoelectrophoresis plasma | Immunoelectrophoresis serum | Effect Ca++ | Bleeding tendency | Comment |
|---|---|---|---|---|---|---|---|---|---|
| Prothrombin Cardeza (Shapiro et al.) | Probably heterozygotes | about 50% | normal | ? | normal band | normal 'propiece' band with abnormal cathodal extension | ? | No (1) | (1) Bleeding manifestations were present in two patients who had Ehlers-Danlos syndrome and (one case) associated factor VIII deficiency |
| Prothrombin Barcelona (Josso et al) | Homozygotes & heterozygotes | 4-13% | normal | normal | anodal band | ? | No effect | Yes | |
| Prothrombin San Juan (Shapiro et al.) | Homozygotes & heterozygotes | 15-20% | normal | normal | anodal band | anodal band | decreased binding capacity | Yes | |
| Prothrombin Padua (Girolami et al.) | Probably heterozygotes | 32-52% | normal | normal | normal band | normal 'propiece' band + 2 abnormal bands (one cathodal and one anodal) | No effect | Yes | |
| Prothrombin Brussels (Kahn et al) | Probably heterozygotes | 35-50% | near-normal | 50% of normal | normal band | two bands in normal 'propiece' area | No effect | Yes | |

222 A. GIROLAMI

## REFERENCES

1. Girolami A., A. Sticchi, M. Lazzarin and R. Scarpa, Congenital hypoprothrombinemia. Case report. *Acta haemat.* 44, 164 (1970).
2. Girolami A., The hereditary transmission of true congenital hypoprothrombinemia. *Brit. J. Haemat.* 21, 695 (1971).
3. Girolami A., G. Bareggi, A. Brunetti and A. Sticchi, Prothrombin Padua: a 'new' congenital dysprothrombinemia. *J. Lab. clin. Med.* 84, 654 (1974).
4. Josso F., J. Monasterio de Sanchez, J. M. Lavergne D. Menachè and J. P. Soulier, Congenital abnormality of the prothrombin molecule (factor II) in four siblings: Prothrombin Barcelona. *Blood* 38, 9 (1971).
5. Kahn M. J. P., *Personal Communication.* March 1974.
6. Pina-Cabral J. M. and B. Justiça, Congenital hypoprothrombinemia in a Portuguese family. *Thrombos. Diathes. Haemorrh.* 30, 451 (1973).
7. Shapiro S., J. Martinez and R. H. Holburn, Congenital dysprothrombinemia: an inherited structural disorder of human prothrombin. *J. clin. Invest.* 48, 2251 (1969).
8. Shapiro S. S., M. Maldonado and J. Fradera, *Prothrombin San Juan: a third congenital dysprothrombinemia.* Abstracts, Meeting Int. Soc. Thromb. Haemost., pag. 227. Vienna (1973).

# PROTHROMBIN BRUSSELS

M. J. P. KAHN

## INTRODUCTION

Antibodies to normal human prothrombin can recognize two groups in congenital hypoprothrombinemia: with and without an immunologically reactive protein (1, 2, 3). This protein has common antigenic determinants with normal prothrombin but lacks the capacity to be converted into thrombin. Prothrombin Cardeza (4) and prothrombin Barcelona (5) were the first congenitally abnormal protein to be described. A congenital defective prothrombin was found in a Brussels family. This family (fig. 1) involves the parents and eleven children; none of them but the propositus ($II_3$), has any clinical hemostasis disorder. The parents are known to be related but the extent of this consanguinity was impossible to determine.

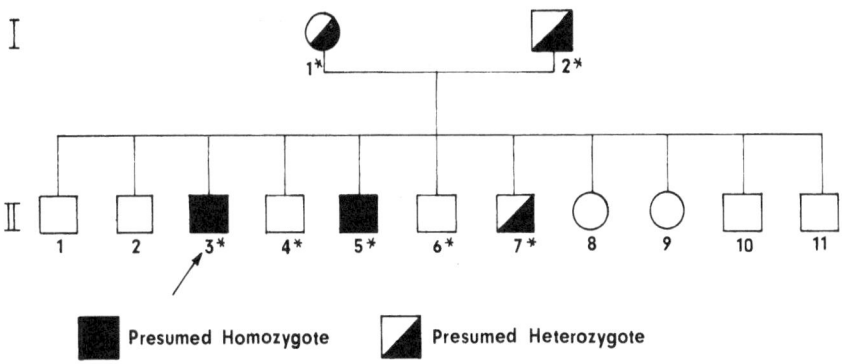

*Fig.* 1. Pedigree of a family with congenital dysprothrombinemia. The propositus is marked by an arrow. The asterisks indicate the members of the family who were studied.

## Materials and methods

The one stage and two stage measurements were carried out according to Hemker et al. (6, 7, 8, 9).

*The immunochemical methods* were performed according to Shapiro (10) and Laurell (11). In our hands, the electroimmunoassay showed a reproducibility of $\pm 16\%$.

*Staphylocoagulase reactive material* was assayed according to the method proposed by Josso et al. (12), using reagents obtained from the Stago Laboratories. This method has a reproducibility of $\pm 3\%$, in our laboratory.

## CLINICAL MATERIAL

The propositus, a 22 year old male was referred with a traumatic haemarthrosis which needed surgical care. The coagulation factors I, V, VII, VIII, IX, X, XI, and XII, assessed by one stage determinations were within normal range but prothrombin showed an abnormally low value. Tests of liver function were within the normal limits. Surgery was carried out under constant infusion of a concentrated prothrombin complex prepared according to Soulier (13). This substitution therapy was continued for 10 days and recovery was uneventful.

*Table* 1. Prothrombin estimations in propositus' plasma.

|  | Normal range value | Propositus |
|---|---|---|
| One stage clotting assay (sec.) |  |  |
| Prothrombinase | 24,8—26,3 | 40,2 (20%) |
| Echis carinatus venom | 14,2—18,6 | 63,9 (10%) |
| (500 µg/ml) |  |  |
| Taipan snake venom | 18,8—22,6 | 35,9 (27%) |
| (5 µg/ml) |  |  |
| Staphylocoagulase | 36,9—40,7 | 46,5 (50%) |
| (250 U CNTS/ml) |  |  |
| Two stage clotting assay (NIH U Thrombin/ml) |  |  |
| Prothrombinase | 246—273 | 119 (48%) |
| Echis carinatus venom | 60,5—66,5 | 20 (32%) |
| (500 µg/ml) |  |  |
| Taipan snake venom | 245—270 | 160 (64%) |
| (5 µg/ml) |  |  |
| Staphylocoagulase | 297—338 | 300 (93%) |
| (250 U CNTS/ml) |  |  |
| Trypsin (1 mg/ml) | 480—517 | 510 (100%) |
| Immunochemical assay % of normal | 52—110 | 71 |

RESULTS

The results of different prothrombin estimations are shown in table 1. The one stage prothrombin assays (prothrombinase, Echis carinatus venom, Taipan snake venom and staphylocoagulase) reveal about half the normal amount of prothrombin. The two stage prothrombin assays with prothrombinase, Echis carinatus venom and Taipan snake venom reveal about half the normal amount of prothrombin but a normal amount of prothrombin was found when the propositus' prothrombin was activated by staphylocoagulase or trypsin.

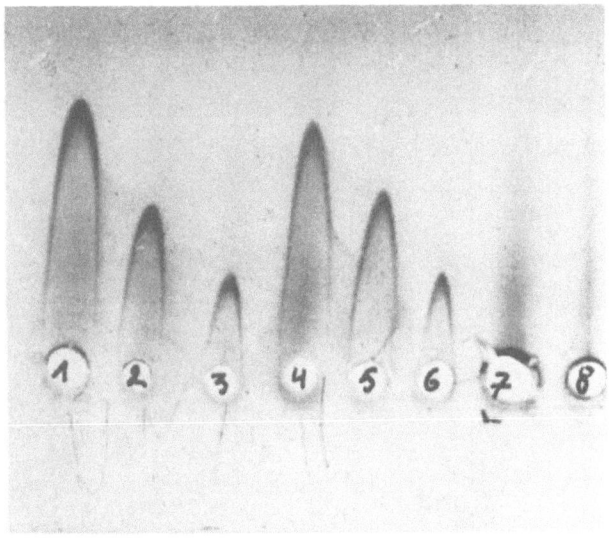

*Fig.* 2. Immunoassay of the propositus' plasma prothrombin by Laurell's quantitative method. Sample volumes were 8 μl. Wells 1→3 normal pooled plasma and wells 4→6 propositus' plasma undiluted and diluted 1:2 and 1:4. Wells 7 and 8 normal and propositus' plasma after adsorption with 10% BaSO₄ (W/V) undiluted.

Laurell's electrophoresis technique using an antibody against a normal human prothrombin showed 71% of the normal amount of precipitating molecule (fig. 2). No immunochemically reactive protein could be demonstrated in the propositus' plasma adsorbed with 2.5% (W/V) Al (OH)₃ or 10% (W/V) BaSO₄ (fig. 2).

Qualitative double diffusion experiments and immunoelectrophoresis (fig. 3) of the propositus' plasma demonstrated identity between the propositus' and normal prothrombin. Table 2 indicates that the clotting process

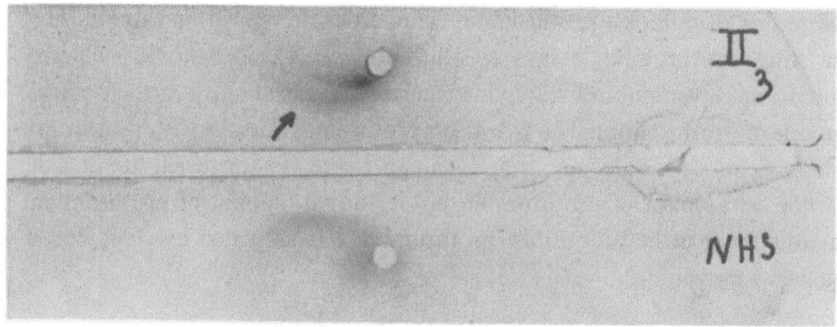

*Fig.* 3a.

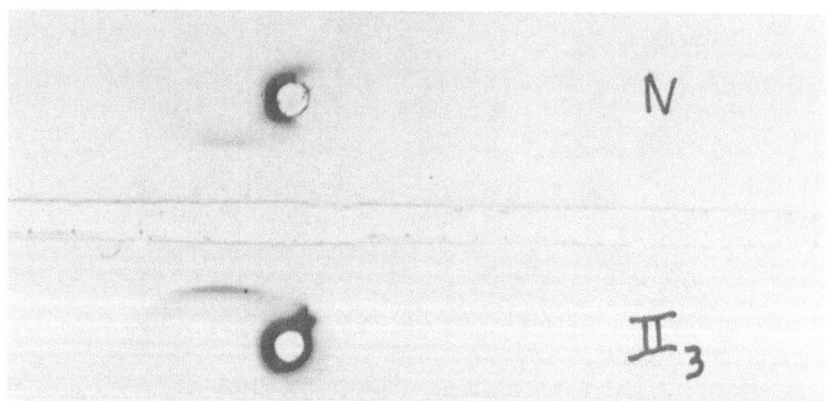

*Fig.* 3. Immunoelectrophoresis performed with antiserum to human prothrombin, of normal and propositus' serum (NHS), the propositus' (II₃) serum in presence of Ca⁺⁺ (2.5 mM calcium lactate).

seems to change the abnormal prothrombin molecule, it enables seric derivatives of prothrombin to produce thrombin-coagulase. In the serum, obtained by spontaneous clotting, the ratio of the staphylocoagulase reactive material to the prothrombin concentration, estimated in the one or two stage tests with prothrombinase, Echis carinatus venom or Taipan snake venom, increases significantly (table 2).

Immunoelectrophoresis of the propositus' serum against antiprothrom-

*Table* 2. Prothrombin activity in propositus' serum

| | One stage (sec.) | | Two stage (NIH U Thrombin/ml) | |
|---|---|---|---|---|
| | Propositus | Normal | Propositus | Normal |
| Prothrombinase | 48 (5%) | >95 (<0,5%) | 7,2 (3%) | <2,5 (<0,9%) |
| Echis carinatus venom (500 µg/ml) | 212 (1,2%) | >143 (<2%) | 1,2 (0,5%) | <1 (<0,5%) |
| Taipan snake venom (5 µg/ml) | 38 (2,3%) | >48 (1%) | 9 (3,6%) | <5 (<2%) |
| Staphylocoagulase (250 U CNTS/ml) | 45 (57%) | >140 (3%) | 130 (52%) | <2,5 (<1%) |

Serum was obtained by spontaneous clotting and incubation for 24 h at 37 °C.
One stage assays were performed on sera diluted 1:2. Figures in brackets indicate activities relative to normal pooled plasma.

bin antiserum in the presence of Ca ions shows a double line in the prothrombin region (fig. 3).

The *study of the family* revealed that one brother ($II_7$) has a low (56%) and another ($II_5$) a very low prothrombin level (27%).

The Laurell technique showed variable but normal amounts of the precipitable molecule in other family members.

Immunoelectrophoresis, with antiserum to human prothrombin, of sera from the parents ($I_1$, $I_2$) and a brother ($II_5$) showed a second but weak line of precipitation. The staphylocoagulase reactive material as estimated in serum using the one stage test, was significantly increased in the mother $I_1$ (32%) and the two brothers $II_5$ (14%) and $II_7$ (16%).

DISCUSSION

The propositus' disorder was suspected of being a prothrombin deficiency because of the low level of factor II and normal levels of the other factors.

The one stage determinations of factors II, V, VII, IX and X showed a slightly higher activity when tested at high dilutions than at lower dilutions. This indicates a small inhibitor effect. This effect was neither of the progressive type nor of the immediate type. Clotting times plotted against dilutions indicated that the observed inhibition was most likely competitive (14).

The propositus' plasma contained 71% cross-reacting material in an assay against prothrombin antiserum as compared to a pooled normal standard. This result based on 6 assays was not significantly different from values found in repeated assays of normal plasma (n = 6, t = 1.47, P = 0.20-0.10). However, the 50% staphylocoagulase one stage clotting assay mean value (n = 12) for plasma prothrombin activity is significantly lower than that of the pool of normal plasma (n = 22) (t = 13.7 P < 0.001). But an incubation of 30 min. at 37°C of staphylocoagulase with the propositus' plasma demonstrated a normal level of staphylocoagulase reactive material. This indicated that the abnormal prothrombin had a low sensitivity to staphylocoagulase activation.

Immunoelectrophoresis of the propositus' serum against anti human prothrombin antibodies revealed an abnormal pattern: a double line was observed in the prothrombin region in the presence of calcium ions only. The abnormal pattern of the propositus' serum immunoelectrophoresis indicates the presence of abnormal prothrombin seric derivatives (10) because the prothrombin antiserum used recognizes common antigenic sites in the prothrombin seric derivatives and in prothrombin.

Techniques used do not indicate that the propositus' plasma contains normal and abnormal prothrombin molecules as is the case with patients having prothrombin Cardeza (4). The fact that the parents $(I_1, I_2)$ have some prothrombin abnormalities suggests that the propositus is homozygous for the defect. The inheritance of the defect seems then to be autosomal recessive. The family members $(I_1, I_2, II_7, II_5)$ are clinically normal but their sera contain abnormally high amounts of staphylocoagulase reactive products $(I_1, II_5, II_7)$ and present an abnormal electrophoretic pattern similar to that of the propositus $(I_1, I_2, II_5)$.

The properties of this abnormal prothrombin molecule can be summarized as follows: it presents a low sensitivity to prothrombinase, Echis carinatus venom and Taipan snake venom but a normal sensitivity to trypsin activation. Only after a long incubation time is the activation by staphylocoagulase of this prothrombin normal. Its concentration in the plasma as judged by immunoprecipitation is normal. The seric derivatives of this prothrombin have an abnormal pattern demonstrated by immunoelectrophoresis in presence of calcium ions.

## REFERENCES

1. Girolani, A., A. Sticchi, M. Lazzarini and R. Scampa, Congenital hypoprothrombinemia. *Acta haemat.* 44, 164 (1970).
2. Baudo, F., F. de Cataldo, F. Josso and L. Silvello, Hereditary hypoprothrombinemia. *Acta haemat.* 47, 243 (1972).
3. Kattlove, H. E., S. S. Shapiro and M. Spivack, Hereditary prothrombin deficiency. *New Engl. J. Med.* 282, 57 (1970).

4. Shapiro, S. S., J. Martinez and R. R. Holburn, Congenital dysprothrombinemia and inherited structural disorder of human prothrombin. *J. clin. Invest.* 48, 2251 (1969).
5. Josso, F., J. Monsaterio de Sanchez, J. M. Lavergne, D. Menache and J. P. Soulier, Congenital abnormality of the prothrombin molecule in four siblings. Prothrombin Barcelona. *Blood* 38, 9 (1971).
6. Hemker, H. C., A. C. W. Swart and A. J. M. Alink, Artificial reagents for factor VII and factor X, a computer programme for obtaining reference tables for one stage determination in the extrinsic system. *Thrombos. Diathes. haemorrh.* 27, 205 (1972).
7. Hemker, H. C., A. D. Muller and E. A. Loeliger, Two types of prothrombin in vitamin K deficiency. *Thrombos. Diathes. haemorrh.* 23, 633 (1970).
8. Hemker H. C., P. W. Hemker, K. van der Torren, P. P. Devilee, W. Th. Hermens and E. A. Loeliger, The evaluation of the two stage prothrombin assay. *Thrombos. Diathes. haemorrh.* 25, 545 (1971).
9. Hemker, H. C., E. A. Loeliger and J. J. Veltkamp, *Human blood coagulation.* Leiden University Press, Leiden p. 152 (1969).
10. Shapiro, S. S., Human prothrombin activation immunochemical study. *Science* 162, 127 (1968).
11. Laurell, C. B., Quantitative estimation of proteins by electrophoresis in agarose gel containing antibodies. *Anal. Biochem.* 15, 45 (1966).
12. Josso, F., J. M. Lavergne, M. Gouault, O. Prou Wartelle and J. P. Soulier, Différents états moléculaires du facteur II (prothrombine). Leur étude à l'aide de la staphyloco-agulase et d'anticorps anti-facteur II. I. Le facteur II chez les sujets traités par les antagonistes de la vitamine K. *Thrombos. Diathes. haemorrh.* 20, 88 (1968).
13. Soulier, J. P., D. Menache, M. Steinbuch, C. Blatrix and F. Josso, Preparation and clinical use of P.P.S.B. (factor II, VII, X and IX concentrate). *Thrombos. Diathes. haemorrh.* 35, 61 (1969).
14. Hemker, H. C. and A. D. Muller, Kinetic aspects of the interaction of blood-clotting enzymes VI. Localisation of the site of blood-coagulation. Inhibition by the protein induced by vitamin K absence (PIVKA). *Thrombos. Diathes. haemorrh.* 20, 78 (1968).
15. Engel, A. M. and B. Alexander, Molecular changes during prothrombin activation. *Biochim. biophys. Acta,* 320, 687 (1973).
16. Engel, A. M. and B. Alexander, Studies of thrombin formation with an insoluble derivative of prothrombin. *J. biol. Chem.* 246, 1213 (1971).
17. Seegers, W. H., G. Murano and L. McCoy, Structural changes in prothrombin during activation: A theory. *Thrombos. Diathes. haemorrh.* 23, 26 (1970).
18. Tishoff, G. H. Proteolytic digestion of purified bovine prothrombin: formation of active fragments. *Thrombos. Diathes haemorrh.* 10, 390 (1964).

# FACTOR X FRIULI[1]

ANTONIO GIROLAMI

Classical factor X deficiency was first recognized in 1956 and in 1957 (22, 25).

A congenital coagulation disorder due to the presence of an abnormal factor X was described by us in 1969-1970 (4, 5, 6). Since all original patients came from an isolated valley of the northeastern italian region called Friuli, it was attached to the condition as an eponym (6, 9, 16). Friuli inhabitants are both of celtic and latin extraction.

Recently a patient with a different geographical background was described bringing the total to 11 homozygote cases (14). About 60 heterozygotes have been studied too (17). The disease is transmitted, like classical factor X deficiency, as an autosomal incompletely recessive trait (6, 7, 8, 21, 23, 24). All homozygous patients show invariably a moderate bleeding tendency, bleeding manifestations are minor and rare in the heterozygote population, however (17). Factor X Friuli may not be activated or may be activated only very slowly by tissue thromboplastins complete as well as partial whereas it may still be normally activated by Russell's viper venom (RVV). Consequently partial thromboplastin and prothrombin times are both prolonged whereas the Stypven-Cephalin clotting time is normal in these patients. The thromboplastin generation test is abnormal even when a RVV-Cephalin solution is included in the generation mixture. This suggest that the RVV is capable of compensating for the defect only as far as the conversion of prothrombin to thrombin is concerned but not for the genesis of intrinsic thromboplastin (fig. 1) (4, 5, 6, 9).

Factor X in Friuli patients is low when assayed using a tissue thromboplastin, whereas it is normal when assayed using a RVV-Cephalin mixture (12).

Other 'Thromboplastins' such Trypsin, Bothrops atrox venom and vipera aspis venom seem to activate factor X Friuli to an intermediate level (table 1).

It is interesting to note that all these activating agents seem to be capable

1. This study was supported in part by a grant from the C.N.R. (grant CT 73.00599.04)

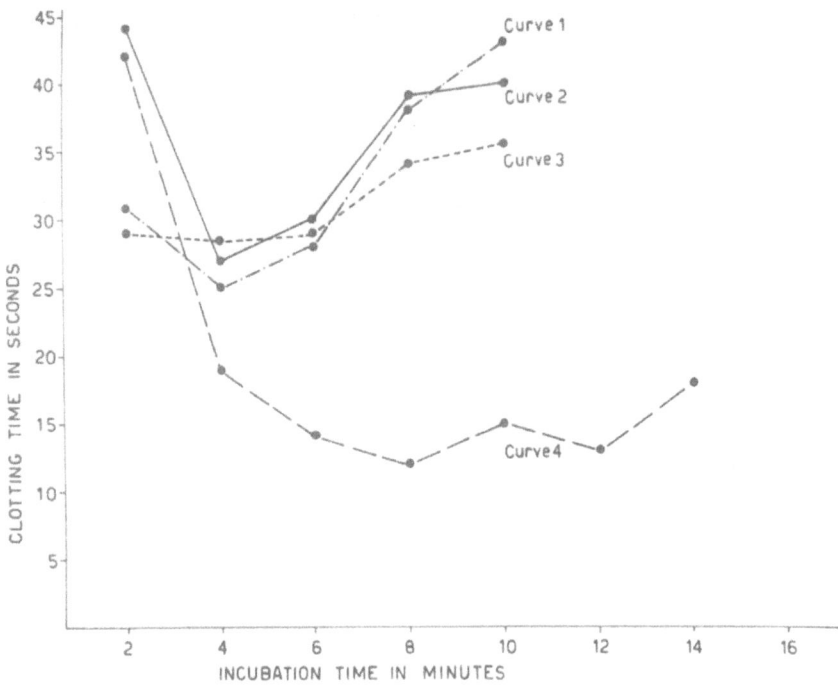

*Fig.* 1. Thromboplastin generation test in a patient with the factor X Friuli coagulation disorder. The composition of the generation mixtures were as follows:

| Curve | Adsorbed plasma | Serum | Phospholipid |
|---|---|---|---|
| 1 | normal | patient | platelin |
| 2 | patient | patient | platelin |
| 3 | patient | patient | Stypven-Cephalin |
| 4 | patient | normal | platelin |

*Table* 1. Factor X level in Friuli patients as determined using different 'thromboplastins'.

| Thromboplastins | Factor X level | Comment |
|---|---|---|
| Tissue complete Thromboplastins | 3,5-14% | Extremes of several determinations carried out using different thromboplastins. |
| Tissue partial Thromboplastins | 4-10% | idem |
| Stypven-Cephalin mixture | 60-100% | idem |
| Trypsin | 35-40% | |
| Vipera Aspis | 40-45% | Kindly supplied by Dr. Boquet |
| Bothrops atrox (thromboplastin fraction) | 43-50% | Kindly supplied by Stago Laboratories. |
| Thermolysin | 35-45% | |

of activating factor X Friuli to a similar extent. Values of about 45% activity have been obtained in all instances. The nature of the defect lies in an abnormal activation of factor X via the extrinsic and intrinsic pathways. No concomitant abnormalities or defects are present in the plasma of these patients. Specifically factors II, VII and IX are normal both as activity and as antigen.

However, prothrombin results in a two-stage system are normal only after the addition of an aliquot of normal serum to the system (fig. 2) (10).

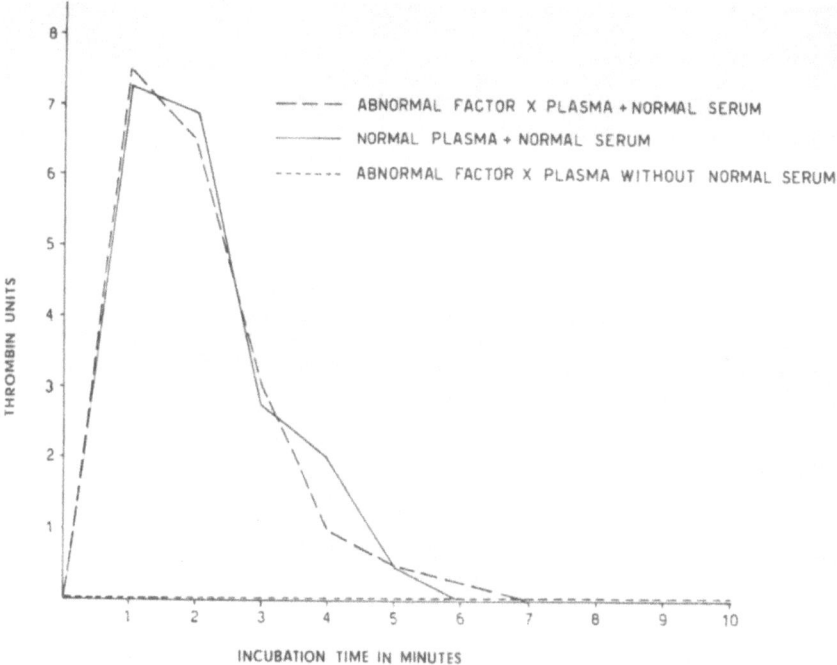

*Fig.* 2. Oxford two-stage prothrombin assay in Friuli plasma. If no normal serum is added to the system no thrombin is generated. After the addition of normal serum a normal curve is obtained.

The Thermolysin factor X activation is abnormal too. In a specific activation experiment both a delayed activation and a defective yield is obtained (fig. 3). However, as activation proceeds the difference between normal and Friuli plasma seems to decrease. These results are of interest since it seems that thermolysin, a non-specific broad enzyme, acts on amide substitution rather than on the carboxyl side of the peptide bond (1).

Factor X Friuli has a peculiar behavior when assayed in serum. Using tissue thromboplastins, factor X is approximately as low as in plasma; using a

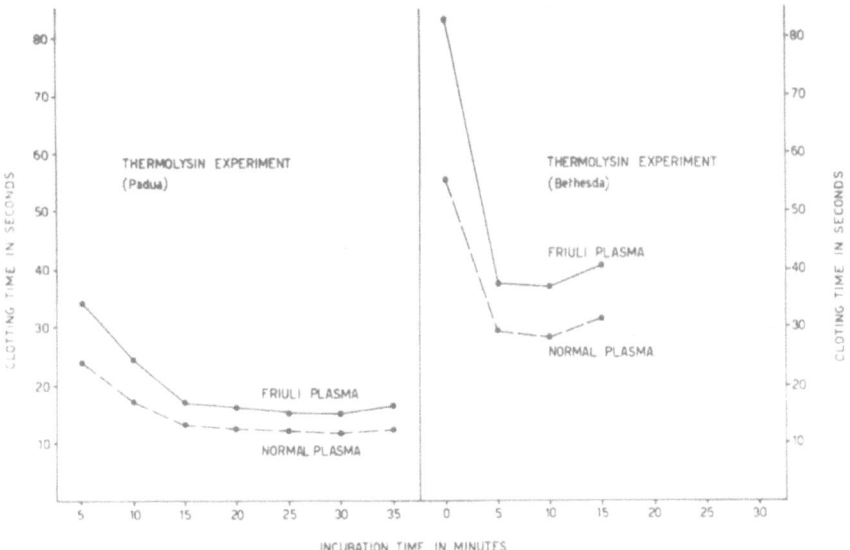

*Fig.* 3. Thermolysin activation of factor X Friuli. Two experiments were carried out, one in Bethesda by Dr. Aronson and one in Padua by us. The results are similar save for the clotting times which were shorter in the Padua experiment. This was due to the fact that in the Bethesda experiment the aliquots obtained from the incubation mixture were diluted 1:5 before assaying for activated factor X.

Thermolysin activation of factor X Friuli is both delayed and defective.

RVV-Cephalin mixture, factor X in the serum appears to be lower as compared with the values found in plasma, in which essentially normal amounts of factor $X_a$ can be generated (table 2).

*Table* 2.  Factor X levels in Friuli plasma and serum.

|  | Rabbit brain | human brain | Stypven-Cephalin mixture | Comment |
|---|---|---|---|---|
| Friuli plasma | 12% | 6,5% | 88% | Average of several determinations |
| Friuli serum | 15% | 10% | 28% | Average of at least three determinations |

This seems to suggest that the Stypven-Cephalin mixture is unable to further activate the clotting-modified factor X Friuli and that, once activated, factor X is normal in Friuli serum. The modifications induced by clotting are similar both after whole blood coagulation in a glass tube and after plasma recalcification.

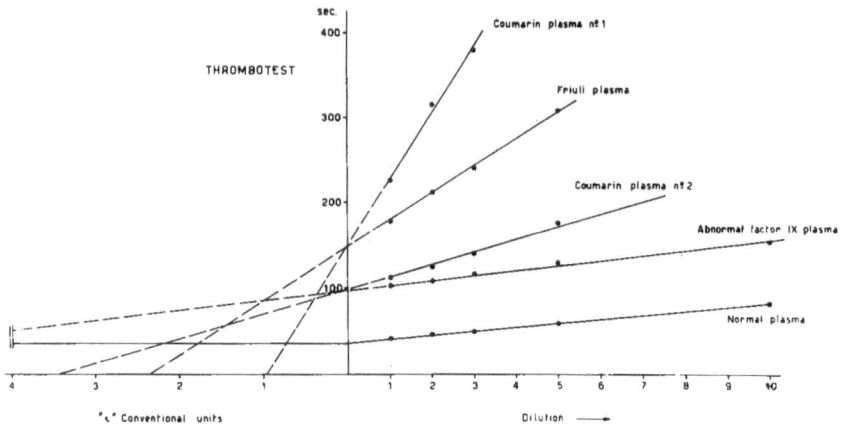

*Fig.* 4. Thrombotest dilution curve studies in the factor X Friuli and in other acquired and congenital disorders. The prolongation of the line obtained with Friuli plasma does not meet the prolongation of the line obtained with normal plasma at or about the y axis. The same is true for the other conditions taken into consideration.

The Thrombotest dilution curve would seem to suggest the presence of an inhibitor in Friuli plasma (fig. 4). However, this has been demonstrated not to be the case. The Thrombotest results are probably secondary to the fact that in single factor congenital deficiencies or abnormalities the dilution curve kinetics is no longer valid (13).

A similar pattern is seen in congenital isolated factor II, factor VII and factor X deficiencies besides hemophilia $B_M$ (19). By mixing increasing quantities of Friuli plasma with normal plasma one observes the same pattern obtainable by mixing increasing quantities of factor X deficient plasma with normal plasma, namely a parallel prolongation of the clotting times. On the contrary by mixing increasing quantities of hemophilia $B_M$ plasma with normal plasma one obtains a pattern completely different from that obtainable by mixing increasing quantities of factor IX deficient plasma with normal plasma. The ox-brain thromboplastin clotting times of the first serial mixtures become progressively longer in accordance with the percentile increase of patient plasma in the mixture (fig. 5).

In a specific PIVKA experiment it was also shown that no PIVKA like effect is present in Friuli plasma. The inhibitory activity was practically equal to zero (fig. 6).

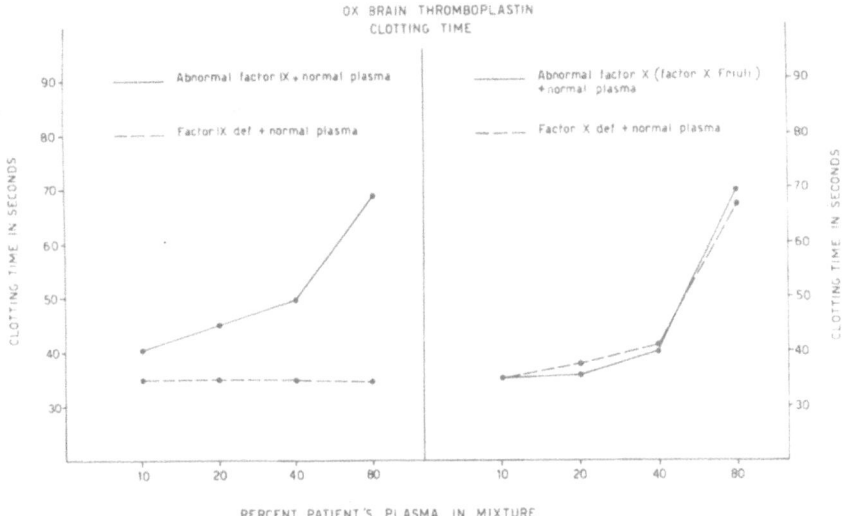

*Fig.* 5. Mixing experiment in Friuli plasma and in Hemophilia $B_M$ plasma. By mixing increasing aliquots of Friuli plasma with normal plasma one observes a progressive lenghtening of the ox brain thromboplastin clotting times similar to that obtainable by mixing factor X deficient plasma with normal plasma. On the contrary, a different pattern is observed by mixing increasing aliquots of Hemophilia $B_M$ plasma with normal plasma and factor IX deficient plasma with normal plasma.

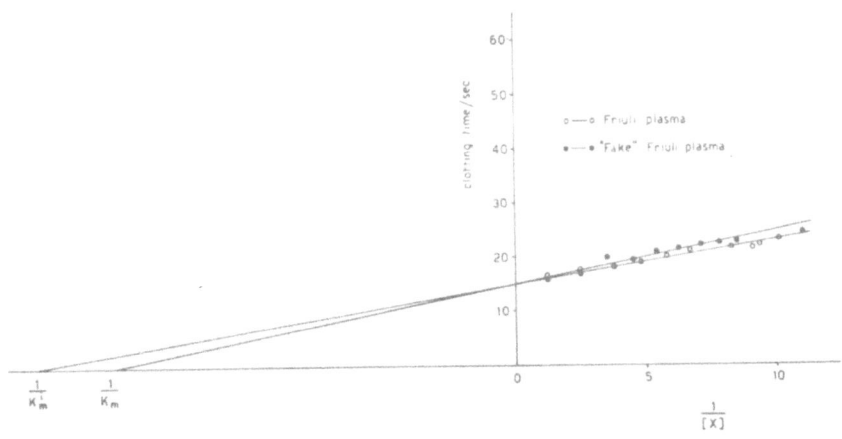

*Fig.* 6. Lack of PIVKA effect in Friuli plasma. No difference is noted between Friuli plasma (circles) and 'fake' Friuli plasma (dots). 'Fake' Friuli plasma is an artificial mixture containing the same amount of known clotting factors as Friuli plasma. Inhibitory capacity 'i' is practically equal to zero. These experiments were carried out in collaboration with Dr. H. C. Hemker and Miss A. Muller of the Academisch Ziekenhuis, Leiden.

Furthermore no inactivation of transfused exogenous factor X occurs in Friuli patients since a normal factor X survival half-life has been obtained on several occasions in three patients (fig. 7) (18).

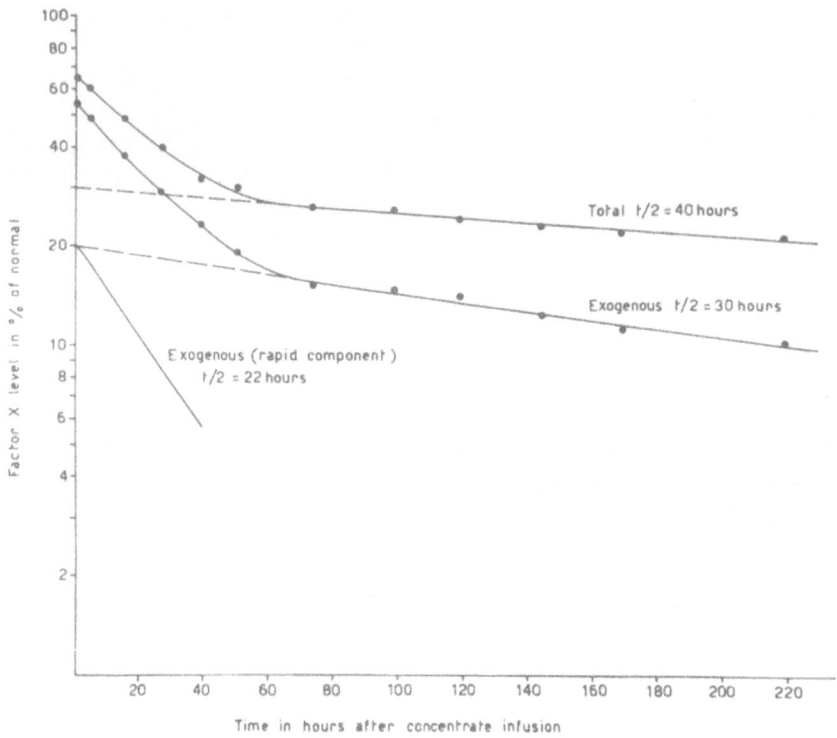

*Fig.* 7. Factor X survival studies in a patient with the Friuli abnormality. The half-life of the exogenous component is 30 hours. This is in good agreement with known survival times obtained in classical factor X deficiency and suggests that no inactivation of exogenous factor X occurs in Friuli patients.

Immunologically, factor X Friuli behaves as normal factor X in the neutralization test, in immunodiffusion studies and in the cross-over electrophoresis system. Using this latter method it is also possible to show that factor X Friuli has the same mobility as normal factor X and a different one as compared with Coumarin-induced abnormal factor X (11, 15, 20) (fig. 8, 9). Only one major band is present in Friuli plasma and in normal plasma whereas two distinct factor X bands are seen in Coumarin plasma (15). The first of these two bands is equivalent in position to its normal counterpart, the second one is an abnormal, more cathodal band not present in normal plasma. No factor X band is visible in Mr Stuart's plasma and in the plasmas of the other patients with classical factor X deficiency (fig. 8). In Friuli serum as in normal serum, only one factor X band, is visible.

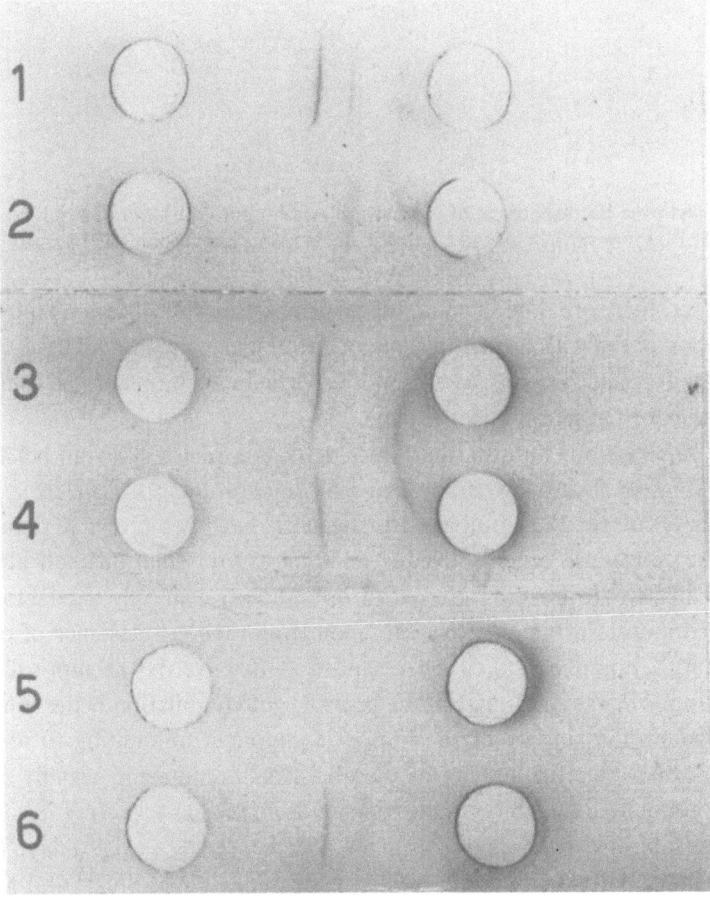

*Fig.* 8. Cross-over electrophoresis (electrosyneresis) of: I) factor X Friuli plasma; 2) mr. Stuart's plasma; 3) pooled normal plasma; 4) heterozygote for Friuli abnormality; 5) another factor X deficient plasma; 6) a second Friuli plasma.
A clear factor X band is evident in: 1), 3), 4) and 6). No factor X band is present in Mr. Stuart's and in the other factor X deficient plasma.
Lighter or minor bands are seen in most plasmas. They are due to secondary activities of the antiserum used and may be disregarded.
The antiserum used in this and in the following experiments was kindly supplied by Dr. D. Aronson, of the National Institutes of Health, Bethesda, USA.

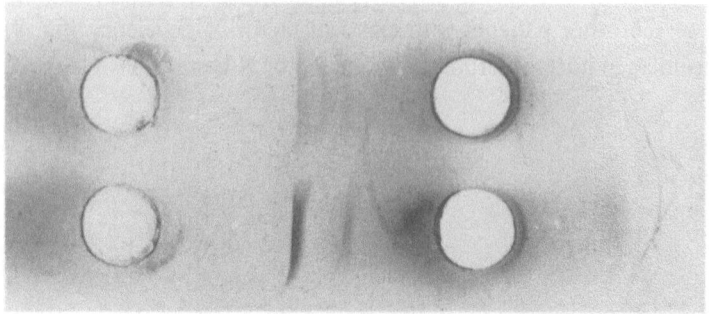

*Fig.* 9. Cross-over electrophoresis of coumarin plasma (upper run) and of Friuli plasma (patient M.P.; lower run). A second factor X band is visible in the coumarin plasma.

However, there are differences in the position of the Friuli serum factor X band as compared with normal plasma or Friuli plasma factor X (fig. 8).

The Friuli serum factor X band is more anodic in position and the same is true for the normal serum factor X band.

These observations indicate that, once activated, factor X Friuli behaves in the cross-over electrophoretic system as normal serum.

Heterozygotes for the Friuli abnormality may have two factor X populations: one active and one inactive, or one factor X population: half active and half inactive. In the cross-over electrophoretic system only one factor X band is seen even in the heteroxygote, indicating that the existence of only one factor X population, half active and half inactive, is the more likely explanation. The factor X level in the heterozygote population is the sum of two activities: the activity of the normal component amounting to about 50% of normal plus the activity of the abnormal component, usually 50% of the level found in the homozygote (namely 2-7%).

Three established variants of the factor X defect seem to exist today. The classical index patients for factor X deficiency, namely Mr. Stuart and Miss Prower, are 'per se' two different variants. Mr. Stuart has very low factor X activity regardless of the assay method used and very low or no factor X antigen. Miss Prower, on the contrary, has low factor X assay (about 8% of normal) in both assay system but normal factor X antigen (3). Mrs. Minin, the index patient with the Friuli disorder, has low factor X activity in the tissue thromboplastin assay, normal factor X activity in the Stypven-Cephalin assay method and normal factor X antigen (table 3).

It is likely that many other intermediate cases may exist. Some of the

*Table* 3. Main genetic variants of factor X defect.

| Index patient | Factor X level (tissue thromboplastin) | Factor X level (S-Ceph. mixture) | Factor X antigen |
|---|---|---|---|
| Miss Prower | Low | Low | Normal |
| Mr. Stuart | Very Low | Very Low | Absent |
| Mrs. Minin (Factor X Friuli) | Low | Normal | Normal |

patients described by others may indeed represent these variants (2, 3). Genetic polymorphism of coagulation disorders surely applies to the factor X defect too.

In conclusion it may be stated that factor X Friuli has the following main characteristics (table 4). These features are compatible only with the assumption that the defect is a genetically transmitted abnormality of factor X protein synthesis.

*Table* 4. Main features of Factor X Friuli.

1. It may not be activated by tissue thromboplastins.
2. It may be normally activated by RVV.
3. It may be partially activated by trypsin, thermolysin, etc.
4. It has no inhibitory effect on the ox-brain thromboplastin + factor VII reaction.
5. It is not accompanied by factor II, VII and IX deficiences or abnormalities.
6. Immunologically it behaves as normal factor X and is different from coumarin-induced abnormal factor X.
7. The factor X band seen in normal and Friuli serum is slightly more anodic in position as compared with the normal or Friuli plasma factor X band.
8. No PIVKA- like effect is present in Friuli plasma.
9. No in vivo inhibitory effect on transfused factor X is noted in Friuli plasma.-

As a person born and raised in Friuli I am very proud that my region has somehow contributed to the understanding of the prothrombin complex factors.

The purpose of future research will rest mainly on the attempt to elucidate the nature of the factor X structural abnormality.

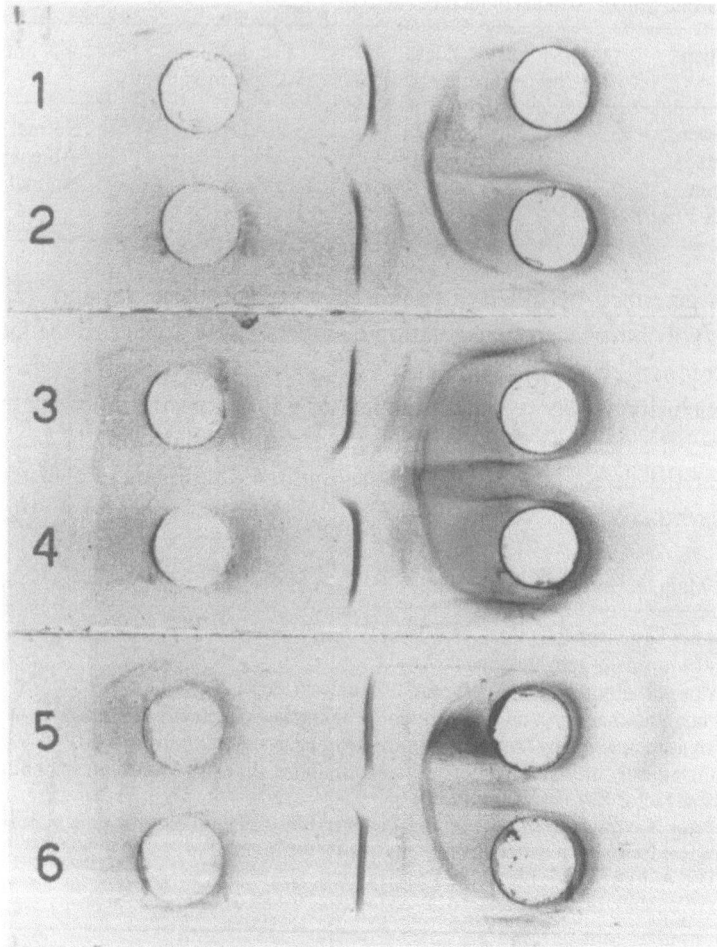

*Fig.* 10. From top to bottom cross-over electrophoresis of: 1) pooled normal plasma; 2) pooled normal serum; 3) factor X Friuli serum; 4) pooled normal serum; 5) factor X Friuli plasma; 6) factor X Friuli serum.

Note that the factor X band both in Friuli serum and in normal serum is slightly more anodic in position as compared with the normal or Friuli plasma factor X band.

REFERENCES

1. Aronson, D. L., *Personal communication.*
2. Chodosch, B. T., S. S. Shapiro and D. L. Aronson, Immunological investigation of two patients with congenital factor X deficiency. *Clin. Res.* 17, 599 (1969).
3. Denson, K. W., A. Lurie, F. De Cataldo and P. M. Mannucci, The factor X defect: recognition of abnormal forms of factor X. *Brit. J. Haemat.* 18, 317 (1970).

4. Girolami, A., G. Molaro, M. Lazzarin and R. Scapra, Una nuova coagulopatia emorragica congenita probabilmente dovuta alla presenza du un fattore X abnorme. Studio preliminare. *Minerva med.* 60, 4939 (1969).

5. Girolami, A., G. Molaro, M. Lazzarin, R. Scarpa and A. Brunetti, Congenital hemorrhagic condition similar but not identical to factor X deficiency. A hemorrhagic state due to an abnormal factor X. *Scand. J. Haemat.* 7, 91 (1970).

6. Girolami, A., G. Molaro, M. Lazzarin, A. Brunetti and R. Scarpa, A 'new' congenital hemorrhagic condition due to the presence of an abnormal factor X (factor X Friuli). A study of a large kindred. *Brit. J. Haemat.* 19, 179 (1970).

7. Girolami, A., G. Molaro and B. Orazi, L'ereditarietà della coagulopatia emorragica da fattore X abnorme (fattore X Friuli). *Policlinico, Sez. med.* 77, 103 (1970).

8. Girolami, A., G. Molaro, A. Galligaris and G. De Luca, Severe congenital classical factor X deficiency in a 5 month old child. *Thrombos. Diathes. haemorrh.* 24, 175 (1970).

9. Girolami, A., M. Lazzarin, R. Scarpa and A. Brunetti, Further studies on the abnormal factor X (factor X Friuli) coagulation disorder: report of another family. *Blood* 37, 534 (1971).

10. Girolami, A., A. Sticchi and A. Brunetti, Prothrombin level and activity in the abnormal factor X (factor X Friuli) coagulation disorder. *Thrombos. Diathes. haemorrh.* 25, 147 (1971).

11. Girolami, A., A. Sticchi and G. Bareggi, Cross-over electrophoresis (electrosyneresis) visualization of the abnormal factor X (factor X Friuli). *J. Lab. clin. Med.* 80, 740 (1972).

12. Girolami, A., M. Lazzarin and G. Molaro, The effect of several tissue thromboplastins on the activation of abnormal factor X (factor X Friuli). *Thrombos. Diathes. haemorrh.* 27, 535 (1972).

13. Girolami, A., A. D. Muller and H. C. Hemker, Lack of PIVKA effect in the abnormal factor X (factor X Friuli) coagulation disorder. *Haemostasis* 1, 23 (1972).

14. Girolami, A., R. Nicolini, P. Furlani and G. Bareggi, Abnormal factor X (factor X Friuli) coagulation disorder. First report of patient outside Friuli. *Acta haemat.* 49, 114 (1973).

15. Girolami, A., G. Bareggi and D. Fioretti, Different cross-over electrophoresis (electrosyneresis) mobility of factor X Friuli and coumarin-induced abnormal factor X. *Haemostasis* 1, 229 (1972/73).

16. Girolami, A., R. Falomo, A. Carli and L. De Marco, Factor X Friuli coagulation disorder. First report of a patient born in Friuli after the description of the disease. *Blut* 27, 151 (1973).

17. Girolami, A., A. Brunetti, G. Bareggi and G. Cella, Abnormal factor X (factor X Friuli) coagulation disorder. The heterozygote population. A Study of 57 subjects. *Acta haemat.* 51, 40 (1974).

18. Girolami, A., G. Molaro and L. de Marco, Factor X survival studies and hemostatically effective factor X levels in abnormal factor X (factor X Friuli) coagulation disorder. *Acta haemat.* 52, 223 (1974).

19. Girolami, A., A. Brunetti, L. de Marco and L. Virgolini, Dilution curve studies in prothrombin complex factors deficiencies or abnormalities. *Blut* 29, 134 (1974).

20. Girolami, A., G. Bareggi and N. Borstato, *Factor X Friuli coagulation disorder. An immunological study. Blut* (in press).

21. Graham, J. B., E. M. Barrow and C. Hougie, Stuart clotting defect. II. Genetic aspects of a new hemorrhagic state. *J. clin. Invest.* 36, 497 (1957).

22. Hougie, C., H. M. Barrow and J. B. Graham, Stuart clotting defect. I. Segregation of an hereditary hemorrhagic state from the heterogeneous group heretofore called

'stable factor' (SPCA, proconvertin, factor VII) deficiency. *J. clin. Invest.* 36, 485 (1957).

23. Lechler, E., W. P. Webster, H. R. Roberts and G. D. Penick, The inheritance of Stuart disease: investigation of a family with factor X deficiency. *Amer. J. med. Sci.* 249, 191 (1965).

24. Roos, J. and J. Huizinga, Genetic investigation of the Stuart coagulation defect. *Acta genet.* 9, 115 (1959).

25. Telfer, T. P., K. W. Denson and D. R. Wright, A new coagulation defect. *Brit. J. Haemat.* 2, 308 (1956).

PART FOUR

# PIVKA VII, IX AND X

# SYNTHESIS OF FACTOR VII

H. PRYDZ

Factor VII is the only plasma protein which we know to be specific for the extrinsic coagulation system. The importance of this system for the rapid generation of thrombin following exposure to tissue thromboplastin after trauma is the background for the current interest in factor VII and its activation.

Like the other coagulation factors present in plasma, factor VII is a glycoprotein. Our data suggest that plasma contains a few µg of this protein per ml.Calculations on the data of Nemerson (1) suggest that the content may be one order of magnitude lower. The molecular weight has been estimated to be 56000-59000 by SDS-gel electrophoresis and sucrose gradient centrifugation when factor VII is isolated in the unactivated form.

There are probably three different ways in which factor VII can be activated from its normal circulating state in plasma and they lead to two different states of activation.

The three ways are:

1. by tissue thromboplastin, the classical mechanism for the extrinsic pathway;
2. possibly by kallikrein or factor XIIa. This is the mode of action recently described by Gjønnaes (2, 3), its mechanism is unknown but may involve proteolysis;
3. and finally, it is possible that the activation of factor VII seen in serum after spontaneous clotting is due to a third way of activation. Johnston & Hjort (4) reported that factors VIII, IX, XI and XII were necessary for the full increase of factor VII activity during intrinsic coagulation. Factor X was apparently not necessary.

The activation during intrinsic coagulation is probably caused by factor IXa, since homogeneous preparations of human factor IXa activate purified factor VII in vitro, albeit slowly. The activation during intrinsic coagulation is accompanied by a reduction of the molecular weight of factor VII when isolated from serum 4-5 h after coagulation, from about 56000-59000 down to about 45000, and a concommitant reduction in Stoke's radius from 35 Å to 30 Å (5). Neither the intrinsic nor the factor XII-kallikrein induced activation enables factor VII alone to activate factor X, but they activate probably by increasing the affinity of factor VII for tissue thromboplastin.

The activation by tissue thromboplastin has been more closely studied. Tissue thromboplastin is a protein-phospholipid complex. The protein part has been purified to homogeneity and shown to have a M.W. of about 52000 (6). Both the protein and phospholipid parts are necessary for procoagulant activity. Purified, unactivated factor VII from plasma is activated by purified tissue thromboplastin in the presence of calcium ions.

Earlier, it was generally held that factor VII had to be bound in a complex with tissue thromboplastin to be activated, as studied in great detail by Hjort (7). It is possible, however, to filter activated factor VII through a 0.1 $\mu$ Millipore filter, whereas this filter completely retains tissue thromboplastin (8). The activity in the filtrate is not inhibited by antibodies to tissue thromboplastin.

This filtrable form of factor VIIa is probably a smaller complex with phospholipid, since prolonged treatment with phospholipase C reduces the activity to the starting value. Factor VII can be reactivated again by a new exposure to tissue thromboplastin and has thus probably not undergone any permanent changes during activation by tissue thromboplastin and inactivation by phospholipase C (9).

Hence, it is possible to observe in vitro factor VII activated by contact with tissue thromboplastin and remaining activated after being separated from tissue thromboplastin. We have postulated (9) that factor VII is activated in the reaction with tissue thromboplastin by a conformational change induced by the contact of factor VII with the phospholipid-protein complex. The active state is maintained by the binding of some phospholipid from tissue thromboplastin to factor VII. The physiological significance of this activation mechanism is presently unknown and we are trying to establish an experimental model to study this.

Turning now to the real subject of this communication, factor VII is one of the four vitamin K-dependent factors, the biosynthesis of which is blocked by the peroral anticoagulants of the warfarin/dicumarol type. It is synthesized mainly in the liver, but may be synthesized in other organs as well, such as kidney (10, 11). The biosynthesis has been studied in whole animals (12, 13) by organ perfusion (11), in single cell suspensions (10, 14), in rat hepatoma cell cultures (15) and in subcellular systems (16, 17). Being a glycoprotein, factor VII follows the normal biosynthetic pathway for glycoproteins. This implies that the polypeptide chain is formed more or less completely on the polyribosomes in the rough endoplasmic reticulum in the ordinary way before the carbohydrate residues are added in stepwise fashion.

Polypeptides associated with the polyribosomes contain very little or no carbohydrate; in the rough endoplasmic reticulum membranes most of the residues closer to the polypeptide chains are added. The outermost residues are added in the smooth endoplasmic reticulum, in the Golgi region and in some cases possibly in the plasma membrane in connection with the secretory process (18, 19, 20, 21). The internal transport of the precursor from the rough endoplasmic reticulum to the Golgi region may be coupled to the glycosylation process, since when this process is inhibited, certain polypeptide precursor chains (for instance immunoglobulin precursor chains) are not transported into the cisternae of the rough endoplasmic reticulum and further into the smooth reticulum.

The carbohydrate precursors are nucleotide-carbohydrate compounds and they seem to transfer the carbohydrate residue to a polyprenol phosphate intermediate, dolichol phosphate, which has a structure reminiscent of the side chain of vitamin K.

There are thus three or four possible intracellular 'pools' of varying size for various glycoproteins intended for export out of the cell:

1. Growing or unreleased complete polypeptide chains on membrane-bound polyribosomes.
2. Molecules containing 'core' carbohydrates, localized in the rough membranes.
3. Molecules containing nearly complete or complete carbohydrate structures localized in the smooth membranes, in the Golgi region, in secretory vesicles or even in the plasma membrane itself.

By studying the time intervals between the injection of various inhibitors and the decline in factor VII activity in plasma and in a smooth endoplasmic reticulum fraction from rat liver, a flow chart for the biosynthesis of factor VII may be constructed, based on the general scheme for glycoprotein synthesis (12). The time relationship established suggest that warfarin acts later than cycloheximide, i.e., after the completion of the polypeptide chain. There appears from these data to be at least two intracellular precursor pools for factor VII, one prior to the step where vitamin K is necessary (Finalization step I) and one after the vitamin K and warfarin sensitive step (Finalization step II). This latter pool can be isolated and located to a smooth microsomal fraction (16, 17), and the reaction will be seen as a temperature-dependent warfarin and cycloheximide resistant increase of factor VII activity upon incubation of whole cells or this microsomal fraction. This is probably part of the release reaction to which we will return briefly later.

Through studies from several laboratories, mainly by immunological methods, it is now firmly established that plasma PIVKAs as well as intracellular precursors exist. Plasma from patients or animals deficient in vitamin K or treated with anticoagulants contains substances without or with reduced or abnormal procoagulant activity. These substances crossreact with antibodies against the respective normal factors. It has also been shown that the liver microsomal fraction from warfarin-treated rats contains a precursor of factor VII. This precursor may be converted to active factor by vitamin K up to 40 min after protein synthesis has been blocked 95% (13).

A rat liver microsomal fraction is also apparently able to activate rat plasma PIVKA-VII. Plasma from warfarin-treated rats was treated with $BaSO_4$ to remove the small amount of normal factor VII present and subsequently incubated with a crude microsomal fraction from rat liver. To prevent interference from factor VII precursor in the microsomal fraction, the animals from which the microsomes were prepared, were given cycloheximide and vitamin K 120 min before removal of the liver. These results (table 1) are preliminary, but they suggest a way of studying the reaction mechanism and enzymology of the vitamin K dependent step. We are currently studying this reaction using the isolated PIVKA-II as a substrate.

Table 1. Incubation* of rat liver microsomal fraction with $BaSO_4$ treated rat warfarin plasma as source of PIVKA-VII.

Coagulation time (sec)**

| Incubated | Control |
|-----------|---------|
| 82.6 | 40.4 |
| 81.1 | 45.2 |
| 80.2 | 39.1 |
| 76.2 | 41.0 |
| 69.6 | 46.2 |

\* 120 min/37°C.
\*\* In factor VII test system, buffer control 75-80 sec.

The changes induced in the factor VII molecule by the vitamin K-dependent step are less studied than those for factor II and factor X. There must, however, be a certain difference between factor II on one hand and the factors VII, IX and X on the other. It has become quite clear that in the case of factor II and X, the vitamin K-induced modification of the precursor molecules imparts the $BaSO_4$- and $Ca^{2+}$-binding capacity upon them. If we assume the same to be the case for factor VII and IX a difference is evident. The vitamin K-induced modification takes place in the N-terminal part of prothrombin which is split off during its activation, since the activated form of prothrombin, i.e. thrombin, is not adsorbed to $BaSO_4$ and does not take part in a reaction involving binding to calcium. Moreover, the prothrombin fragment that is split off has been shown directly to be adsorbed to $BaSO_4$ and to bind $Ca^{++}$ both in bovine and human material. On the other hand, factor VII (molecular weight 45000) (5), factor Xa (molecular weight 25000 and 46000) (22) and factor IXa (molecular weight 44000) (23) all take part in reactions involving $Ca^{2+}$ binding and they are adsorbed to $BaSO_4$ also after activation. In these factors, the vitamin K-induced modification must therefore be retained in the molecule which carries the activity after the proteolytic activation.

Since there are no data on the nature of the vitamin K-induced modification in factor VII, I will not discuss it further.

Finally, I will describe briefly some experiments where we have been looking at the last phase of the biosynthetic pathway, the transport out of the cells. The system we used is a clonal strain of rat hepatoma cells grown in vitro as monolayers in Dulbecco's modification of Eagle's medium with 15% horse and 2.5% fetal calf serum. We have previously shown that they produce at least 12 different immunologically detectable rat serum proteins (24). They produce factor VII and respond to warfarin and vitamin K (15).

Such cells were treated with colchicine and cytochalasin B (and dimethyl sulphoxide as one control) to study the influence on their excretion of factor VII during a 6 h incubation.

Colchicine had no marked effect, the factor VII activity was reduced to 88-91% of the untreated controls and DMSO had no effect at all (factor VII activity 97% of control).

In the presence of 5 µg/ml of cytochalasin B, however, a very rapid release of factor VII appeared, but no further increase was found (fig. 1).

The incorporation of radioactive alanine into protein during the same interval was hardly reduced (97% of control) even in the presence of 25 µg/ml of cytochalasin.

These observations suggest that the microfilaments may be involved in the excretion of factor VII.

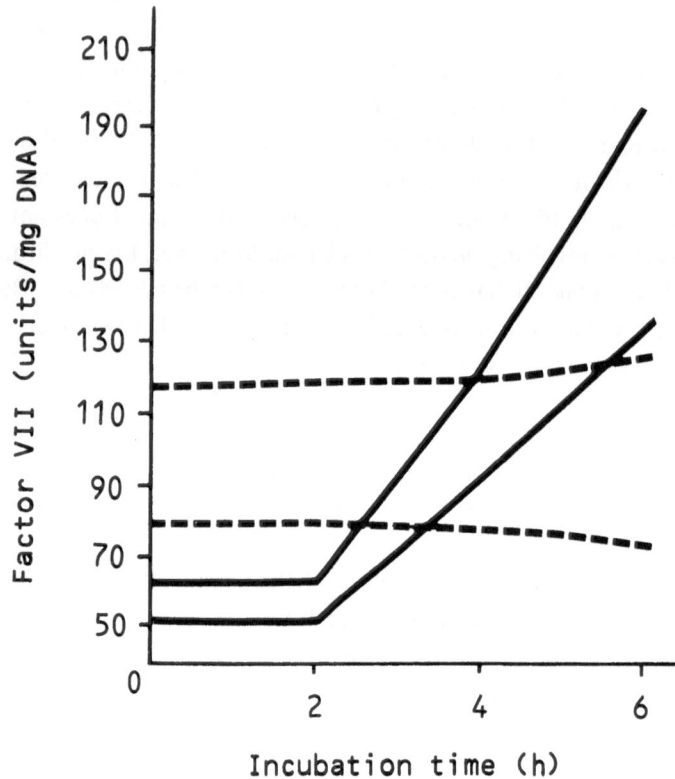

*Fig.* 1.

REFERENCES

1. Jesty, J. and Y. Nemerson, *J. biol. Chem.* 249, 509 (1974).
2. Gjønnaess, H. and H. Stormorken, *Thrombos. Diathes. haemorrh.* 24, 308 (1970).
3. Gjønnaess, H., *Kallikrein Activation of Factor VII.* Thesis. Oslo University Press (1973).
4. Johnston, C. L. and P. F. Hjort, *J. clin. Invest.* 40, 743 (1961).
5. Gladhaug, Å. and H. Prydz, *Biochim. biophys. Acta* 215, 105 (1970).
6. Bjørklid, E., E. Storm and H. Prydz, *Biochem. biophys. Res. Commun.* 55, 969 (1973).
7. Hjort, P. F., *Scand. J. clin. Lab. Invest.* 9, suppl. 27 (1957).
8. Hvatum, M. and H. Prydz, *Biochim. biophys. Acta* 130, 92 (1966).
9. Østerud, B., Å. Berre, A.-B. Otnaess, E. Bjørklid and H. Prydz, *Biochemistry* 11, 2853 (1972).
10. Prydz, H., *Scand. J. clin. Lab. Invest.* 17, 143 (1965).
11. Dodds, W. J., *Amer. J. Physiol.* 217, 879 (1969).
12. Prydz, H. and G. Gaudernack, *Biochim. biophys. Acta* 230, 373 (1971).
13. Rez, G. and H. Prydz, *Biochim. biophys. Acta,* 244, 495 (1971).

14. Prydz, H., *Scand. J. clin. Lab. Invest.* 16, 540 (1964).
15. Rugstad, H. E., H. Prydz and B. Johansson, *Exp. Cell. Res.* 71, 41 (1972).
16. Gaarder, A. and H. Prydz, *Biochim. biophys. Acta* 140, 545 (1967).
17. Gaarder, A. and H. Prydz, *Biochim. biophys. Acta* 184, 220 (1969).
18. Helgeland, L., T. B. Christensen and T. L. Janson, *Biochim. biophys. Acta* 286, 62 (1972).
19. Melchers, F., *Biochemistry*, 11, 2204 (1972).
20. Melchers, F., *Biochemistry* 12, 1471 (1973).
21. Redman, C. M. and M. G. Cherian, *J. Cell Biol.* 52, 231 (1972).
22. Berre, Å. G., B. Osterud, T. B. Christensen, T. Holm and H. Prydz, *Biochem. J.* 135, 791 (1973).
23. Østerud, B., K. Laake and H. Prydz, *Thrombos. Diathes. haemorrh.* (1975) (in press).
24. Gaudernack, G., H. E. Rugstad, I. Hegna and H. Prydz, *Exp. Cell Res.* 77, 25 (1973).

# FACTOR VII IN PATIENTS ON ORAL ANTICOAGULANTS

MILICA BROZOVIC AND D. J. HOWARTH

In patients on oral anticoagulants the levels of prothrombin, factor IX and factor X determined by immunological techniques invariably exceed the levels estimated by coagulation assays (Ganrot and Nilehn, 1968; Josso et al., 1968; Larrieu and Meyer, 1970; Denson, 1971; Brozovic and Gurd, 1973). In the case of factor VII, however, the relationship between the immunologically reactive and biologically active material is less clear cut. Prydz (1965) found no excess of antibody neutralizing material in the plasma of patients on phenindione; Goodnight et al. (1971) and Denson (1971) demonstrated the presence of inactive factor VII in the patients on oral anticoagulants they studied. Levanon et al (1972) reported an excess of antibody neutralizing material in short term anticoagulation, whereas both immunologically reactive and biologically active factor VII were reduced by equal amounts in long term treatment.

In an effort to clarify the situation for factor VII, we measured biological (clotting) and immunoreactive factor VII estimates in a random sample of men and women in an industrial population and in a group of patients stabilized on anticoagulants (Howarth et al., 1974). Values in the industrial group may be considered as an estimate of the distribution of factor VII levels in the population as a whole, against which the findings from the patients on oral anticoagulants may be compared. In addition, we followed the behaviour of factor VII in two volunteers given a single dose of warfarin and in three patients starting long term anticoagulant treatment.

Factor VII levels in plasma were measured using an automated one stage assay on ELECTRA 600 D. Artificial factor VII deficient plasma and freeze dried human brain thromboplastin were used throughout (Brozovic et al, 1974); the results were expressed as percentages of freeze dried reference plasma 72/244, containing 0.8u of factor VII per ampoule.

*Immunoreactive factor VII* was measured by the antibody neutralization test according to Denson (1971). The antiserum against factor VII was raised in rabbits injected with a purified preparation obtained from a concentrate of factor VII, kindly given by Dr. Bidwell and Mr. Dike, Plasma Fractionation Laboratory, Oxford Haemophilia Centre. The concentrate was further purified using large scale preparative polyacrylamide gel electrophoresis (Brownstone, 1969). Figure 1 shows the polyacrylamide gel separations of

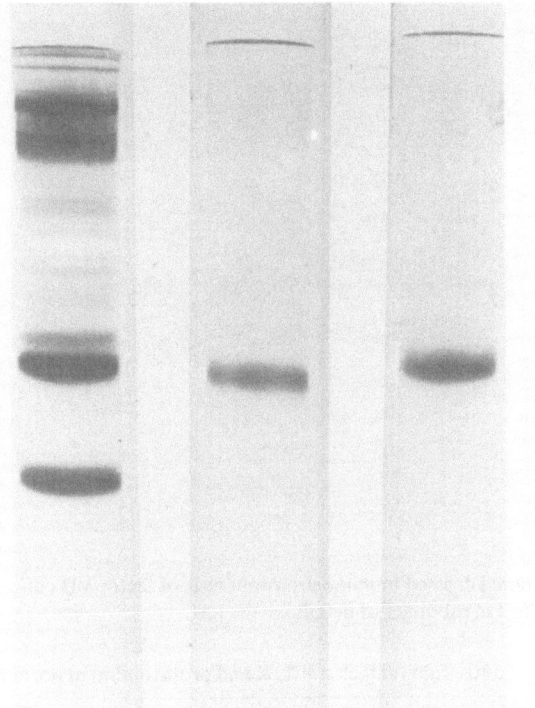

*Fig.* 1. Polyacrylamide gel separations of starting factor VII concentrate (a) and after preparative gel electrophoresis (b and c) Factor VII activity is associated with the major protein component.

the starting material and the purified factor VII. Factor VII activity was associated with the major component of the purified preparation. This material contained 86u of factor VII activity per mg of protein. Two rabbits were given three injections at weekly intervals of 2 mg of this protein with Freund's adjuvant. The antiserum obtained did not show any precipitin lines on immunodiffusion or on immunoelectrophoresis against starting factor VII concentrate, purified material, normal plasma or normal serum. The antiserum displayed strong anti-factor VII activity and weak anti-factor

X and anti-prothrombin activity (table 1); anti-factor IX activity was weak and variable. After concentration, the antiserum showed two peaks (one of which was very faint) on Laurell crossed immunoelectrophoresis against the starting material, and the purified material (fig. 2); and one peak against normal serum, and against plasma and serum of a patient on long term warfarin treatment.

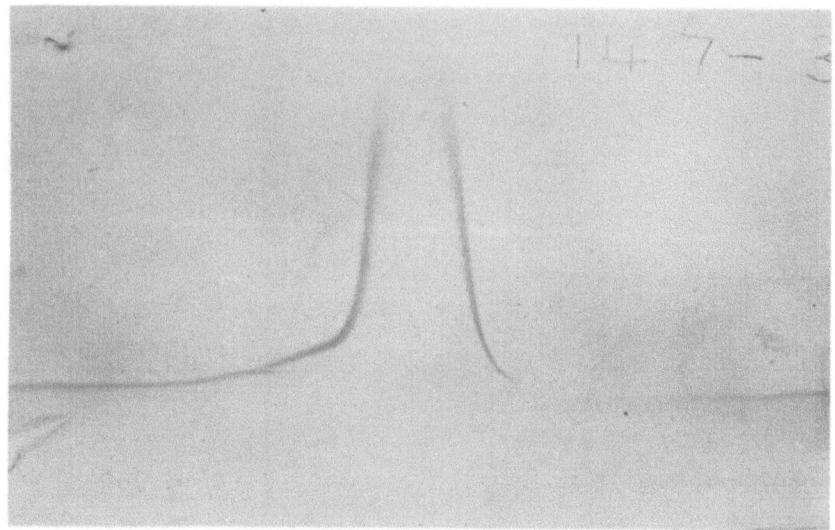

*Fig.* 2. Two dimensional crossed immunoelectrophoresis of factor VII concentrate against the antiserum obtained in rabbits. For details see the text.

*Table* 1. The effect of antiserum on factor VII, X and prothrombin in normal plasma.

| Clotting factor | Control | Residual activity % after 60 min. incubation | |
| --- | --- | --- | --- |
| | | Untreated serum | Absorbed serum |
| VII | 100 | < 1 | < 1 |
| X | 100 | 60 | 92 |
| Prothrombin | 100 | 75 | 100 |

The antiserum obtained was pepsin-treated according to Denson (1967). and then absorbed to remove traces of anti-II, anti-XI and anti -X. The absorbed antiserum was used to estimate the levels of immunoreactive factor VII using a modified antibody neutralization assay. The coefficient of variation of the assays was between $\pm$ 8 and $\pm$ 15% (Howarth et al., 1974).

## FACTOR VII IN THE INDUSTRIAL GROUP

The group studied were employees of H. J. Heinz Co. Ltd., and consisted of 47 men (mean age 47.2) and 44 women (mean age 47.8), members of a larger group participating in a long term prospective study of arterial disease (Meade, 1973). Of the women 27 were pre-menopausal and 17 post-menopausal. None of the women had ever taken oral contraceptives.

*Table 2.* Factor VII activity in men and women in an industrial group.

| | | Factor VII activity* | | | | | |
| | | Clotting assay | | | Antibody neutralization assay | | |
| Subjects | No. | Mean | Range | Coeff. of Variation % | Mean | Range | Coeff. of Variation % |
|---|---|---|---|---|---|---|---|
| All | 91 | 130.4 | 63-227 | 26.98 | 124.9 | 60-936 | 42.29 |
| Men | 47 | 122.2 | 70-227 | 26.68 | 131.6 | 61-936 | 48.57 |
| Women | 44 | 139.9** | 63-216 | 25.78 | 118.6** | 60-197 | 34.05 |

* % reference plasma 72/244 (N.B. M. Brozovic et al, 1974, reference plasma 71/11 was used).
** p < 0.01.

Table 2 shows factor VII estimates obtained by the two methods in the industrial group. The difference between the biological (clotting) and immunoreactive factor VII for all 91 subjects was not significant. However, the difference between the estimates obtained by the two methods was significant for the women, though not for men, the women having an excess of clotting over immunoreactive factor VII. The women had higher mean clotting factor VII than men and this difference was significant (P < 0.02), whereas men had higher mean immunoreactive factor VII levels than women, but this difference was not statistically significant.

## FACTOR VII IN PATIENTS STABILIZED ON LONG TERM WARFARIN TREATMENT

Factor VII was estimated in 46 patients attending the anticoagulant clinic at Northwick Park Hospital; 33 were men (mean age 60.3) and 13 were women (mean age 57.2). The prothrombin ratios using British comparative throm-

boplastin ranged from 2.0 to 3.0. All the patients had been on warfarin for
6 weeks or longer at the time of study.

*Table*. 3. Factor VII activity in an industrial group and patients on long-term warfarin
treatment.

| | No. of subjects | Factor VII activity* | | | | | |
| | | Coagulation assay | | / | Antibody Neutralisation assay | | |
| | | Mean | Range | Coeff. of Var. | Mean | Range | Coeff. of Var. |
| Industrial group | 91 | 130.4 | 63-227 | 26.98% | 124.9 | 60-936 | 42.29% |
| Warfarin treated | 46 | 38.8** | 4-72 | 52.25% | 51.70** | 19-83 | 25.40% |

  * expressed as % of reference plasma 72/244
** $p < 0.001$.

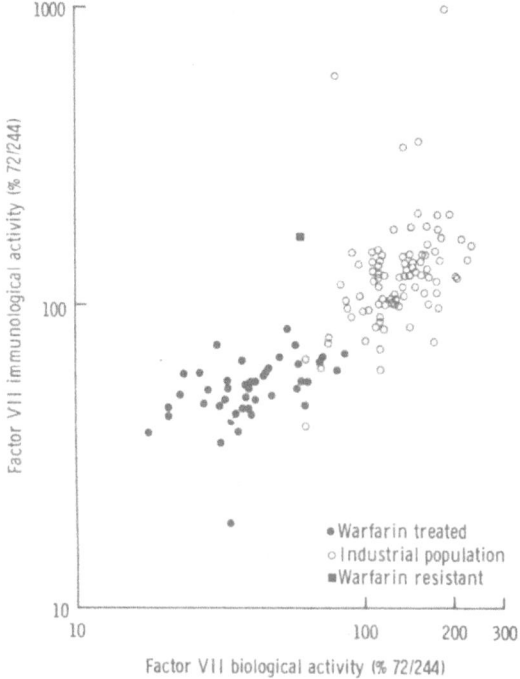

*Fig*. 3. The relationship between factor VII estimated in the clotting assay and by the
antibody neutralization assay. ○ Controls ● Warfarin treated patients.

Factor VII was, as expected, markedly reduced in warfarin-treated patients (table 3). The means of the factor VII estimates were 38% and difference is highly significant (P < 0.001). No difference in the immunoreactive factor VII levels between men and women was detected.

The plot of factor VII estimates determined in coagulation assays against the estimates measured in the antibody neutralization test is shown in figure 3. The coefficient of correlation is 0.40 for healthy subjects and 0.51 for warfarin treated patients; both correlations are highly significant (P < 0.001). It is of interest that the individual denoted with a square in figure 3 is warfarin resistant; his immunoreactive factor VII was higher than clotting factor VII on all occasions tested.

## FACTOR VII LEVELS IN TWO HEALTHY VOLUNTEERS GIVEN A SINGLE ORAL DOSE OF WARFARIN

A single 15 mg oral dose of warfarin was given before a meal to two healthy

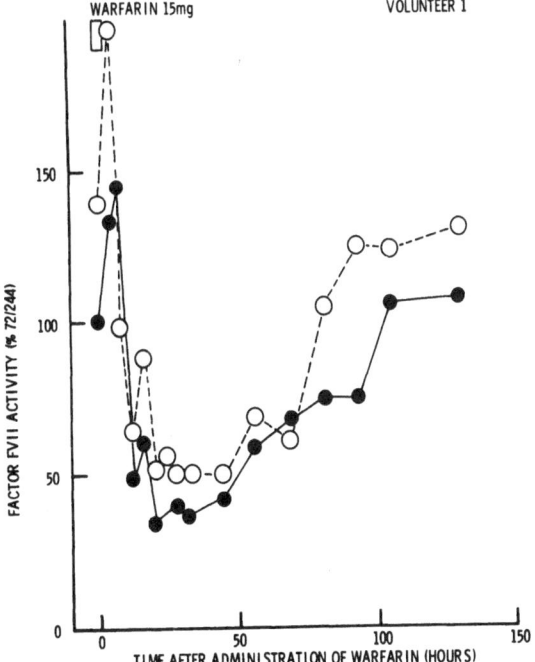

*Fig.* 4. Factor VII is volunteer 1 after a single dose of Warfarin.
●——● Factor VII estimated in the clotting assay.
○----○ Factor VII estimated in the antibody neutralization assay.

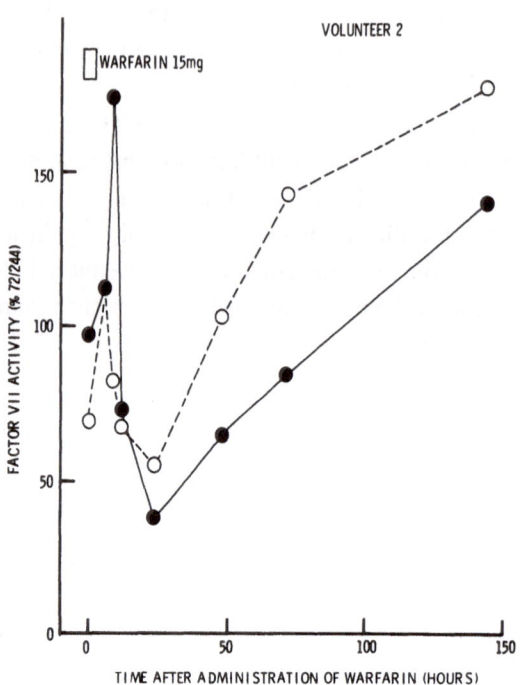

*Fig.* 5. Factor VII in volunteer 2 after a single dose of warfarin. Legend as for Fig. 4.

male volunteers, and factor VII levels were followed serially for 6 days. As shown in figure 4 and 5 factor VII levels rose three hours after warfarin administration, the peak of factor VII detected by the antibody neutralization assay preceding the peak in clotting activity. The levels of factor VII then fell to a minimum after 24 hours and returned towards the initial value over the next 48 hours. During this time, levels detected by the antibody neutralization test almost invariably exceeded the values detectable by the one stage clotting assay.

## FACTOR VII LEVELS IN PATIENTS STARTING LONG TERM WARFARIN TREATMENT

In patient 1 (fig. 6), a young woman treated with warfarin for deep vein thrombosis, the levels of factor VII fell after 80 hours of treatment and then remained low during the next few weeks. Initially, the biological activity of

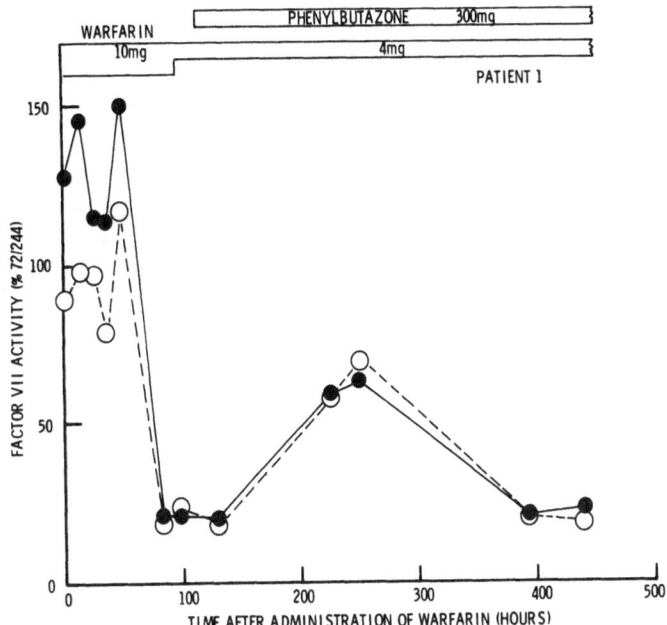

*Fig.* 6. Factor VII in patient 1 starting Warfarin treatment. Legend as for Fig. 4.

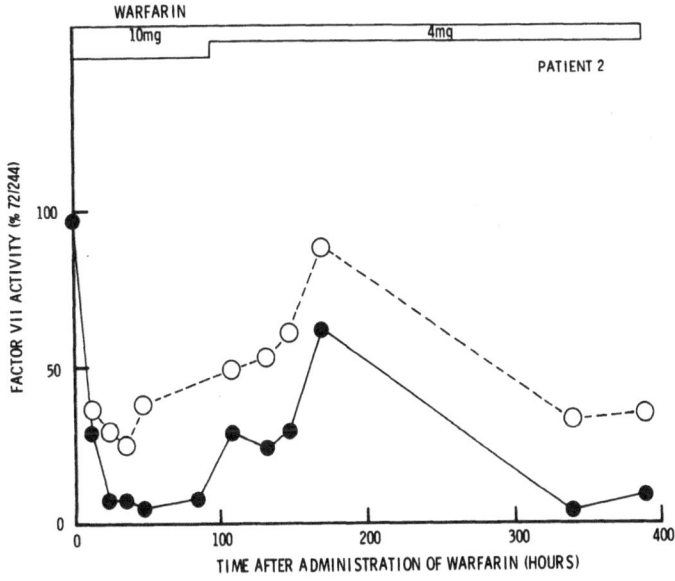

*Fig.* 7. Factor VII in patient 2 starting Warfarin treatment. Legend as for Fig. 4.

factor VII exceeded that obtained by antibody neutralization. In the course of treatment, levels of factor VII measured by both methods were lowered equally and no excess of immunoreactive material was observed (fig. 6).

In patients 2 and 3, both men treated with warfarin after myocardial infarction, factor VII levels fell to below 20% within 24 hours of starting treatment. In patient 2 (fig. 7) excess immunoreactive over clotting factor VII was present throughout the period of observation. In patient 3 (fig. 8), although an excess of antibody neutralizing activity was detected during the first 10 days of treatment, both immunoreactive and biological activity were at a similar level after 24 days of treatment.

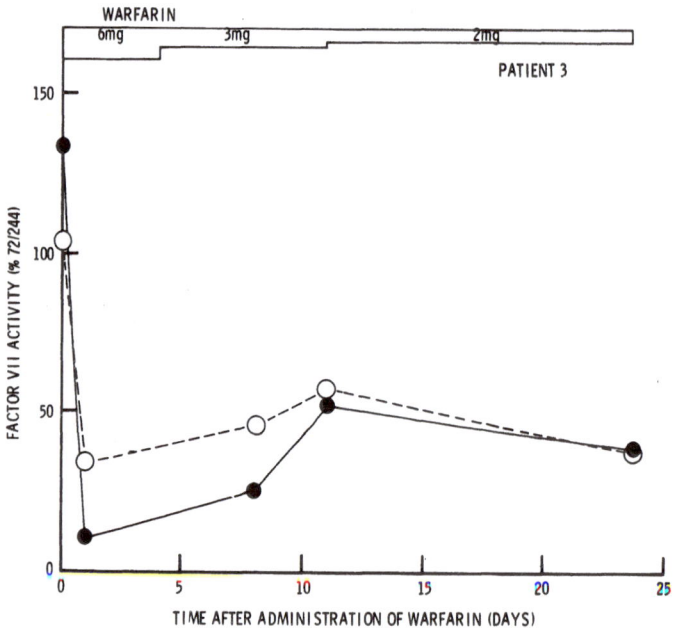

*Fig.* 8. Factor VII in patient 3 starting Warfarin Treatment. Legend as for Fig. 4.

## DISCUSSION AND CONCLUSIONS

The results obtained in the industrial group indicate that in women, factor VII estimated by a clotting assay exceeds the immunoreactive factor VII. In men, although mean immunoreactive factor VII was higher than in women, this difference is not significant. Studies of larger numbers may clarify the situation. Although every care was taken to avoid contact or cold promoted activation of factor VII the results may indicate that factor VII is more easily activated in plasma from women than men, as already suggested by the work of Gjønnaess (1972, 1973). In addition, the increase in factor VII levels with age is greater in women than in men (the rise being 1.1% and 0.45% per year of age for women and men, respectively) (Chakrabarti et al., 1974). Factor VII levels measured in plasma are affected by different *in vivo* factors (such as age and sex) and *in vitro* effects such as contact and cold-promoted activation.

Additional variables possibly affecting factor VII levels can be seen in the follow-up of the two volunteers given a single oral dose of warfarin after the evening meal. Three hours later a peak of immunoreactive factor VII was observed, whereas the clotting activity was at its maximum at 6 hours. Whether these rises were due to the administration of warfarin, or circadian rhythm, or were a result of the meal remains to be established. In the pre-liminary 48 hour studies on two subjects and the warfarin resistant indivi-dual no definite circadian rhythm was observed, although very high values for the immunoreactive factor VII were observed in some midnight samples (fig. 9). Further studies will clarify this point.

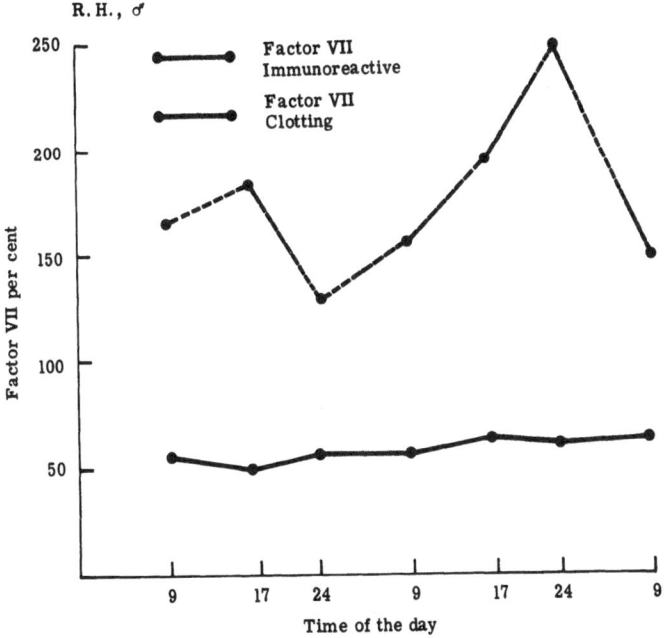

*Fig.* 9. Factor VII in a Warfarin resistant subject, off Warfarin for 4 months. Legend as for Fig. 4.

In 37 out of 47 patients on long term warfarin treatment there was an excess of immunoreactive material over the biologically active. Of the three patients serially followed, one never had an excess of immunoreactive material, one had more immunoreactive than 'biological' factor VII at the beginning of treatment only, and one had an excess of the immunoreactive factor VII throughout the period of observation.

The complicated interplay between different *in vivo* and *in vitro* phenomena affecting factor VII make it difficult to interpret the relationship between immunoreactive and biologically active factor VII during warfarin treatment. Nevertheless, there is an excess of immunoreactive factor VII in most patients at some time during warfarin treatment. It is possible that the use of an antiserum obtained against factor VII purified in a different way and therefore directed against other antigenic determinants on factor VII may reveal higher concentrations of inactive factor VII in patients on oral anticoagulants.

### REFERENCES

1. Brownstone, A. D., A versatile system for preparative electrophoresis in polyacrilamide gel. *Analyt. Biochem.* 27, 25-38 (1969).
2. Brozovic, M., L. J. Gurd, Prothrombin during warfarin treatment. *Brit. J. Haemat.*, 24, 537-582 (1973).
3. Brozovic, M., Y. Stirling, C. Harricks, W. R. S. North and T. W. Meade, Clotting factors in healthy industrial population. I. Factor VII. *Brit. J. Haemat.* In press.
4. Chakrabarti, R., M. Brozovic, W. R. S. North, Y. Stirling, T. W. Meade, Effects of age on fibrinolytic activity, and factor V, VII and VIII. *Proc. roy. Soc. Med.* In press (1974).
5. Davis, J. B., Disc. Electrophoresis. II Method and application to human Serum proteins. *Ann. N.Y. Acad. Sci.*, 121, 404-427 (1964).
6. Denson, K. W. E., The specific assay of Prower Stuart factor and factor VII. *Acta haemat. (Basel)* 25, 105-112 (1961).
7. Denson, K. W. E., The levels of factors II, VII, IX and X by antibody neutralisation techniques in the plasma of patients receiving phenindione treatment. *Brit. J. Haemat.*, 20, 643-648 (1971).
8. Dike, G. W. R., E. Bidwell and C. R. Rizza, The preparation and clinical use of a new concentrate containing factor IX, prothrombin and factor X and of a separate concentrate containing factor VII. *Brit. J. Haemat.*, 22, 469-490 (1972).
9. Ganrot, P. O. and J. E. Nilehn, Plasma prothrombin during treatment with dicoumarol. Demonstration of an abnormal prothrombin fraction. *Scand. J. clin. Lab. Invest.*, 22, 23-29 (1968).
10. Gjønnaess, H., Cold promoted activation of factor VII. I. Evidence for the existence of an activation. *Thrombos. Diathes. Haemorrh.* 28, 155-169 (1972).
11. Gjønnaess, H., Cold promoted activation of factor VII, *Gynec. Invest.*, 4, 61-72 (1973).
12. Goodnight, S. H., D. I. Feinstein, B. Sterud and S. I. Rapaport, Factor VII antibody neutralizing material in hereditary and acquired factor VII deficiency. *Blood* 38, 1-8 (1971).

13. Hemker, H. C., J. J. Veltkamp, A. Hensen and E. A. Loeliger, Nature of prothrombin biosynthesis. Preprothrombinaemia in vitamin K deficiency. *Nature* 200, 589-590 (1963).
14. Howarth, D. J., M. Brozovic, Y. Stirling and M. Reed, Factor VII during Warfarin treatment. *Scand. J. Haemat.* In press. (1974).
15. Josso, F., J. M. Lavergne and J. P. Soulier, Les dysprothrombinaemies constitution-elles et acquises. *Nouv. Rev. Franc. Haemat.* 10, 633-644 (1970).
16. Larrieu, M. S. and O. Meyer, Abnormal factor IX during anticoagulant treatment. *Lancet* 11, 1085 (1970).
17. Levanon, M., S. Rimon, M. Shani, B. Ramot and E. Goldberg, Active and inactive factor VII in Dubin Johnson syndrome with factor VII deficiency, hereditary factor VII deficiency and on coumadine administration. *Brit. J. Haemat.* 23, 669-677 (1972).
18. Meade, T. W., The epidemiology of thrombosis. *Thrombos. Diathes. Haemorrh.* In press (1973).
19. Nilehn, J. E. and P. O. Ganrot, Plasma prothrombin during treatment with dicumarol I. Immunochemical determination of its concentration of plasma. *Scand. J. clin. Lab. Invest.* 22, 17-23 (1968).
20. Prydz, H., Studies on proconvertin (Factor VII). VI. The production in rabbit of an antiserum against factor VII. *Scand. J. clin. Lab. Invest.* 17, 66-72 (1965).

# STUDY OF HUMAN FACTOR IX VARIANTS
# WITH AN IMMUNOADSORPTION TECHNIQUE

D. MEYER, E. FRESSINAUD, M. DREYFUS
AND M. J. LARRIEU

There is good evidence that in some patients with congenital or acquired Factor IX deficiency, immunologically detectable Factor IX is present in higher amounts than the biological activity, indicating the presence of abnormal molecules or precursor forms of active Factor IX. The existence of inactive Factor IX has been demonstrated either in the plasma of patients with Haemophilia B+ [1-6] or in the absence of vitamin K[7-10]. These Factor IX variants have been detected using homologous or heterologous antibodies to Factor IX and an inhibitor neutralization technique, since no precipitating anti human Factor IX antiserum has been obtained yet.

Factor IX activity was measured by a one-stage assay[11] and inhibitor-neutralizing activity by a two-stage procedure[6], using two types of antibodies to Factor IX: either homologous, developed in a polytransfused Haemophilia B patient, or heterologous, obtained in rabbits following immunization with semi-purified human Factor IX[6]. Inactive Factor IX was immunologically detected in the plasma of 21 out of 22 Haemophilia B patients using a rabbit antibody to Factor IX, and in the plasma of 9 of these patients using a human antibody (table 1).

*Table* 1. Detection of Factor IX-cross reacting material in 22 patients with Haemophilia B.

| Source of antibodies to Factor IX | Haemophilia | |
| --- | --- | --- |
| | B- | B+ |
| Homologous | 13 | 9 |
| Heterologous | 1 | 21 |

In vitamin K deficiency or intake of vitamin K antagonists, it is well established that the synthesis of Factors II, VII and X is blocked, resulting in decreased values of activity but higher levels of antigen.

Using homologous specific antibodies to Factor IX, inhibitor neutralizing activity (INA) was studied in the plasma of 103 controls (undiluted and diluted 1/2 and 1/4) and of 43 patients under coumarin therapy. Results demonstrate that the INA is higher than Factor IX activity in most cases under coumarin therapy (fig. 1). However the mean amount of antibody neutralizing material was decreased in treated patients (1.20 ± 0.39 units) compared to normals (1.56 ± 0.31 units). From these data, as well as others

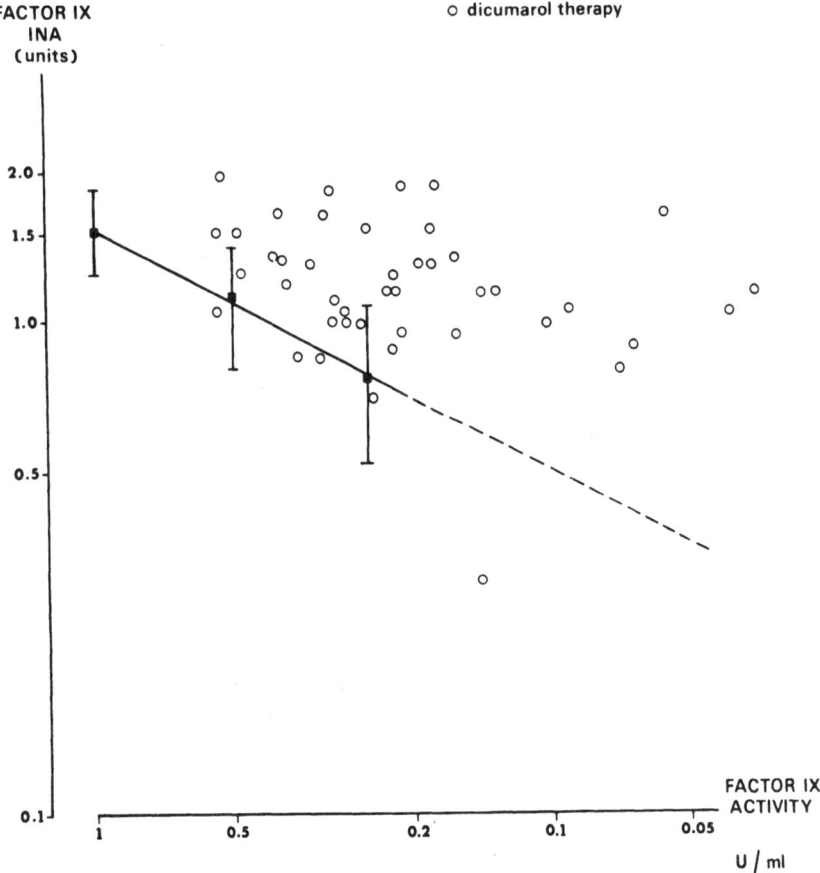

*Fig.* 1. Results of Factor IX inhibitor neutralizing activity versus Factor IX activity in 43 patients under coumarin therapy. Results are compared to those of 103 controls (■) studied at different dilutions and represented by the mean ± 1 SD.

related to prothrombin and Factors VII and X it may be speculated that the molecule of Factor IX which is synthesized in an inactive form in the absence of vitamin K has a more rapid turnover than the biologically active Factor IX molecule; Similar results were obtained in patients under coumarin therapy using heterologous antibodies to Factor IX and our findings, with both types of antibodies, are in agreement with those of others[8-10]. In patients with liver cirrhosis, Factor IX INA corresponded to Factor IX activity or was even lower in some cases[7].

Further progress has been developed using an immunoadsorption technique. Antibodies were obtained from the serum of a patient with Haemophilia B known to have circulating antibodies specifically directed against Factor IX. The antibodies from 5 ml serum were partially purified, before coupling, using 0.47 M octanoic acid. 60 mg IgG containing specific antibodies to

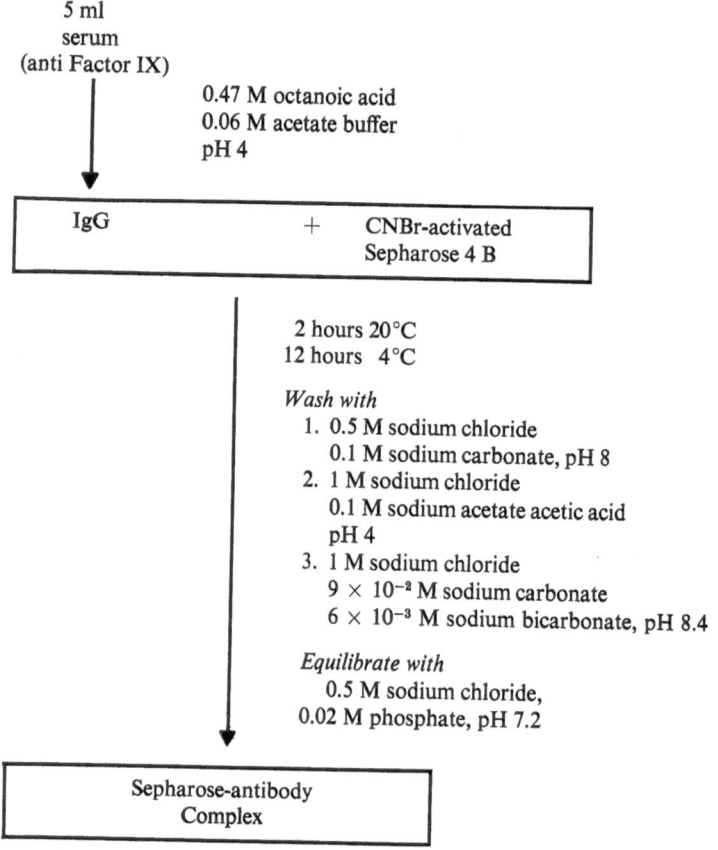

Fig. 2. Preparation of Sepharose – antibody to Factor IX complex.

Factor IX, were unsolubilized by coupling to Sepharose 4 B activated with cyanogen bromide[12] (fig. 2). The yield of coupling was 96%. The same anti Factor IX immunoadsorbent was reutilized throughout the study. Immunoadsorbents containing normal human IgG coupled to activated Sepharose 4 B were used as control.

When normal citrated plasma (pH 7.2) was applied at 20°C to the column of the immunoadsorbent previously equilibrated with 0.5 M sodium chloride, 0.02 M phosphate buffer, pH 7.2, Factor IX was specifically bound (fig. 3). 20 ml of normal plasma were required to saturate 60 mg IgG coupled to Sepharose. Thus 0.33 U Factor IX is bound per mg IgG. Normal human IgG coupled to activated Sepharose did not bind Factor IX.

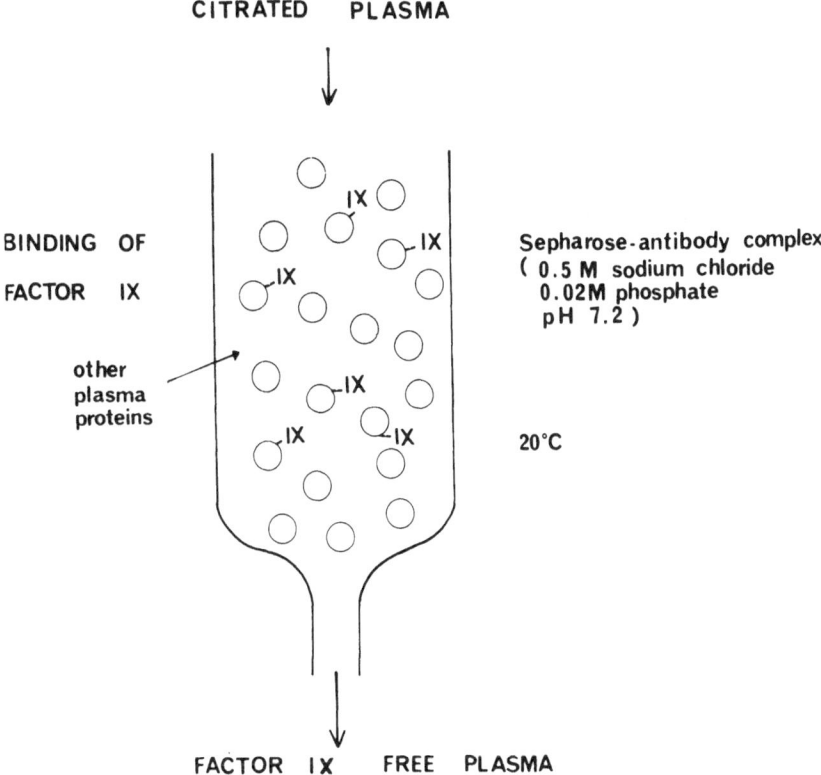

*Fig.* 3. Binding of Factor IX from normal plasma to Sepharose-antibody (anti F. IX) complex.

The effluent of the 20 ml normal plasma applied to the immunoadsorbent contained less than 1% Factor IX and normal levels of Factors II, VII and X

(fig. 4). In some experiments there was a slight decrease in the levels of
Factors II, VII and X which could be accounted for by non specific adsorption since these activities were recovered in the washing fluids (0.15 M
sodium chloride, $6 \times 10^{-3}$ M trisodium citrate, pH 7.2) prior to elution.

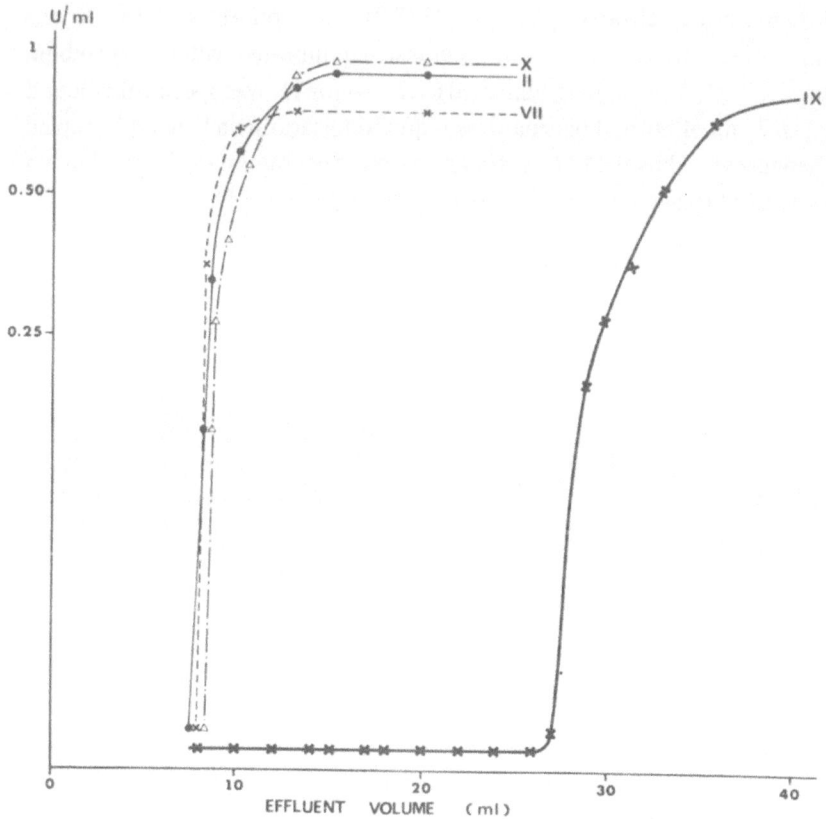

*Fig.* 4. Measurement of Factors II, VII, IX and X in the effluent volume of 20 ml normal
plasma applied to the immunoadsorbent.

Biologically active Factor IX adsorbed from 20 ml normal plasma was
recovered following elution using 2.5 M magnesium chloride pH 7.2 (fig. 5)
and dialyzed against 0.154 M sodium chloride, $6 \times 10^{-3}$ M sodium citrate,
pH 7.2.

When normal plasma, containing 0.013 Factor IX U/ml, was applied
to the immunoadsorbent, the major elution peak contained Factor IX
activity (fig. 6), partially in activated form, and was devoid of Factors II,

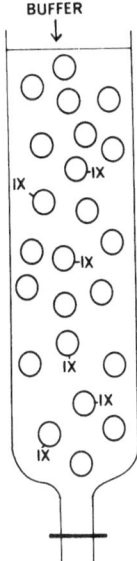

*Fig.* 5. Method of elution of Factor IX from the immunoadsorbent.
1. Wash with 0.15 M sodium chloride 6.10⁻³ M trisodium citrate pH 7.2.
2. Elute Factor IX with 2.5 M magnesium chloride pH 7.2.

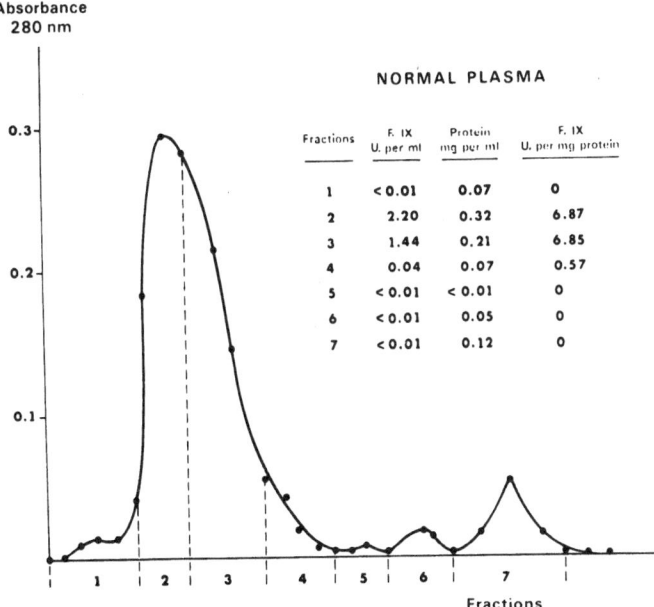

*Fig.* 6. Elution of Factor IX from normal plasma following binding to the immunoadsorbent.

VII and X. Purification of Factor IX was 550 ×. This fraction, containing Factor IX activity, produced 4 bands following application of 20 μg protein and electrophoresis on 7% acrylamide gels in 0.1% SDS[13] (fig. 7). Two of these bands corresponded in relative migration to IgG and albumin. When gels containing 100 μg protein were sliced at 2 mm intervals, Factor IX activity could be qualitatively detected only in the two minor bands with an intermediate migration between IgG and albumin.

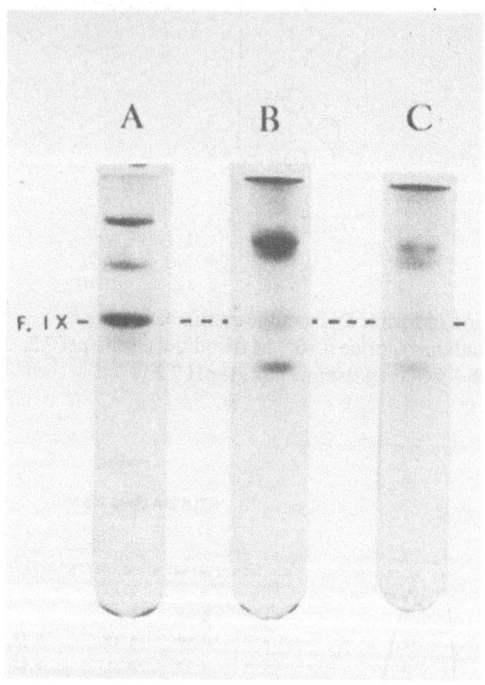

*Fig.* 7. Polyacrylamide gel electrophoresis.
A. Factor IX concentrate₁
B. Fraction 2 eluted from normal plasma (Figure 6).
C. Fraction 2 eluted from coumarin plasma (Figure 9).

Similarly, plasma from patients receiving coumarin therapy was studied by the same technique, using the same immunoadsorbent column, and an identical profile of elution, was observed with normal and coumarin plasma (fig. 8). In the latter case Factor IX like antigen in coumarin plasma (measured by inhibitor neutralizing activity) could be recovered following elution from the immunoadsorbent (fig. 9) and the purification obtained was 440 ×. The eluted fraction containing Factor IX antigenic material produced

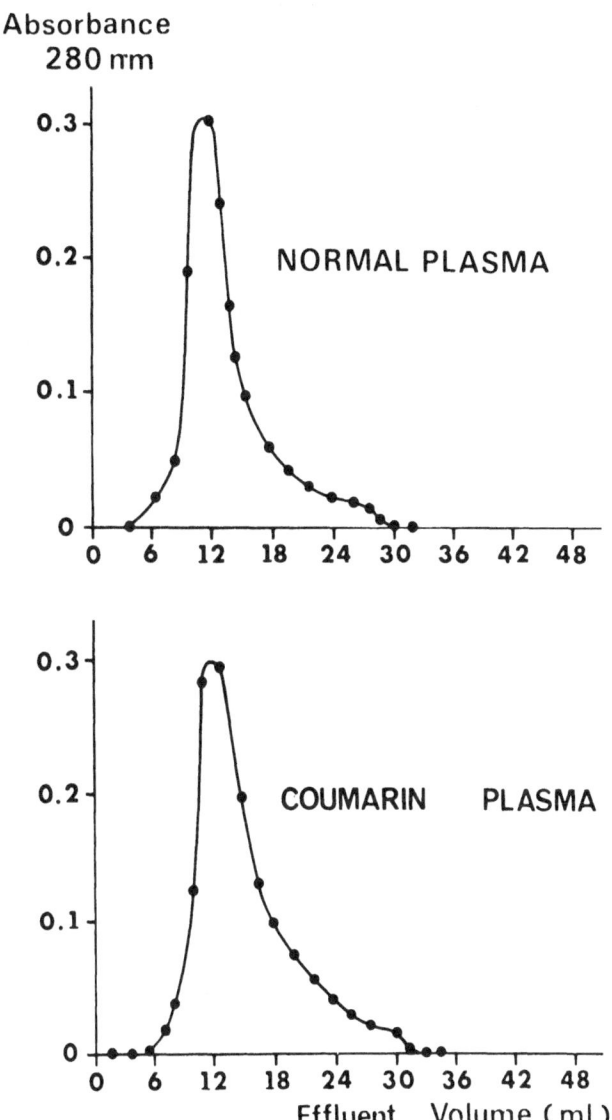

*Fig.* 8. Comparison of the profile of elution from the immunoadsorbent of normal and coumarin plasma.

the same 4 bands following electrophoresis on polyacrylamide as the fraction eluted from normal plasma (fig. 7).

Plasma from one patient with Haemophilia B + B$_M$ (with 1% Factor IX activity) was applied to the same immunoadsorbent and Factor IX antigen

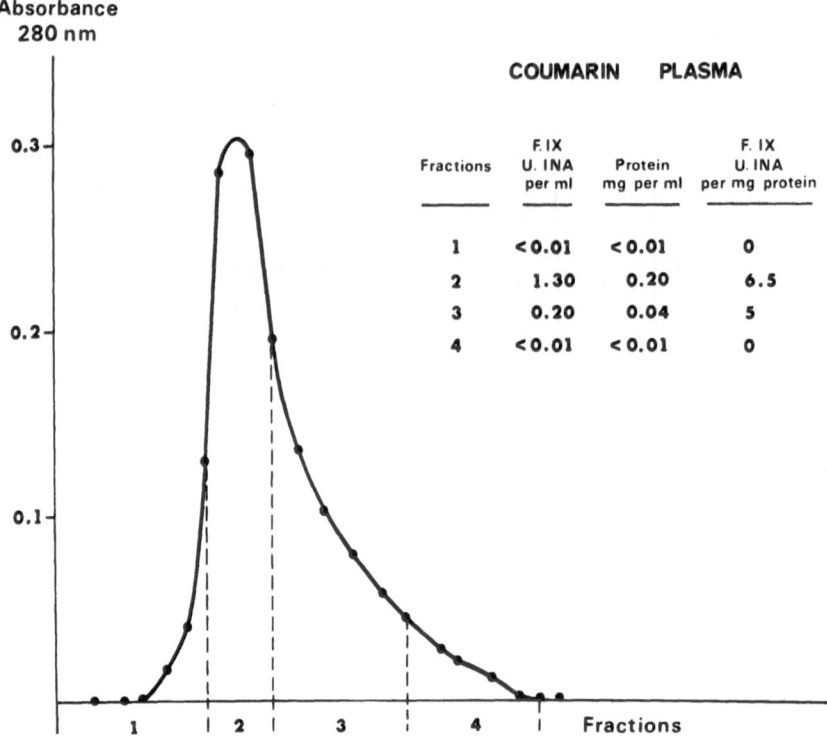

*Fig.* 9. Elution of Factor IX antigen from coumarin plasma following binding to the immunoadsorbent.

was also bound and then eluted (fig. 10). The corresponding fraction also showed 4 bands following electrophoresis on polyacrylamide, with relative mobilities comparable to those obtained with normal or coumarin fractions.

In conclusion the immunoadsorption method has provided a means to isolate and characterize normal and inactive Factor IX (PIVKA Factor IX and Haemophilia B+ variant) which were bound to the specific immunoadsorbent and demonstrated following elution the same profile on polyacrylamide gels. The technique used is similar to that of Reekers[14] and Neal et al[15] except for different immunoadsorbent and eluant. Normal Factor IX and Factor IX variants have been used for the preparation of heterologous antisera and this work is in progress. Moreover the immunoadsorption technique allows the obtainment of Factor IX-free plasma (fig. 3) which may be used for Factor IX assay and following lyophilisation, for adsorbing heterologous antisera.

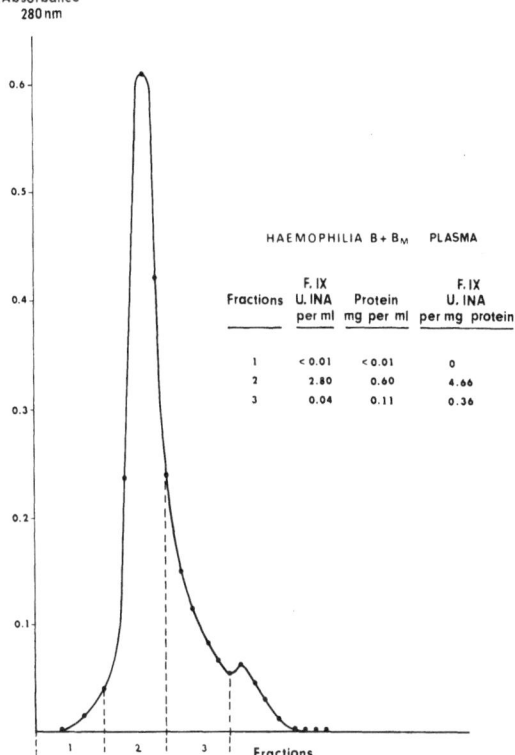

*Fig.* 10. Elution of Factor IX antigen from Haemophilia B + B_M plasma following binding to the immunoadsorbent.

### REFERENCES

1. Fantl, P., R. S. Sawers and A. G. Marr, *Aust. Ann. Med.* 5, 163 (1956).
2. Denson, K. W. E., R. Biggs and P. M. Mannucci, *J. clin. Path.* 21, 160 (1968).
3. Roberts, H. R., J. E. Grizzle, W. D. McLester and G. D. Penick, *J. clin. Invest.* 47, 360 (1968).
4. Pfueller, S., J. B. Somer and P. A. Castaldi, *Coagulation* 2, 213 (1969).
5. Meyer, D. and M. J. Larrieu, *Europ. J. clin. Invest.* 1, 425 (1971).
6. Meyer, D., E. Bidwell and M. J. Larrieu, *J. clin. Path.* 25, 433 (1972).
7. Larrieu, M. J. and D. Meyer, *Lancet* 2, 1085 (1970).
8. Denson, K. W. E., *Brit. J. Haemat.* 20, 643 (1971).
9. Veltkamp, J. J., H. Muis, A. D. Muller, H. C. Hemker and E. A. Loeliger, *Thrombos. Diathes. haemorrh.* 25, 312 (1971).
10. Lechner, K., *Thrombos. Diathes. haemorrh.* 27, 19 (1972).
11. Langdell, R. D., R. H. Wagner and K. M. Brinkhous, *J. Lab. clin. Med.* 41, 637 (1953).
12. Porath, J., R. Axen and S. Ernback, *Nature* 215, 1491 (1967).
13. Weber, K. and M. Osborn, *J. biol. Chem.* 244, 4406 (1969).
14. Reekers, P. P. M., *Thesis*, Leiden (1972).
15. Neal, W. R., D. T. Tayloe jr., A. I. Cederbaum and H. R. Roberts, *Brit. J. Haemat.* 25, 63 (1973).

# PROTEINS INDUCED BY VITAMIN K
# ANTAGONISTS (PIVKAs)

M. J. LINDHOUT AND B. H. M. KOP-KLAASSEN

## INTRODUCTION

The occurrence of an inactive precursor of a prothrombinlike protein in vitamin K deficient plasma (either absolute or induced by vitamin K antagonists) has first been reported by Hemker et al. (1, 2).

Studies on the synthesis of prothrombin in the liver of vitamin K deficient rats treated with vitamin K and inhibitors of protein synthesis give evidence that vitamin K does act at a postribosomal step in prothrombin synthesis (3, 4).

Direct evidence of the existence of a prothrombin precursor in vitamin K deficient humans as well as in the vitamin K deficient cow was obtained with an immunochemical technique (5-9). It has been shown that after the start of oral anticoagulant treatment the abnormal protein increases concomitantly with the decrease of normal prothrombin, but direct evidence for the occurrence of precursors related to the other vitamin K dependent coagulation factors VII, IX, and X in vitamin K deficient plasma is still scarce. Antibody neutralization tests and coagulation kinetics on plasmas from vitamin K deficient humans suggest the existence of proteins induced by vitamin K antagonists corresponding to each of the normal factors IX and X (10-12) which can be designated PIVKA-IX and PIVKA-X, respectively.

In several laboratories abnormal prothrombin (PIVKA-II) produced by dicoumarol-treated cows has been extensively purified and characterized (8, 13, 15). It is clear from these results that the vitamin K sensitive step involves the modification of several glutamic acid residues in a calcium binding site on the precursor by introduction of $\gamma$-carboxyl glutamic acid residues (14). The absence of strong Ca-binding sites in PIVKA-II and the presence of such sites in the N-terminal part of prothrombin has been demonstrated by several authors (15-18). Recently, we found a considerably lower affinity

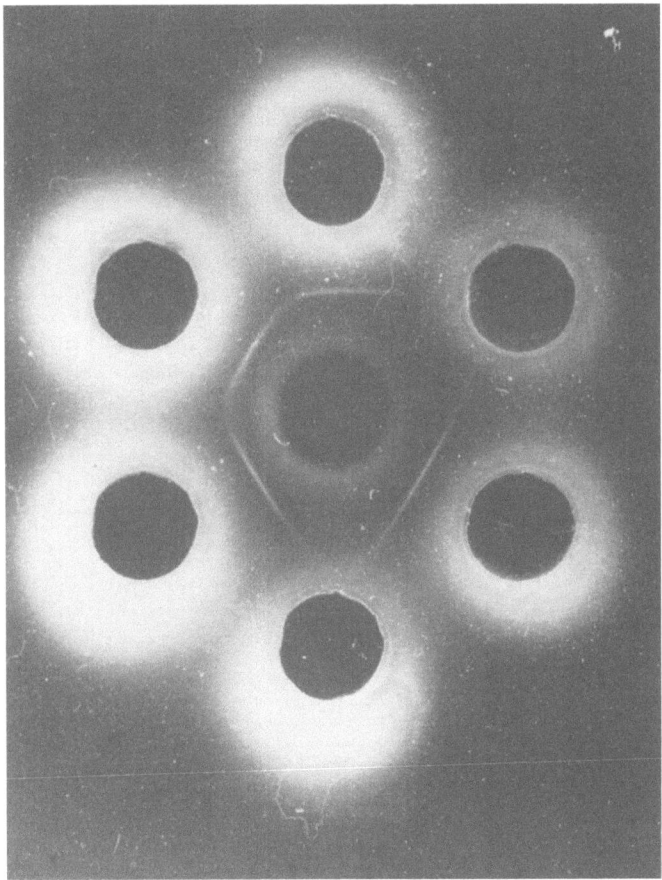

*Fig.* 1. Double immunodiffusion.
Centre well contains anti-bovine factor IX-antiserum.
1. Normal bovine plasma. 2. Coumarin bovine plasma. 3. Al(OH)₃ adsorbed coumarin bovine plasma. 4. Al(OH)₃ adsorbed normal bovine plasma. 5. Al(OH)₃ adsorbed coumarin bovine serum. 6. Al(OH)₃ adsorbed normal bovine serum.
(Numbering starts at the top and is counterclockwise).

of PIVKA-IX and PIVKA-X to $Ca^{++}$-ions compared to that of factors IX and X (19).

Abnormal factor II (PIVKA-II) is inactive in the normal prothrombin assay system after treatment with physiological activators. However, PIVKA-II can be activated to thrombin in a nonphysiological way for in-

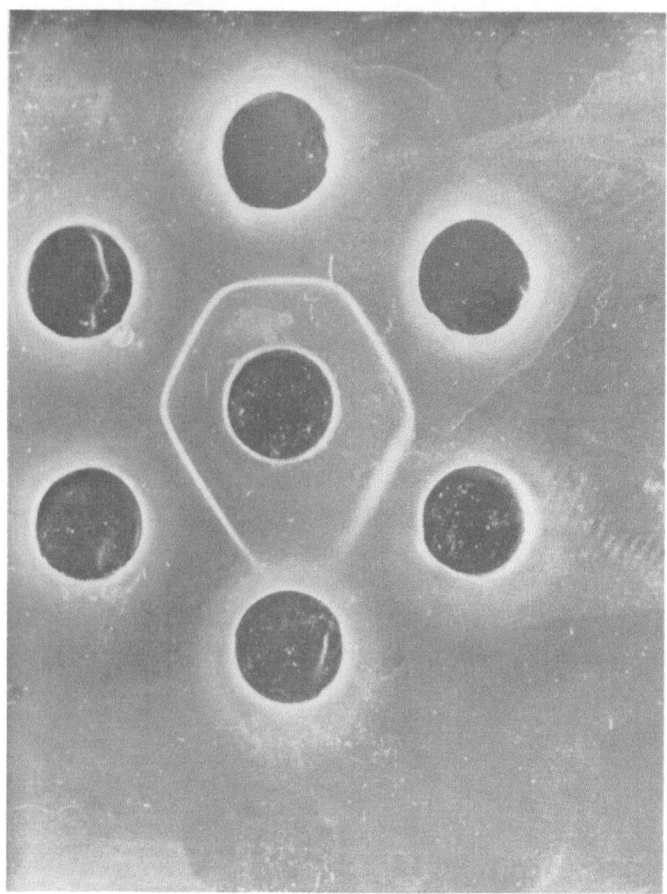

*Fig.* 2. Double immunodiffusion.
Centre well contains anti-bovine factor X-antiserum.
1. Normal bovine plasma. 2. Coumarin bovine plasma. 3. Al(OH)$_3$ adsorbed coumarin bovine plasma. 4. Al(OH)$_3$ adsorbed normal bovine plasma. 5. Al(OH)$_3$ adsorbed coumarin bovine serum. 6. Al(OH)$_3$ adsorbed normal bovine serum.
(Numbering starts at the top and is counterclockwise).

stance with trypsin and Echis carinatus venom (20) and by complex formation with staphylocoagulase (21). This indicates that the active site of PIVKA-II (the thrombin part of the protein) is intact and that a lack of Ca$^{++}$-binding sites accounts for the absence of a physiological activation process.

In the light of these findings we tried to demonstrate an intact active centre in the precursor of factor X (PIVKA-X). This is especially interesting because the Ca-binding site in factor X forms part not only of the proenzyme (as in prothrombin) but of the active enzyme (factor $X_a$) as well.

In order to prove the presence of PIVKAs IX and X in the plasma of anticoagulated cows we used a procedure analogous to that described by Ganrot (5). We purified bovine factors II, IX, and X, with a method developed in our laboratory (23) and injected the purified factors into rabbits. In a double immuno diffusion test, antibovine factor IX antiserum revealed single and completely identical precipitation lines against normal bovine plasma, bovine plasma with less than 5% factor IX activity obtained after oral anticoagulation of the cow, the same coumarin bovine plasma adsorbed onto 0.5% Al(OH)$_3$ and serum of an anticoagulated cow adsorbed

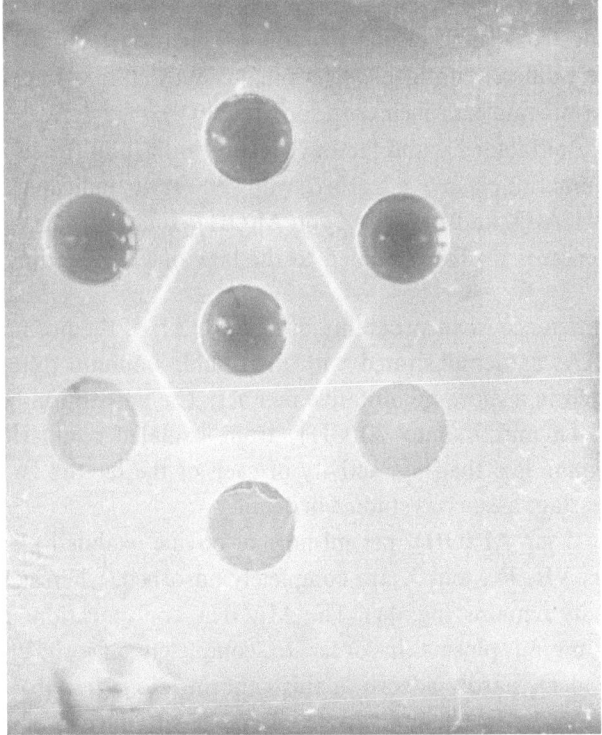

*Fig.* 3. Double immunodiffusion.
Centre well contains normal bovine plasma.
1. Anti-bovine factor II-antiserum. 2. Anti-bovine factor IX-antiserum. 3. Anti-bovine factor X-antiserum. 4. Anti-bovine factor II-antiserum. 5. Anti-bovine factor IX-antiserum. 6. Anti-bovine factor X-antiserum.
(Numbering starts at the top and is counterclockwise).

onto 0.5% Al $(OH)_3$. No precipitation line is seen with normal plasma and normal serum when the coagulation factors are removed by adsorption onto 0.5% Al $(OH)_3$ (fig. 1).

The same results are found with immunodiffusion of antibovine factor X antiserum against normal bovine plasma, coumarin bovine plasma with less than 5% factor X activity, the same plasma adsorbed onto 0.5% Al $(OH)_3$ and coumarin bovine serum adsorbed onto 0.5% Al $(OH)_3$. No precipitation line is seen with normal bovine plasma after adsorption onto 0.5% Al $(OH)_3$ (fig. 2).

Precipitation patterns characteristic of non-identity were obtained between anti-bovine factor II, anti-bovine factor IX and anti-bovine factor X antiserum in a double immuno diffusion test against normal bovine plasma (fig. 3).

We conclude from these results that the coagulation factors IX and X have completely different antigenic determinants but that they have common antigenic determinants with their corresponding PIVKAs.

The presence of factor IX and factor X related antigen in the supernatant of bovine coumarin plasma adsorbed with Al$(OH)_3$ indicates a lower affinity of PIVKA-IX and PIVKA-X for Al$(OH)_3$ than the normal factors. This phenomenon is probably related to the lack of $Ca^{++}$-binding sites on the PIVKAs.

The great difference in adsorbability onto Al $(OH)_3$ of the normal factors and the PIVKAs as demonstrated with the double immuno diffusion test was investigated in a more quantitative manner. The adsorption behaviour of PIVKA-II, IX and X onto Al$(OH)_3$ from oxalated coumarin bovine plasma containing less than 5% activity of each of the factors II, VII, IX, and X in a one-stage assay was studied in detail.

When using 5 mg Al $(OH)_3$ per ml normal bovine oxalated plasma, the normal factors VII, IX, and X are completely adsorbed, whereas still 40% factor II activity remains (fig. 4a). The Al $(OH)_3$ concentration should be raised to 10 mg/ml plasma in order to completely adsorb PIVKA-X. PIVKAs II and IX hardly adsorb at this concentration (fig. 4b). In these experiments PIVKAs II, IX, and X were estimated with the one-dimensional immuno electrophoresis method according to Laurell (27).

Because of the great difference in adsorbability between factor X and PIVKA-X, we could follow the appeerence of PIVKA-X during coumarin treatment in a quantitative way with one-dimensional immuno electrophoresis.

We anticoagulated a cow with 600 mg phenprocoumon the first day and

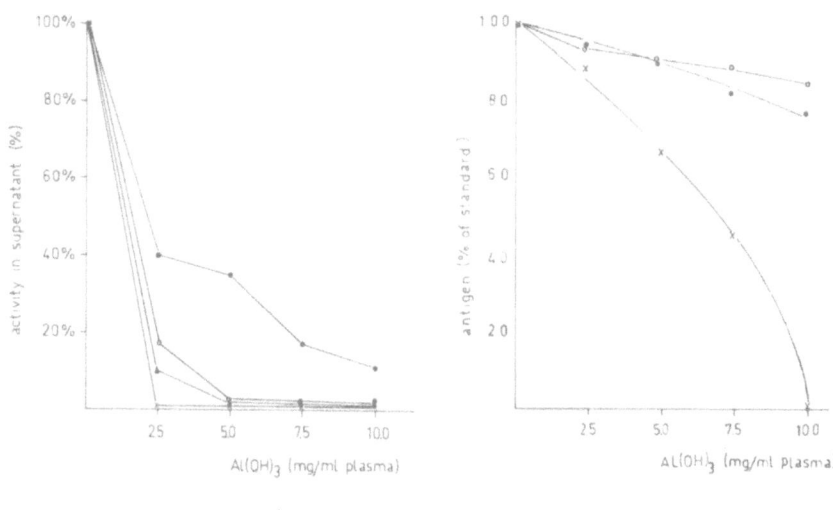

*Fig.* 4a. Adsorption of the coagulation factors II ( ●— ● ), VII ( ▲—▲ ), IX ( ○— ○ ) and X (x—x) from oxalated normal bovine plasma onto various Al(OH)$_3$ concentrations. Activity in the supernatant was determined by one-stage assays.

*Fig.* 4b. Adsorption of PIVKA-II ( ●— ● ), PIVKA-IX ( ○— ○ ), and PIVKA-X (x—x) from oxalated coumarin bovine plasma with less than 5% normal factor II, IX, and X activity onto various Al(OH)$_3$ concentrations. The concentrations of the PIVKAs in the supernatant were determined with one-dimensional immunoelectrophoresis.

thereafter 200 mg phenprocoumon daily. The factor X activity decreased after starting the anticoagulant treatment. Treatment with phenprocoumon has no effect on the immunochemically determined concentration of factor X in the plasma. However, after adsorption of these plasmas onto 0.2% Al (OH)$_3$ an increasing amount of factor X related antigen is observed in the supernatant (fig. 5). We conclude that the complete blocking of factor X synthesis results in the appearence of PIVKA-X parallel to the disappearence of factor X.

We were able to confirm the existence of two populations of factor X-like molecules in an anticoagulated cow with the aid of antifactor X-antiserum in a two-dimensional immunoelectrophoresis (9) in the presence of Ca$^{++}$-ions (fig. 6). The pattern obtained with plasma from a cow treated with phenprocoumon shows a double peaked precipitate; the cathodal peak represents normal factor X, the anodal one represents PIVKA-X.

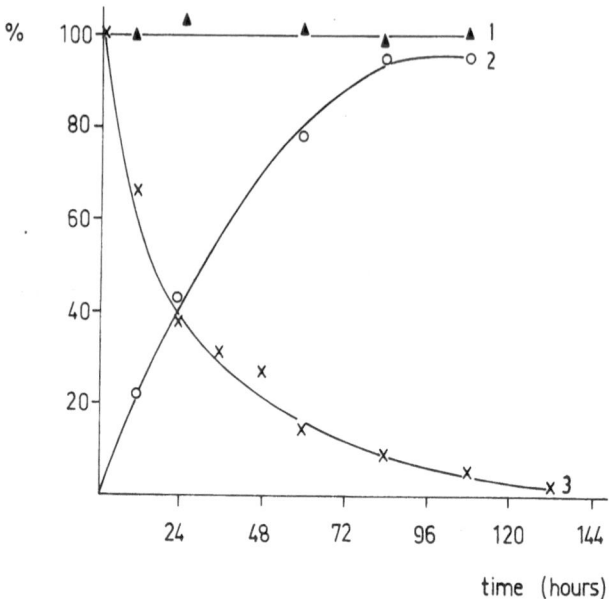

*Fig. 5.* Effect of phenprocoumon treatment on factor X activity. A cow weighing 600 kg was anticoagulated with 600 mg phenprocoumon the first day, and 200 mg daily. Factor X activity (x—x) was determined with the one-stage assay. Factor X concentration (▲—▲) was determined in plasma with one-dimensional immuno electrophoresis. PIVKA-X concentrations were immunochemically determined in plasma after adsorption onto 0.2% Al(OH)$_3$. PIVKA-X concentration is given in percentage of coumarin bovine plasma standard with less than 5% factor X activity.

Comparable results are obtained with anti factor IX-antiserum; we did not succeed in making precipitating antibodies against factor VII.

Under anticoagulant treatment a second species of factor IX, exhibiting a higher anodic mobility in the presence of Ca$^{++}$-ions is induced. With an immunologic and a one-stage assay we observed that the amount of PIVKA-IX increases concomitantly with the decrease of the normal factor IX.

We carried out a two-dimensional immunoelectrophoresis in the presence of Ca$^{++}$-ions with a mixture of the three antibodies present in the second dimension (fig. 8) to demonstrate the existence of the three different PIVKAs (PIVKA-II, PIVKA-IX, and PIVKA-X) unequivocally, each of them immunologically identical to the normal factor but not identical to each other.

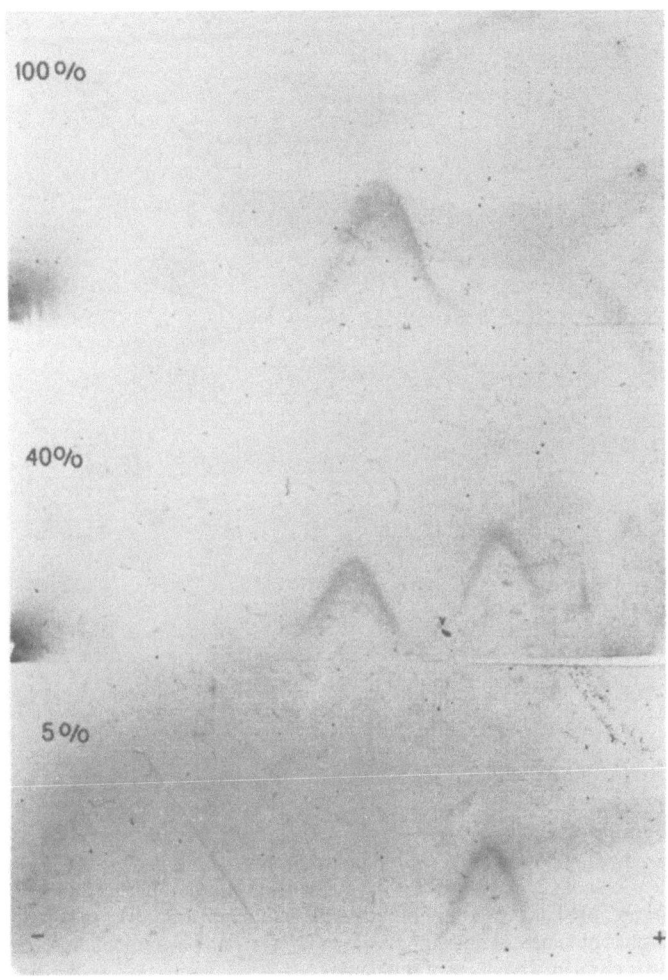

*Fig.* 6. Crossed immunoelectrophoresis pattern of bovine plasma in 1% agarose gel. Second dimension contained 1% anti bovine factor X antiserum. Barbital buffer 0.075 M, 2 mM Ca-lactate, pH 8.6. A: Pattern obtained before administration of phenprocoumon; B and C: plasmas obtained 24 hours and 5 days after starting phenprocoumon administration. Factor X activity is given in percentage of standard.

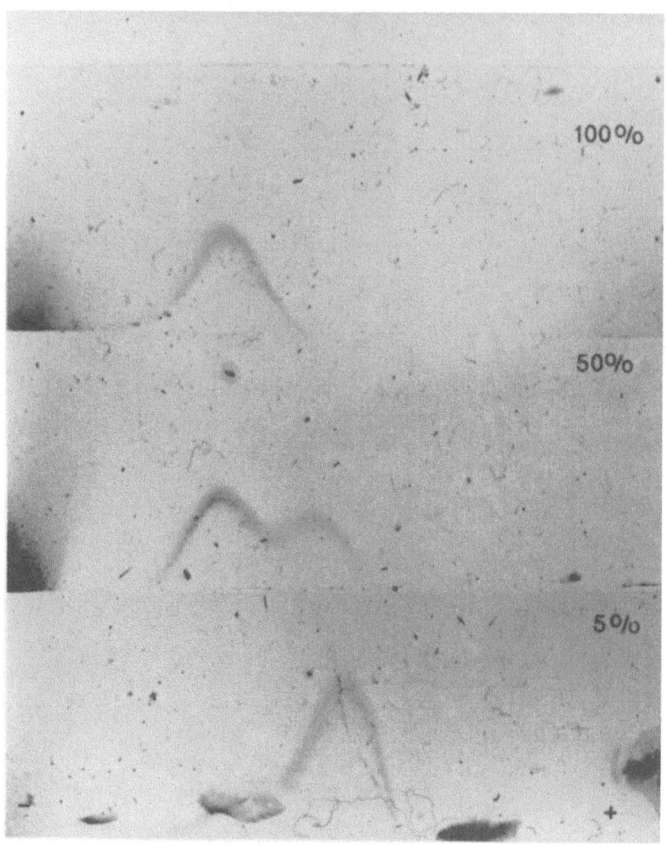

*Fig.* 7. Crossed immunoelectrophoresis pattern of bovine plasma in 1% agarose gel. Second dimension contained 1% anti bovine factor IX antiserum. Barbital buffer 0.075 M, 2 mM Ca-lactate, pH 8.6. A: Pattern obtained before administration of phenprocoumon; B and C: plasmas obtained 24 hours and 5 days after starting phenprocoumon administration. Activity is given in percentage of standard.

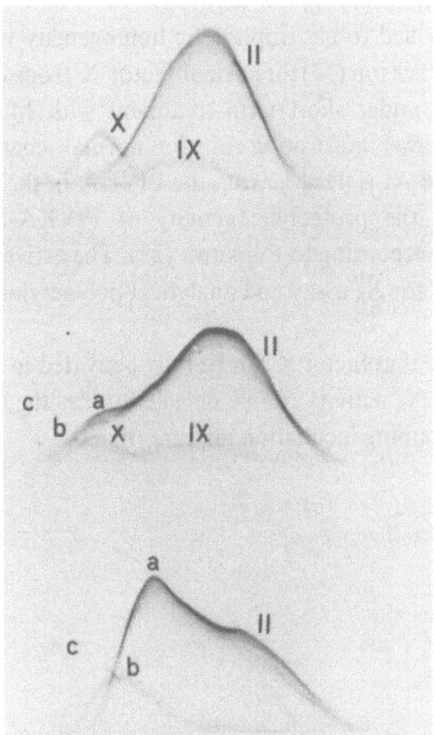

*Fig.* 8. Crossed immunoelectrophoresis pattern of bovine plasma in 1% agarose. Second dimension contained a mixture of the antibovine factor II, IX, and X antiserum. A: Pattern obtained before administration of phenprocoumon; B and C: plasmas obtained 24 hours and 100 hours after starting of the phenprocoumon treatment. II: prothrombin; X: factor X; IX: factor IX; a: PIVKA-II; b: PIVKA-IX; c: PIVKA-X.

## STUDIES ON THE ACTIVE CENTRE OF PIVKA-X

Several nonphysiological mechanisms for the activation of factor X with different proteolytic enzymes have been described (24-29). The activation reaction by a protein present in Russell's Viper Venom (RVV) involves the splitting of a glycopeptide from the amino terminal end of the heavy chain in factor X (28). Once factor X is activated it has proteolytic action on prothrombin (29-33). The rate of factor $X_{a \, RVV}$ catalyzed activation of prothrombin is accelerated in the presence of $Ca^{++}$, phospholipds and factor V.

However, the products of prothrombin activation are the same under conditions of activation with factor $X_{a\,RVV}$ only (33).

PIVKA-X was purified to electrophoretic homogeneity with a procedure analogous to that of Jackson (34) for normal factor X from oxalated plasma obtained from cows under short term treatment with Marcoumar[R]. The major modification was adsorption of the normal coagulation factors from the plasma onto Al $(OH)_3$, leaving the PIVKA in the supernatant. In order to investigate the proteolytic activity of PIVKA-X we activated PIVKA-X with RVV according to Fujikawa (28). The activation of PIVKA-X is followed by a factor $X_a$ assay and analytical polyacrylamide gel electrophoresis (28).

The results indicate that factor X can be fully activated in a time course of 5 minutes. No factor $X_a$ activity can be detected under the same conditions in the PIVKA-X containing incubation mixture (fig. 9).

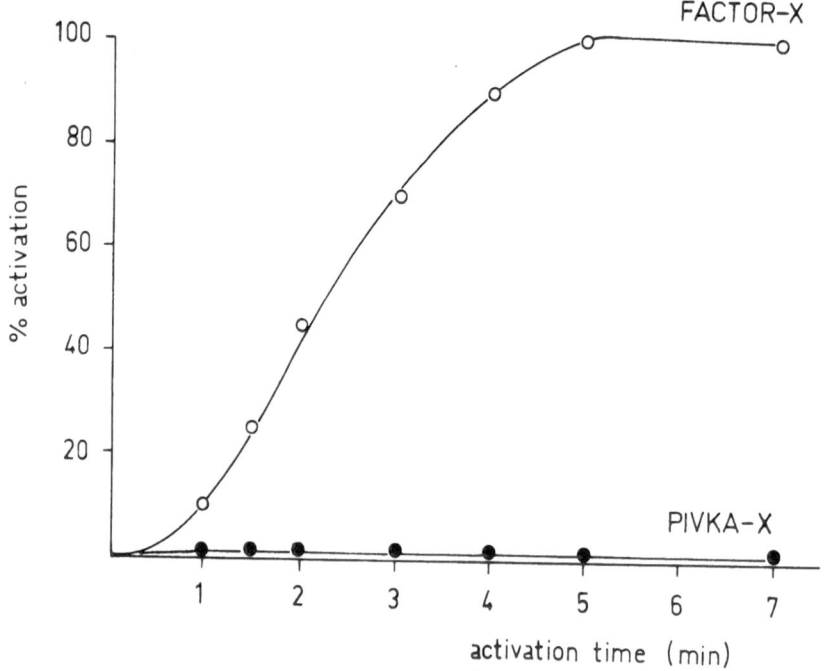

*Fig.* 9. Time curve for the activation of factor X (O—O) and PIVKA-X (●—●) with a protein from Russell's Viper Venom.

Following the activation of PIVKA-X on polyacrylamide gel electrophoresis a protein with a higher mobility appears within 5 minutes (fig. 10).

It seems that a partial activation could be achieved. However, the presence of a contaminating protein in the PIVKA-X preparation is more likely.

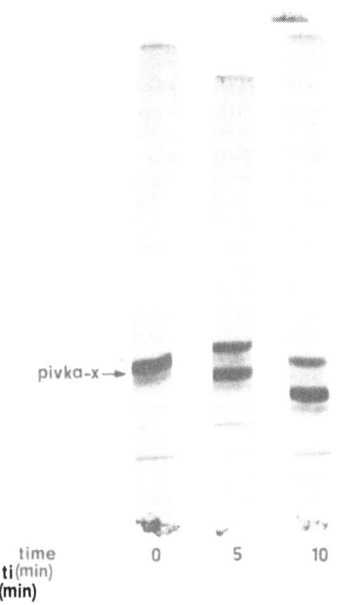

pivka-x →

time
ti(min)        0        5        10
(min)

*Fig.* 10. Polyacrylamide gel electrophoresis pattern of samples removed from the incubation mixture containing PIVKA-X and Russell's Viper Venom.

Under favourable conditions p-nitrophenyl-p-guanidinobenzoate (p-NPGB) reacts essentially stoichiometrically with activated factor X. The active site of factor $X_a$ is acylated by p-guanidino-benzoate and p-nitrophenol equivalent to the concentration of active sites, is released.

A sample of PIVKA-X incubated for 30 min with RVV was titrated with the procedure of Smith (35) and found to be 49% active. Active site titration of PIVKA-X before activation with RVV had a negative result.

We also demonstrated esterase activity in the PIVKA-$X_{RVV}$ sample using tosylarginine-methylether as a substrate (36). The specific esterase activity was calculated as 6 μeq/min/mg protein. Under the same conditions the specific esterase activity was found to be 12 μeq/min/mg protein in a factor $X_a$ sample.

Although PIVKA-$X_{RVV}$ has no activity in a one-stage factor $X_a$ assay, it seems that the active site is intact as was estimated by active site titration and esterase activity. However, the non-specificity of the substrate used makes it compulsory to look at the proteolytic activity of PIVKA-X$_{RVV}$ on prothrombin.

Prothrombin (2,0 mg/ml) isolated with the method of Owren (33) was incubated with 10 µg/ml of PIVKA-X$_{RVV}$ at 37°C. The proteolytic action of PIVKA-X$_{RVV}$ was monitored by sodium dodecyl sulfate gel electrophoresis (37) and thrombin assays (38). The time curve of prothrombin activation with PIVKA-X$_{RVV}$ as obtained with gel electrophoresis is shown in fig. 11. Lysozyme was taken as a marker protein.

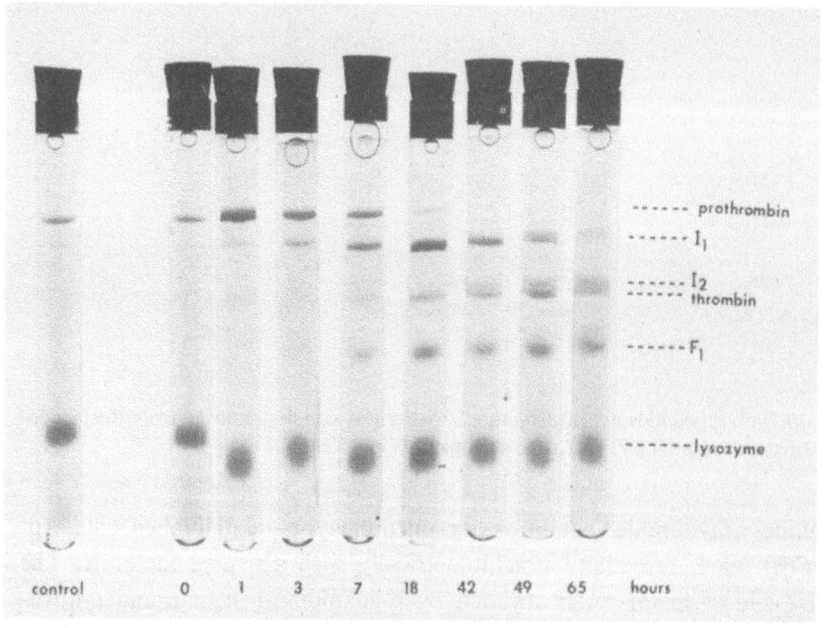

*Fig.* 11. SDS polyacrylamide gel electrophoresis pattern of samples removed from the incubation mixture containing prothrombin and PIVKA-X$_{RVV}$.

Prothrombin (molecular weight 72,000-74,000) disappeared from the reaction mixture and a transient component, which is designated intermediate 1 (molecular weight 48,000-50,000) appears. At the same time a stable component (fragment 1-molecular weight 22,000-24,000) arises. Intermediate 1 is subsequently converted into intermediate 2 (molecular weight 37,000-38,000) and fragment 2 (molecular weight 12,800) is not seen in the gel. Intermediate 2 is only partially converted into an active thrombin (molecular weight 37,000).

A similar experiment was done with factor $X_{aRVV}$ (not illustrated). The maximum formation of thrombin in the activation experiment with factor $X_a$ and PIVKA-$X_{RVV}$ was achieved after incubation for 25 and 45 hours, respectively. The specific activity of the thrombin generated in the time indicated was 850 NIH units/mg protein and 85 NIH units/mg protein, respectively.

In control experiments where PIVKA-$X_{RVV}$ is replaced by RVV or PIVKA-X a trace amount of thrombin could be measured after incubation for 40 hours. SDS electrophoresis of the control samples shows that prothrombin is partially converted into intermediate 1.

From these preliminary results we conclude that the active centre of PIVKA-$X_{RVV}$ seems to be intact with respect to the esterase activity when it is compared to factor $X_a$ but that there is in addition to or as a consequence of the lack of $Ca^{++}$ binding sites, another defect, resulting in a lower rate of activation of prothrombin by PIVKA-$X_{RVV}$.

REFERENCES

1. Hemker, H. C., J. J. Veltkamp, A. Hensen and E. A. Loeliger, *Nature* 200, 589 (1963).
2. Hemker, H. C., A. D. Muller and E. A. Loeliger, *Thrombos. Diathes. haemorrh.* 23, 633 (1970).
3. Suttie, J. W., *Nutr. Rev.* 31, 105 (1973).
4. Woolf, I. L. *Ann. J. Med.* 53, 261 (1972).
5. Ganrot, P. O. and J. E. Nilehn, *Scand. J. clin. Lab. Invest.* 22, 23 (1968).
6. Josso, F., J. M. Lavergne, M. Gouault, O. Prou-Wartelle and J. P. Soulier, *Thrombos. Diathes. haemorrh.* 20, 28 (1968).
7. Brozovic, M. and L. Gurd, *Lancet* 2, 427 (1971).
8. Stenflo, J. and P. O. Ganrot, *J. biol. Chem.* 247, 8160 (1972).
9. Laurell, C. B., *Anal. Bioch.* 10, 358 (1965).
10. Hemker, H. C., *Thrombos. Diathes. haemorrh.* Suppl. XLV, 119 (1971).
11. Veltkamp, J. J., H. Muis, A. D. Muller and H. C. Hemker, *Thrombos. Diathes. haemorrh.* 25, 312 (1971).
12. Denson, K. W. E., *Brit. J. Haemat*, 20, 643 (1971).
13. Stenflo, J., *J. biol. Chem.* 247, 8167 (1972).
14. Stenflo, J., *J. biol. Chem.* 249, 5527 (1974).
15. Nelsestuen, G. L. and J. W. Suttie, *Biochemistry* 11, 4961 (1972).
16. Stenflo, J. and P. O. Ganroth, *Bioph. Res. Comm.* 50, 98 (1973).
17. Nelsestuen G. L. and J. W. Suttie, *Proc. nat. Acad. Sci.* 70, 3366 (1973).
18. Benson. B. J., W. Kisiel and D. J. Hanahan, *Biochim. biophys. Acta* 329, 81 (1973).
19. Reekers, P. P. M., M. J. Lindhout, B. H. M. Kop-Klaassen and H. C. Hemker, *Biochim. biophys. Acta* 317, 559 (19??).
20. Nelsestuen, G. L. and J. W. Suttie, *J. biol. Chem.* 247, 8176 (1972).
21. Hemker, H. C., *Nouv. Rev.franc. Hémat.* 10, 645 (1970).
22. Reekers, P. P. M. and H. C. Hemker, *Haemostasis* 1, 2 (1972).
23. Laurell, C. B., *Anal. Biochem.* 15, 45 (1966).

24. Esnouff, M. P. and W. J. Williams, *Biochem. J.* 84, 62 (1962).
25. Papahadjoupoulos, D., E. T. Yin and D. J. Hanahan, *Biochemistry* 3, 1931 (1964).
26. Macfarlane, R. G., *Brit. J. Haemat.* 7, 496 (1961).
27. Pechet, L. and B. Alexander, *Fed. Proc.* 19, 64 (1960).
28. Fujikawa, K., M. E. Legaz and E. W. Davie, *Biochemistry* 11, 4892 (1972).
29. Hemker, H. C., M. P. Esnouff, P. W. Hemker, A. C. W. Swart and R. G. Macfarlane, *Nature* 215, 248 (1967).
30. Mann, K. G., C. M. Heldebrant and D. N. Fass, *J. biol. Chem.* 246, 6106 (1971).
31. Stenn, K. S. and E. R. Blout, *Biochemistry* 11, 4502 (1972).
32. Gitel, S. H., W. J. Owen, C. T. Esmon and C. M. Jackson, *Proc. Nat. Acad. Sci.* 70, 1344 (1973).
33. Owen, W. J., C. T. Esmon and C. M. Jackson, *J. biol. Chem.* 249, 594 (1974).
34. Jackson, C. M., T. F. Johnson and D. J. Hanahan, *Biochemistry* 7, 4492 (1968).
35. Smith, R. L., *J. biol. Chem.* 248, 2418 (1973).
36. Schwert, J. W., H. Neurath, S. Kaufman and J. E. Snoke, *J. biol. Chem.* 172, 221 (1948).
37. Weber, K. and M. Osborn, *J. biol. Chem.* 244, 4406 (1969).
38. Hemker, H. C., A. D. Muller and E. A. Loeliger, *Thrombos. Diathes. haemorrh.* 23, 633 (1970).

# INDEX OF SUBJECTS